RAWSOME!

Maximizing Health, Energy, and Culinary Delight with the Raw Foods Diet

BRIGITTE MARS

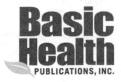

Basic Health PUBLICATIONS, INC.

This book in not intended to cure or give medical advice. Its intention is to educate, inform, and empower readers to make their own decisions on health and well-being. Each person will have unique reactions to changes in diet. If you have concerns about your health or diet, consult with your healthcare practitioner.

The publisher does not advocate the use of any particular healthcare protocol but believes the information in this book should be available to the public. The publisher and author are not responsible for any adverse effects or consequences resulting from the use of the suggestions, preparations, or procedures discussed in this book. Should the reader have any questions concerning the appropriateness of any procedures or preparation mentioned, the author and the publisher strongly suggest consulting a professional healthcare advisor.

Basic Health Publications, Inc.
28812 Top of the World Drive
Laguna Beach, CA 92651
Phone: 949-715-7327 • www.basichealthpub.com

Library of Congress Cataloging-in-Publication Data

Mars, Brigitte.
    Rawsome!: maximizing health, energy, and culinary delight with the raw foods diet / Brigitte Mars.—1st ed.
        p. cm.
Includes bibliographical references and index.
    ISBN-13: 978-1-59120-060-4
    ISBN-10: 1-59120-060-1
    1. Nutrition. 2. Raw foods. 3. Cookery (Natural foods) I. Title.

    RA784.M355   2004
    613.2'6—dc22

                                                    2003022901

Editor: Nancy Ringer
Typesetter/Book design: Gary A. Rosenberg
Cover design: Mike Stromberg

Printed in the United States of America

18   17   16   15   14   13

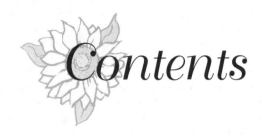

Contents

Acknowledgments, vii

Preface, ix

INTRODUCTION: The Raw Advantage, 1

1. What Is Raw—And What Is Not?, 3

2. Why Go Raw?, 9

3. Raw Foods Encyclopedia, 25

4. The Raw Kitchen, 117

5. Raw Recipes, 135

6. Eating Raw with Family and Friends, 251

7. Using Food for Healing, 261

APPENDIX: Nutrients and Source Foods, 281

Glossary, 315

Bibliography, 320

Resources, 326

Index, 345

About the Author, 355

Dedicated to
The Children of the Future
and to making the world
a better place right now.

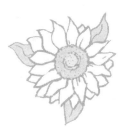

Acknowledgments

I would like to express my heartfelt thanks to all those who have inspired us on the raw path. Thanks to my publisher, Norman Goldfind, who thought *Rawsome!* would be a great project, for all his support of my work. Thanks as well to editor Nancy Ringer and copyeditor Kate Herman. Gratitude to Carol and Gary Rosenberg for all their help.

Juliano, I'm so glad we met. Thank you for feeding your wonderful food to Rainbeau, and for enhancing her health. You are truly a beautiful, generous spirit and your message will resonate worldwide. David Wolfe, you rock, you inspire, you are a man on fire. Jeremy Safron, as soon as I met you, I wanted to know, "What's this man about?" Thank you, Victoria and Igor Boutenko, for the great workshops, clear message, and loving light. Anyone who thinks raw people are frail should try a massage from Igor.

Tom Pfeiffer, thank you so much for taking this journey with me. Had I gone raw all by myself, it would have been a lonely path. Having you to make beautiful food for, your generous help in the kitchen and my classes, and your endearments and praise about all of it make my life truly blessed. I love you more than ever and find you amazingly beautiful, after twenty-five years.

Sunflower Sparkle Mars, beloved firstborn, thanks for being open to trying this new way of eating. Thanks for keeping an open mind and for staying on a healthy path yourself.

Rainbeau Harmony Mars, amazing daughter, I only went raw to support you and make sure that you were going to be okay. Did I learn a lot!

Tamara Kerner, thanks for all your girlfriend support and spirit of adventure. Laura Lamun, I am so grateful to you for always being with me at the right time. Debra St. Clair, Richard Rose, and Alana—you all inspire. Double Dose, beautiful twins, thank you for your music that brings us together.

Woody Harrelson, did you know the day you spent here would change my life? Michael Shulgin, Peter Kizer, Alex Ferrara, Chad Sarno, Elaina Love, Roz Greuben, Doug Graham, Robert Snaidach, Art Baker, Matthew Becker, Steve Meyerowitz, and Elsa Markowitz, thank you all for answering my questions. Carol Giambri, thank you for bringing the raw community in Boulder together, and for all your helpfulness to all who know you. Merci to Tehya and Steve MacIntosh, Martina Hoffmann, and Roberto Venosa. John Hay, you have always been a mentor.

Thanks so much to all the friends who come to our "salons" and are willing to be part of this great human experience. Bill Brennan, you are a video wizard!

Ariana Saraha and Kari diPalma, I am so grateful for your friendship and creativity. Love to the great people of Boulder's raw group.

Thank you, God. Thank you, Universe. Thank you, Universal Mother Spirit. Blessed be. *Om shanti.*

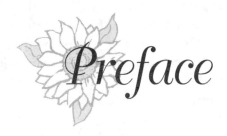

Preface

While living in Miami, I first tried going on a raw diet in the mid-1970s, having been inspired by Viktoris Kulvinskas's *Survival into the Twenty-First Century*, one of the earliest books to advocate raw foods. But back then, the only organic produce widely available was carrots and apples, and most natural foods stores didn't carry produce at all. After moving to Colorado, when I would talk about being raw, people would look at me with blank expressions. Most had never heard of it, and they didn't think it was a good idea. "It's too cold in Colorado," they protested. "You can't live on uncooked food during the winter. You need hot, cooked food to warm you up." So, after a few months, I let go of the idea.

Over the following years, I studied macrobiotics, herbal medicine, Oriental medicine, vitamin therapy, flower essences, and homeopathy. Eventually, I began to teach classes on natural medicine at institutions such as Naropa University, Boulder College of Massage, and Esalen. I became the herbalist for one of the nation's largest natural foods stores, and for thirteen years I promoted multitudes of remedies, potions, pills, and tinctures. I began a private practice and wrote scores of magazine articles and several books.

During all this time, my family—my husband, Tom, and my two daughters, Rainbeau and Sunflower—followed what I thought was a healthy vegetarian lifestyle. We ate organic food whenever possible, though almost all of it, with the exception of the occasional salad, was cooked. As the years went by, my lovely children became complicated teenagers. I surrendered to serving whole-wheat bagels, pasta dishes, veggie burgers, home-cooked vegetarian chili, and other things I was glad they would eat. "At least it's organic!" I would say to myself.

When Sunflower and Rainbeau admitted to me that they were some-times eating meat at their friends' houses, I wasn't pleased, but I appreciated their honesty and decided that it would be better if I prepared an organically raised, free-range chicken once a week than for my daughters to eat lord-knows-what lord-knows-where. Although I had then been vegetarian for twenty-three years, I actually felt energized consuming some animal protein.

My children grew up and moved out. Middle-aged and pudgy, I found myself making organic cakes and chocolate-chip cookies (with organic sugar), meat, and quick-cooking rice once a week. We had some wild greens with many meals and felt healthy about that. The truth was, however, that I still struggled with skin breakouts and was getting heavier despite skipping dinners and drinking "natural" diet shakes. Meanwhile, Tom frequently had digestive problems that caused him sleepless nights.

In 1996, Rainbeau, an aspiring actress, was cast in her first movie. She flew to Memphis for the filming and found herself having a great time with Woody Harrelson and his brother Brett, both of whom were into raw foods, yoga, and environmental issues. Rainbeau dropped out of college and soon moved to Hollywood, like many young hopefuls, to pursue dreams of fame and fortune.

On one occasion when I was visiting Rainbeau, we ran into Juliano, an energetic young chef, in a natural foods store in Santa Monica. He gave her a flyer for a raw potluck. Soon after, she called us in Colorado to say, "I've gone raw! Juliano is my new housemate. He has written a book called *Raw* and says, 'Get your mom down here. She'll get raw.'"

"Not very likely," I thought. "I know too much." I had studied way too long and knew all about "cold, damp spleen," "excess *yin*," and how eating tropical fruits can make you "ungrounded and spaced out." My biggest concern was that Rainbeau was going to become anorexic, like some of the models and actresses one reads about.

Tom and I had planned a trip to Los Angeles to attend the Natural Products Expo, the major convention for the natural foods industry. We hoped to talk some sense into Rainbeau. On our first night in L.A., Juliano was hosting one of his huge raw dinners, and we were invited. Tom was apprehensive about how his stomach would handle such fare, and I was worried that the meal would be insubstantial; I told Tom we could always go out for Mexican food afterward if we were still hungry. We were served a raw, vegetarian "meatloaf" with cauliflower mashed potatoes. We drank coconut water. It was all amazingly delicious and satisfying. Tom's stomach was blissfully peaceful, and we had to admit that Rainbeau looked healthier and more beautiful than ever. When we left the dinner, my worries were eased, and I felt grateful for Juliano.

The next day, Rainbeau and I left for Anaheim to attend the convention, while Tom had business to attend to in L.A. Rather than walking through the convention and tasting every free sample of tofu hot dog, organic chocolate bar, and frozen vegan pizza, I noticed that very little of the "health food" was raw, and that one-third of the show was devoted to vitamins and herbal remedies. Did one relate to the other? "Natural" foods might be good, but obviously they had not brought us perfect health! Macaroni and cheese in a box, though whole wheat and organic, was still processed food.

When Tom and I returned to Boulder, I decided that I would be raw for a year to support Rainbeau. Surprisingly, Tom loved the food and would sit down to meals saying, "You're saving me." His digestion improved so much. As for me, after about a month, I felt better than I had in twenty years. After about three months, I experienced a bit of a detox reaction: my skin broke out worse than it had in years, but then it got better than ever. We both felt more energetic. We needed less sleep. We felt infused with positive, vibrant energy.

We sponsored David Wolfe, author of *The Sunfood Diet Success System,* to teach a one-day workshop in our courtyard. We were amazed at how quickly the workshop was filled, with barely any effort on our part. It was also delightful that making lunch for the sixty-five attendees was so easy, when I remembered the stress and toil of cooking a dinner party menu for ten!

As time passed, my teaching of herbal medicine changed. I wanted to talk about raw foods. The raw foods diet seemed to have so much in common with natural medicines. I found that many of my herbal allies, such as dandelion greens and violet blossoms, made great additions to raw salads and fresh green juices. I came to realize that diet—next to spirit—was the most potent healer of all.

I've been completely raw since 2001. When I went to the Natural Products Expo this year, people who knew me saw a real difference. "What have you been doing?" they asked. "You look younger! More slender! Your skin is great!" In the three and a half years of being raw, my bone density has tested at excellent levels, and both my husband and I have tested for having excellent levels of antioxidants. Tom has had his eyeglass prescription reduced three times. His eye doctor is amazed, saying this usually doesn't happen to men in their fifties!

Being raw continues to bring health, happiness, and a multitude of blessings and synchronicities into my life. I am forever grateful for the revelation of raw. I wonder what took me so long. After so many years of searching for remedies for illnesses, I found a beautiful way to prevent them.

It amazes me how something so simple, something that saves time, money, and natural resources, could have such a positive effect in my life. What's more amazing is that everyone isn't doing it! Now a trip to the grocery store yields four bags of groceries, rather than one or two, for $50. We feel great. We're sticking with the program. And with this book, I invite you to revel with us in the beautiful, simple power of raw foods.

INTRODUCTION

The Raw Advantage

*Y*ou may already have heard about the raw foods diet. You may have picked up this book to find out more, because you can't quite believe that the diet is really as good as they say. Or, you may never have heard about the diet, and you've picked up this book because you can't quite believe that anyone would be foolish enough to propose such a thing. Well, fad diets come and go, but the raw foods diet is *not* a fad—it's been around for thousands of years—and it's not going anywhere—especially after you, my friends, have tried it and begun to feel the incredible energizing effect it has on your body and spirit. For the uninitiated, undertaking and sticking with the raw foods diet might seem like a daunting task; but having been raw since 2001, I am convinced that it's one of the best things I've ever done. Every week I discover new reasons to love being raw. Here are a few of the advantages to consider.

The dishes prepared with raw foods recipes are absolutely delicious. The vibrant flavor is inherent to the foods themselves; they require fewer additives such as salt, spices, oils, and sweeteners.

Every major health organization in this country (including the American Cancer Society and the American Heart Institute) recommends that we eat at least five servings of fruits and vegetables daily. On the raw foods diet, five servings is generally just a baseline—you may find yourself eating much more.

Raw foods have more nutrients and fibers than cooked foods do. Enzymes in raw foods are active, not having been deactivated through the application of heat, and they support the overall health of the body. No bottled supplement or prepackaged food can compare with the life force of fresh, raw food.

1

Raw foods are digested easily and quickly, in 24–36 hours as opposed to 48–100 hours for cooked food. Your body's vitality won't be sapped from breaking down hard-to-digest foods.

A raw foods diet strengthens the immune system, thereby preventing illness and helping you overcome nagging ailments. The raw path has been used to improve the health of those with arthritis, asthma, high blood pressure, cancer, diabetes, digestive disturbances, menstrual problems, allergies, obesity, psoriasis, skin conditions, heart disease, diverticulitis, weakened immunity, depression, and hormonal imbalances. On a raw diet, degenerative diseases often disappear. The aging process can slow. Bad breath and body odor can go away. Eyes will become brighter and the voice more clear. Skin and muscle tone will improve. Memory and concentration can become sharper. You'll feel better, have more energy, and need less sleep. (It is also more difficult to camouflage spoilage in raw foods than in cooked foods, so you are much less likely to get food poisoning.)

In addition, by following a raw foods diet, you can easily normalize your weight without restricting food intake. Those extra pounds you've been trying to lose will melt away, without your having to go hungry, and your body will maintain its optimal weight for as long as you stay raw.

Imagine never having to clean the oven! Dirty dishes can simply go in the dishwasher after a simple rinse—no more baked-on grease that requires soaking and scrubbing. Grease won't collect on the walls, stovetop, or ceiling, either, and you'll find that gentle, biodegradable cleansers really work. You'll spend less time in the kitchen and less money in the grocery store. In fact, when you're on a raw foods diet, you'll spend from 25 to 80 percent less money on food.

Less land is required to produce fruits, vegetables, grains, nuts, and other plant-source foods than is required to produce animal products. And by focusing your spending on organic produce, you can encourage good stewardship of the earth. Think of all the energy that would be saved if more people ate raw food: less fuel, packaging, and pollution! Instead of being trash, most of what is now thrown away could be composted and given back to the earth to create new life.

Eating raw food is a manifestation of care for, and consciousness of, the next generation. The raw movement is the future. And if you can experience a higher state of consciousness, have better health, eat more delicious food, and save time, money, and the planet's resources, why not say yes to raw?

1

What Is Raw— And What Is Not?

A raw foods diet is exactly that: raw foods. No cooking, no grilling, no steaming, no application of heat of any kind. Why? Because eating food that is closest to its natural state engenders a tremendous exchange of energy between food and body. The result, over time, is a feeling of buoyant, radiant health.

What is the difference between raw and vegetarian or vegan? A vegetarian is one who abstains from eating meat from any animal, including birds and fish. A vegan is one who abstains from eating any animal product, including meat, eggs, and milk. A raw foods diet is predominantly raw vegan. (Some raw practitioners include raw dairy products. Others even include raw meat, although this book does not encourage that practice.) Raw foods are still "living," in a manner of speaking. They may be dehydrated, frozen, or fermented, but at no time have they been heated to a temperature over 110°F. Their enzymes and nutrients are intact. If you set these foods in their whole form into soil and watered them, many would sprout.

THE DETRIMENTS OF MEAT

Most raw foodists do not eat meat, for both physiological and environmental reasons. The primary reasons are that meat is hard to digest and that it diminishes the vitality of the body.

In nature, true carnivores don't really chew meat much, as their digestive tracts have such high concentrations of hydrochloric acid that meat swallowed whole can be digested. Human digestive systems, however, have much lower levels of hydrochloric acid, which means that meat is harder for us to digest and must be chewed well before being swallowed. The liver and kidneys must work overtime in digesting meat, which can adversely affect their health.

3

Also, the flesh that we consume contains uric acid, and the body must draw upon its alkaline reserves to neutralize this acid. (If not neutralized, uric acid contributes to the development of health problems such as gout and arthritis.) When one eats a meat-heavy diet, the bloodstream and other tissues and organs become more acidic. The body attempts to buffer the acidity by pulling calcium from its bones. This leaching of calcium, in combination with the high levels of phosphorus found in meats, contributes to a loss of bone density. Most flesh foods also contain high levels of fats, which carry toxins and elevate cholesterol levels.

Livestock consume 50 percent of our nation's water supply and 80 percent of our grain. Twenty pounds of fodder (forage and grain) is required to produce 1 pound of meat. That same 1 pound of meat also requires 2,500 gallons of water, compared to only 25 gallons required to produce 1 pound of wheat. Meanwhile, half a million animals are killed for meat every hour in the United States.

At one time, humans needed meat to survive. We did not stay in one place long enough to grow enough food to support ourselves. We did not have the means to preserve fresh foods so that they would last through the winter. We did not enjoy the luxury of global transportation, by which fresh foods are made available all year long. But we have so many more healthful and environmentally conscious options today. Are we to stay bound to the hard realities of the past? Or will we let the evolution of our culture and technology guide our food choices toward a more healthful way of eating?

If you do eat meat, consider purchasing it from farmers and ranchers who raise free-range animals on organic feeds. And you can easily stay open to the health and pleasure of raw foods, incorporating them whenever possible into your meals.

THE DETRIMENTS OF COOKING

What do you think would happen if you fed a gorilla coffee, grilled meat, boiled vegetables, and doughnuts? If you subjected your hand or your garden to torching, boiling, or baking, would it be improved in any way? Intuitively, we understand that fresh foods are necessary for our nutrition, and that the application of heat destroys the vitality of just about every living component. In our day-to-day life, however, we have been trained to think of our meals as being mostly cooked foods. How has that come to be?

The predominance of cooked food harkens back to our nomadic days, when meat was the most important element of our diet. Cooking meat destroyed bacteria, and smoking or curing meat allowed it to be kept for long periods of time. We needed fire for warmth and protection; we grew accustomed to warm foods and hot drinks. These habits have been carried forward through generations to today.

Food industries have little interest in researching and marketing raw foods. Profit margins are lower for foods in their natural state than for foods that are processed and packaged. Did you ever notice that most food advertisements are for junk food? It is rare to see an ad for Vermont apples or California oranges, though we are inundated daily with a media barrage of sugary cereals, fatty burgers, deep-fried chips, and aspartame-filled sodas. We are also subjected to scores of ads for drugs to remedy our ailments. It's funny—many of the ailments that we need these drugs for are caused by the very foods we are encouraged to eat.

The reason that cooked food smells so appealing is that its flavors and nutrients are being evaporated by the heat and are passing from the food into the air. But once the food is cooked, it then requires lots of salt, sweetener, spices, and fat to make it taste better.

Steamed vegetables (ostensibly among the healthiest of cooked foods) are usually heated to about 212°F. Unfortunately, many vitamins lose potency at a mere 130°F. Vitamins A, D, E, and K are destroyed in cooking. High temperatures decrease levels of vitamin C and most of the B-complex vitamins in food. The loss of vitamin B_1 from cooking can be from 25 to 45 percent, and B_2 loss can be from 40 to 48 percent.

Similarly, cooked food loses enzymes, which begin to be destroyed at 116°F. Cooking also causes the minerals in food to leach out into the water in which it is cooked, and causes mineral salts to become degenerated, deanimated, and inorganic. Cooking disrupts the structure of indoles, which are anticancer compounds found in many fresh produce items.

In addition, cooking produces free radicals in foods (and especially in oils). Free radicals are unpaired, charged molecules that cause cellular destruction and are thought to be the primary environmental cause of aging. The higher the cooking temperature, the more free radicals created.

Proteins start breaking down under the application of heat. According to studies in Germany at the Max Planck Institute for Nutritional Research, well-cooked proteins have only 50 percent bioavailability. Proteins start becoming denatured at 161°F. Denatured proteins are not usable by the body and have been linked to disorders including heart disease, cancer, and arthritis. Cooking coagulates the proteins in food and causes them to become deaminated. The amino acids lysine and glutamine are both destroyed by cooking; and when the amino acid methionine is heated, it begins to inhibit the production of hemoglobin (the oxygen-carrying molecule in red blood cells).

When greens that are high in oxalic acid (beet greens, collard greens, rhubarb stalks, Swiss chard, lamb's-quarter, purslane, sorrel, and spinach) are cooked, the oxalic acid combines with calcium, iron, and magnesium; over the long term, ingesting cooked oxalic acid impedes the absorption of calcium and iron by the body. When oxalic acid is consumed in raw rather than cooked foods, however, this effect is minimalized.

Cooking damages fats, changing them into trans-fatty acids that impede cellular respiration and that can be a factor in heart disease and cancer. When heated, the fats in oils adversely affect the skin, leading to clogged pores, acne, and eczema. Excessive use of cooked oils also causes cravings for stimulants like alcohol and caffeine and can lead one to feel unclean, depressed, and heavy.

Cooking softens food fibers, which can hamper intestinal motility. Cooked fibers become demagnetized and leave a slimy coating on the intestines. In fact, you are more likely to have gas, heartburn, and bloating after a cooked meal than after a raw one. Cooked carbohydrates become caramelized and dextrinized, and are known to increase body weight.

A diet of cooked foods requires the body to devote more energy toward digestion and elimination. When you eat cooked foods, you are more likely to feel fatigued, groggy, and hungry the next morning. The eliminative system (the pores, lungs, kidneys, and bowels; see "The Channels of Elimination" on page 15) becomes congested and overworked, leading to states of disease. Because cooking depletes the nutrients in foods, it is more difficult to feel satisfied by eating them; therefore, overeating and obesity become the norm.

Eating cooked food causes an immediate increase in white blood cell production and causes a pathogenic leukocytosis. In addition, after a typical cooked-foods meal, red blood cells tend to clump together. When the clumps reach the capillaries (where blood from the arteries delivers oxygen to the body's cells and enters the veins), circulation in these tiny vessels becomes clogged.

On June 28, 2002, *The Washington Post* reported on a Swedish study finding that acrylamide, a chemical known to cause cancer in animals and listed by the World Health Organization as a probable carcinogen in humans, is produced in foods when certain combinations of fats and carbohydrates (such as the mixture in French fries and potato chips) are heated to temperatures greater than 248°F. "We found the substance at levels [in these foods] that, if it was just one product, we would ask that it be immediately taken off the market," stated Leif Busk, head of the Research and Development Department of the Swedish National Food Administration. Raw and boiled foods, on the other hand, were found not to contain acrylamide.

The free radicals, toxins, and loss of nutrients that result from cooking contribute to aging, bloating, depression, weight gain, cellulite, hair loss, wrinkles, anxiety, and puffiness and dark circles under the eyes. Do you want to feel baked, fried, cooked, and toasted? Or would you rather feel fresh, alive, radiant, and vital?

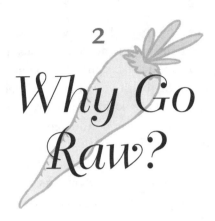

2

Why Go Raw?

A catalyst is a substance that enables a chemical reaction to take place, usually at a faster rate or under different circumstances (such as at a lower temperature) than is otherwise possible. In 1878, the German physician, philosopher, and physiology professor Willy Kuhne coined the word "enzyme" to specify a biocatalyst (a living catalyst) originating outside a living cell. We now know, however, that enzymes exist in all living things and in each of our cells. In fact, enzymes are the "living sparks" needed for every chemical action and reaction in the body. Over 3,000 enzymes have so far been identified, and researchers believe that many thousands more are yet to be discovered.

Minerals, vitamins, and hormones cannot work except in the presence of enzymes; enzymes help synthesize, join, and duplicate entire chains of amino acids. Breathing, sleeping, eating, digestion, nutrient absorption, thinking, moving, working, growing, blood coagulation, immunity, thinking, dreaming, sexual activity, excitement, reproduction, and sensory perception are all dependent on enzymes. Enzyme therapy has been used to treat arthritis, autism, autoimmune disorders, bruises, contusions, cystic fibrosis, fat intolerance, inflammation, multiple sclerosis, pain, pancreatic insufficiency, shingles, sports injuries, varicose veins, and viral infections. Enzymes are cancer's enemy as well: they break away the protective fibrin around cancer cells, make the cells less sticky (thereby preventing metastasis, which is the spread of cancer cells to other parts of the body), and alert the immune system to their presence.

Although enzymes are themselves composed of tiny proteins, which, in turn, are made of amino acids, they cannot be synthetically reproduced. (Most of the pharmaceutical enzymes available are derived from pig pancreas.) Enzymes can be divided into two basic categories: exogenous (introduced from outside the body) and endogenous (produced in the body).

For years, nutritionists were taught that exogenous enzymes in food had no more nutritional or digestive value than their amino acid content because stomach acid would break down the enzymes before they could be absorbed. However, a recent study conducted by W. A. Hemmings of the University College of North Wales indicates that a significant amount of dietary protein (that is, exogenous enzymes) is actually absorbed into the body intact (that is, not broken down into its amino acid components). When food is consumed, acid secretion is very low for the first thirty minutes or so. As food sits in the upper section of the stomach, the exogenous enzymes aid in their own digestion, which enables the body to do less work later. After thirty to forty-five minutes, the bottom portion of the stomach opens, and the body secretes its own endogenous enzymes and acids. Even at that point, exogenous enzymes are not inactivated until the acid level becomes prohibitive, which can take up to an hour.

Decreased enzyme activity has been found to contribute to chronic conditions such as allergies, skin disease, diabetes, and cancer. It also results in weight gain, lethargy, inflammation, digestive impairment, and loss of skin elasticity and muscle tone—which are all symptoms of aging. In 1946, James Summer, M.D., winner of the Nobel Prize in chemistry, claimed that the "middle-aged feeling" was due to diminished enzymes. The author of *Enzyme Nutrition*, Edward Howell, M.D., seemed to offer proof of this theory: Dr. Howell said that by age fifty, people usually have only 30 percent of their endogenous enzymes left.

A decrease in the quantity and quality of our endogenous enzymes is a natural result of aging. The typical Western lifestyle and diet also deplete the body of enzymes, thus rushing us headlong toward premature aging. Alcohol, drugs, tobacco, carcinogenic exposure, radiation, excessive sunlight, chlorine, fluoride, many medications, and stimulants draw enzymes from our limited endogenous supply—but cooked food is the primary culprit in this depletion. Enzymes are fragile: light, heat, and pressure can deactivate them. In fact, many are completely destroyed at temperatures exceeding 118°F, which means that the exogenous enzymes in foods are destroyed by cooking. Because cooked food lacks active enzymes of its own, the body must produce more endogenous enzymes in order to digest it.

When raw food is consumed, on the other hand, its enzymes assist in the preliminary digestive process. Raw foods not only introduce exogenous

Enzyme Activity

We've learned about the two main categories of enzymes, exogenous and endogenous. Endogenous enzymes are further classified into digestive and metabolic subgroups. The functions of these groups can be generalized as follows:

Exogenous Enzymes

In its raw state, each food contains the enzymes needed for its own digestion. These food enzymes are exogenous. They include protease (which breaks protein chains into smaller amino acid chains and finally into individual amino acids), amylase (which breaks carbohydrates into simple sugars), lipase (which breaks fats into free fatty acids and glycerol), lactase (which breaks down milk sugars), and cellulase (which breaks the bonds in fibrous foods).

Endogenous Enzymes—Digestive and Metabolic

Digestive enzymes are endogenous, being produced mainly in the pancreas and to some degree in the stomach and small intestines. They include trypsin, chymotrypsin, and pepsin. Their function is to break down carbohydrates, fats, and proteins into nutrients that are more readily available to the body.

These endogenous enzymes affect the tissues and organs of the body, facilitating functions such as movement and speech. Metabolic enzymes use the nutrients absorbed from food for important bodily processes including tissue repair and regeneration.

enzymes to the body but also provide the nutrients that allow, or trigger, endogenous enzymes to function. Therefore, a large portion of a raw meal is partially digested before it reaches the lower stomach, and fewer endogenous enzymes and acids are needed for its further digestion and absorption. Conserving enzymes contributes to staying youthful—and the raw foods diet is one means of enzyme conservation.

WEIGHT MANAGEMENT

The good news for many of us is that raw foods enable us to eat delicious food and still achieve and maintain our optimal weight. By comparison, the typical Western diet and lifestyle seem to encourage overeating and tend to lead to obesity; in the United States, this has become a national health problem. Overeating has many psychological causes, including stress, emotional insecurity, and depression, but it also can have a physical component: that is, the body's incessant craving for nutritional satisfaction that it never receives from processed foods. Cooking destroys so many nutrients that you have to eat more food in order to get the nutrients you need.

If your food is raw, you can eat eight to ten times less than you would if you were eating cooked food, and still satisfy your body's needs. But that doesn't mean you have to go hungry on a raw foods diet—on the contrary. Raw foods contain so much water, fiber, and general bulk that they fill you up faster than cooked foods do. They also energize you, making it easier to get involved in activities that get you up off the couch and strengthen your muscles and your mind.

In general, a raw foods diet tends to bring body weight to equilibrium, or to its optimal state. When my husband and I started eating raw, he gained weight, and I lost weight—while we were both eating basically the same food and the same portion sizes! You can expect to get healthier and more toned with raw foods. It's important to remember, of course, that optimal weight means different things for different people: we each have a unique, natural shape and size.

Losing Weight

When you're trying to lose weight, a diet of raw foods can certainly help. In general, you'll be consuming fewer fats and starches, which are the main culprits in weight gain, and you'll have more energy, so it will be easier to exercise. Exercise can improve posture, circulation, elimination, and oxygen intake, and is essential in any weight-loss program. Exercising also helps the body produce more endorphins, which can improve your mental outlook.

If weight loss is a goal, eat less of the sweet foods (such as bananas and dates) and more of the cleansing foods (such as apples and carrots). Choose lower-starch vegetables to avoid loading your body with carbohydrates. In addition, any fats you eat should be in raw form. A study at Tufts Medical School found that overweight people were deficient in endogenous lipase, a fat-digesting enzyme, so fat was being stored in the body rather than being broken down. Cooking and refining destroys the lipase in foods (for example, lipase is present in nuts, but not in oils made from nuts). In raw foods, however, the lipase is intact and helps with the metabolism of fats, even high-fat foods such as avocados or sprouted nuts and seeds.

Foods that aid weight loss are those with concentrated nutrients, enzymes, and cleansing ability. These concentrated foods include berries, citrus fruits, leafy green vegetables, melon, pineapple, unpasteurized sauerkraut, sea vegetables, and tomatoes. Using more warming, spicy condiments such as cayenne, cinnamon, garlic, and ginger will improve circulation and help the body metabolize fats. Room-temperature water with some fresh lemon juice squeezed into it is naturally diuretic, and the slightly sour taste will improve liver function and thus aid in fat metabolism as well. Raw celery is also helpful in any weight-loss program because it improves thyroid function, which can energize a sluggish metabolism.

If you experience food cravings between meals, try drinking a green juice or chewing on wheatgrass: either of these will have a stabilizing, alkalinizing effect. Taking a few deep, slow breaths may also help. Most cravings will pass within a few minutes. A craving for sweets may be an indication that the body needs more protein, so you might consider incorporating more protein sources into your diet (spirulina is especially helpful; see page 94). A craving for salty foods may indicate that you need more minerals, which you can get by including mineral-rich sea vegetables like kelp, dulse, or hiziki in your diet.

You may find it helpful to keep a food journal that records what you eat and drink for a week to gain insight into what your diet really looks like. If you do eat something that's not part of your plan, rather than feeling guilty about it, observe and write about the emotional factors that were driving you. Were you tired, bored, or anxious? How did you feel after eating it?

Choosing to lose weight can be an opportunity to pay more attention to yourself and bring better health to all aspects of your person. Clean out the basement, garage, and cupboards: getting rid of unnecessary stuff aids the process of letting go. Set goals for yourself and use the raw foods diet as an opportunity to live a healthier lifestyle that can add years, beauty, and joy to your life.

Gaining Weight

Some people who begin a totally raw diet become thin enough to concern their families and friends. Although this may happen initially, you should then gain back some weight over the course of a few months. Try drinking a smoothie or two between meals, and incorporate foods that encourage weight gain such as avocados, bananas, dried fruits, pumpkin seeds, sunflower seeds, and nut butters into the smoothies. Eventually, your weight should find its balance.

ACHIEVING TRUE HEALTH

In the typical Western lifestyle, we get in the way of our own health by congesting our cells and ourselves with processed and hard-to-digest food. Live food infuses one's being with fresh, vibrant energy, helping us feel invigorated and revitalizing our capability to resist disease.

When we become ill, we must first recognize our illness as a sign that the body is trying to heal itself. Disease is the body's method of cleansing, repairing, and restoring itself. Most often, disease results from the buildup of imbalance or daily "wrongs" against nature. When enough wrongs have occurred, disease manifests itself. And although it may appear to strike suddenly, it is important to remember that disease—or the conditions that allow it to take hold in the body—is, rather, an indicator of long-standing or chronic imbalance.

Causes of imbalance are many, including depletion of vital energy (as from lack of sleep), exposure to toxic substances (like air pollution), and physiological irritation (such as stress). But perhaps the most widespread and damaging cause of imbalance is our diet. "We dig our graves with our forks," says our friend and raw chef Juliano. We eat food that is hard to digest, full of synthetic additives, infused with traces of herbicides or pesticides, allergenic, and nutritionally deficient, and so overprocessed that it sends our systems into wild spirals of hyperactivity.

Simply using remedies to treat the symptoms of disease does nothing to eradicate it. True "medicine" removes the cause of the disease. Rather than inventing new drugs, building more hospitals, training more caregivers, and selling more pharmaceutical products, we should focus on building health in our bodies. Good health is not simply freedom from disease but is also physical, mental, and emotional vitality. All four of these facets of good health are supported and strengthened by the raw foods diet.

When the initial detox reaction (see below) has run its course, you will find that you begin to feel revitalized, invigorated, and fully awake. The raw foods diet cleanses and fortifies the organs, strengthens the immune system, supports emotional stability and mental alertness, and energizes the body. Maintaining your health, physical and mental energy, and positive outlook has never been easier. And to imagine we can do all this just with food!

The Detox Reaction

When you begin a raw foods diet, you may experience a detoxification reaction. This reaction is itself an indicator of the health-endowing powers of raw foods. You'll see for yourself that accumulated toxins in your body are eliminated and physiological imbalances are corrected. You might look worse before you look better; you might feel worse before you feel better. Sometimes we must first get sick in order to get well.

The detox reaction usually kicks in a few months into the raw diet. For me, the reaction began when I was three months into my new lifestyle. Signs of detox can include fatigue, coated tongue, cold or flulike symptoms, muscle soreness, phlegm, low libido, sore throat, headache, bad breath, body odor, cough, sinus congestion, depression, nausea, darkened urine, sweating, fever, skin breakouts, stomachache, diarrhea, and irritability. Rest and sleep facilitate the detox process. Mild exercise such as walking or low-impact aerobics is also helpful, but you should avoid anything strenuous. Drink plenty of water. Focus on supporting the channels of elimination (see below). Spend time in fresh air and sunshine when possible. Soaking in hot mineral springs, going to a sauna, or practicing dry-brush skin massage can assist in the cleansing process. Enemas and colonics can help toxins leave the body through the bowels rather than the skin.

When you embrace a lighter diet, old, repressed emotions (perhaps buried with mounds of cheesecake) can rise to the surface. Cry. Journal. Scream. Pound on pillows. Take a warm bath. Assist the cleansing process rather than suppressing it. Get your "ya-yas" out! This can also be a good time to get some housecleaning and uncluttering done. Let go of "stuck energy" in your physical environment to create more peace in your inner realm.

Research Studies

To date, science has not shown much interest in the benefits of raw foods. Studies are expensive in general and, with no corporate sponsor seeking evi-

The Channels of Elimination

The body has many methods of letting go of what is no longer needed and what needs to be cleansed. The following are the channels of elimination:

- Urine
- Sweat
- Lungs
- Feces
- Secretions from nose, eyes, ears, and throat
- Emotions

dence in support of a new, marketable product, nutrition research can be difficult to fund. A few small studies on raw foods have been done, however, with a range of test subjects, and the results have all been positive, as detailed below. (More studies have been conducted on enzymes. For further information on enzyme research, check out works such as *Enzymes: The Fountain of Life* by D.A. Lopez, R.M. Williams, and K. Miehlke; *Enzyme and Enzyme Therapy* by Anthony J. Cichoke; and *Enzyme Nutrition: The Food Enzyme Concept* by Edward Howell.)

Pottenger

Beginning in 1932, physician Francis M. Pottenger of Monrovia, California, conducted a study that lasted over a decade and included over 900 cats. Two groups of cats were fed identical diets of meat, milk, and vegetables, but the food for one group was cooked and the food for the other group was given raw. The cats of the raw food group had good health, as did their offspring. The cats of the cooked food group, however, all had health breakdowns including hair loss, brittle bones, heartburn, arthritis, pyorrhea, underactive thyroid, liver disorders (cirrhosis, atrophy, and other problems), brain thickening, oozing mucous membranes, skin lesions, allergies, respiratory infections, intestinal parasites, vision problems, and spinal cord degeneration.

The females of the group fed cooked food were aggressive and irritable, while the males were docile and showed little interest in the females. This group of cats did not survive beyond the third generation. Among the first generation, the miscarriage rate was about 25 percent, and among the second generation it was about 70 percent. By the third generation, the cats were sterile and many had congenital deformities. Kittens in the cooked food group weighed an average of 19 grams less than kittens whose mothers ate raw foods.

McCarrison

In the late 1920s and early 1930s, Robert McCarrison, a British officer stationed in India, performed a study with white rats. One thousand rats were fed a partially raw diet consisting of cabbage, carrots, sprouts, bread, milk, and meat. Another 2,000 rats were fed a diet of canned food, boiled vegetables, and milk. The rats of the first group thrived. The rats of the second group began to develop ailments such as tuberculosis, ulcers, hair loss, dental decay, skin diseases, tonsillitis, and arthritis.

Ling and Colleagues

A study published in 1992 in the *Journal of Nutrition* detailed the work of researchers at the University of Kuopio in Finland who studied the effects of a raw, vegan diet on fecal activity. Eighteen participants were divided randomly into a test group and a control group. The test group ate a raw, vegan diet for one month and a conventional diet for a second month, while the control group ate a conventional diet for both months. The researchers measured levels of fecal enzymes and the toxins phenol and p-cresol in the participants' blood serum.

The test group showed declines in the measured substances while on the raw, vegan diet, but then their fecal enzyme levels returned to normal within two weeks of resuming the conventional diet, and their phenol and p-cresol concentrations returned to normal within one month. The control group, on the conventional diet throughout, exhibited no changes in these levels. These results suggest that following a raw, vegan diet causes a decrease in bacterial enzymes and certain toxins that have been shown to contribute to colon cancer risk.

Kaartinen and Colleagues

Another study at the University of Kuopio, published in 2000 in the *Scandinavian Journal of Rheumatology*, detailed the work of researchers who investigated the effects of nutrition on thirty-three female patients (average age fifty-one) suffering from fibromyalgia. For three months, eighteen of the women ate a completely raw diet and the rest ate a vegan diet. At the end of the study, the adherents to the raw foods diet reported less pain, better sleep, and less morning stiffness, whereas the patients on the vegan diet complained of more pain.

Donaldson and Colleagues

A study published in 2001 in *Nutrition and Food Science* presented the results of a survey of followers of a mostly raw, all-vegetarian diet. Self-reported, seven-day dietary records of 141 participants were collected and analyzed for nutrient intake, and the participants also reported on changes in their health and quality of life after adopting the diet. Improvements in health and quality of life were significant: on a scale of 1–100, the group's average rating for general health rose from 61 to 90; for vitality, from 49 to 78; and for mental health, from 71 to 87.

FREQUENTLY ASKED QUESTIONS

For people contemplating a raw foods diet, whether as a possible lifestyle change or when faced with someone who has already made the change, several questions are inevitable. Those questions are addressed here. The answers will, I hope, satisfy your concerns and offer enough information that you can provide an intelligent, heartfelt answer to the curious and the skeptical. Be glad when people ask questions! They give you an opportunity to convey your enthusiasm and spread the word of raw health.

Where Do You Get Protein?

We've been trained to recognize meats, eggs, and dairy products as good sources of protein. However, protein can also be found in many plant-source foods—and some of these foods contain more protein than any food of animal origin.

Proteins are made of amino acids, and twenty-two amino acids are known to be necessary for our physiological health. Eight of these amino acids are termed "essential," because they cannot be produced in the human body and must instead be consumed through the diet. Protein is necessary for tissue growth and repair as well as the formation of blood cells, antibodies, enzymes, hormones, and neurotransmitters. Protein provides the body with energy and plays a role in the body's balancing of water and electrolytes.

While it is imperative to have protein in the diet, it is also important not to overdo it. Excess protein can overload the lymphatic system's ability to cleanse itself. A diet that is excessively rich in protein can contribute to heart disease, high blood pressure, arthritis, gout, kidney, osteoporosis, and liver and prostate disorders. Studies at the Max Planck Institute for National Research have found that too much protein in the diet—even if only a small excess—can decrease the body's ability to transport oxygen, and lack of oxygen is thought to be a contributing factor in the development of cancer.

The amino acids in protein start becoming destroyed at 118°F and are almost completely destroyed by 160°F. In terms of food, this means that cooking causes food proteins to coagulate and become denatured, making them less digestible and more likely to produce inflammation. In fact, cooking food to a temperature just under 200°F causes leukocytosis, a condition wherein leukocytes (white blood cells that attack foreign substances) are called in to help with digestion. After the consumption of a meal including cooked protein, white blood cell levels increase by as much as 600 percent. This immune system response indicates that the body, in striving to maintain homeostasis, is recognizing components of cooked food as invaders that must be neutralized.

Because cooked proteins are at least partially denatured, food that is cooked provides the body with much less protein than the same food in its raw state. As cooked food is predominant in our culture, protein-intake recommendations (currently hovering around 70 grams a day) tend to be based on cooked rather than raw food. But researchers at the Max Planck Institute have found that when protein is consumed in its raw state, a person needs only half as much as when protein is consumed after being cooked. In other words, instead of eating 70 grams of cooked protein a day, you can eat 35 grams of raw protein and still meet your nutritional needs.

Proteins that contain all eight essential amino acids are called complete proteins. These are found in foods including:

- Alfalfa leaf
- Buckwheat
- Clover blossoms
- Fruits (most of them)
- Garbanzo beans
- Leafy green vegetables
- Lentils
- Millet
- Mung beans
- Nuts (all except hazelnuts/filberts)
- Pumpkin seeds
- Quinoa
- Sesame seeds
- Soy foods
- Sunflower greens

Other good protein sources include:

- Apricots
- Avocados
- Bananas
- Beans
- Berries
- Blue-green algae
- Broccoli
- Brussels sprouts
- Cabbages
- Carrots
- Cauliflower
- Cherries
- Coconut
- Corn
- Cucumbers
- Dates
- Durians
- Eggplant

- Grapes
- Hemp seeds
- Melons
- Okra
- Oranges
- Papayas
- Parsley
- Peaches
- Pears
- Peas
- Peppers

- Spirulina
- Sprouts (including sprouted grains)
- String beans
- Summer squash
- Sun-cured olives
- Sweet potatoes
- Tomatoes
- Turnip greens
- Watercress
- Zucchini

Generally speaking, vegetables have a higher percentage of protein per caloric content than nuts, and nuts have a higher percentage of protein per caloric content than fruits, but there are exceptions to these generalizations, of course.

Aren't Raw Foods Hard to Digest?

Many people are plagued with digestive complaints and have had trouble in the past eating raw foods. Some have been told they lack digestive ability and must eat only cooked foods. *Au contraire!* Enzymes are what you need to heal digestion problems, and you're certainly not going to find them in cooked food.

Raw foods work as intestinal brooms, and eating them causes a cleansing reaction; although this may cause gas and/or intestinal discomfort in some people, it is usually only a short-term initial problem. If you find that certain raw foods are difficult to digest, avoid them at first, but don't hesitate to try them in small amounts later, after you've been raw for a couple of months. As your digestion becomes stronger from the intake of enzymes, your food repertoire can increase.

If you have poor digestion or are very ill, help your digestive system by breaking down your food as much as possible before it reaches your stomach. Chew well. Juice or purée vegetables to make soups. Soak dried fruits, and purée them if needed. Make fruit smoothies. Sprout your grains and

The Raw Facts

Here are a few examples of the amount of protein in foods according to their total caloric content:

Almonds	12 percent	Pumpkin	15 percent
Broccoli	45 percent	Spinach	49 percent
Buckwheat	15 percent	Walnuts	13 percent
Cabbage	22 percent	Watercress	84 percent
Honeydew melon	16 percent	Zucchini	28 percent
Kale	45 percent		

nuts. Read the section on food combining. You can also season your food with any of the many herbs and spices that facilitate digestion, including:

- Anise
- Basil
- Cardamom
- Cinnamon
- Cumin
- Fennel
- Ginger
- Rosemary
- Spearmint
- Thyme
- Turmeric

Won't You Be Hungry?

Many people think that a raw foods diet will leave them feeling constantly hungry. Perhaps that's because they equate it with eating only small amounts of raw fruits and vegetables in their plainest form. In truth, as you'll learn through the following chapter, a raw diet is far from the classic stereotype of "rabbit food." It offers a tremendous variety of ingredients, flavors, and preparation methods. Because raw foods are packed with nutrients and fiber, they are satisfying to both the palate and the stomach. They fill you up without giving you that heavy, oily, lethargic, "stuffed" feeling that comes from eating an excess of cooked fats and carbohydrates. And generally speaking, you can eat as much raw food as you like without worrying about weight gain. In fact, as you'll find out, the raw foods diet actually supports the maintenance of your optimal body weight.

Won't You Be Cold in Winter?

For many years, I resisted the raw foods path in the belief that eating raw food would cause a "cold, damp spleen" (as it's described in Oriental medicine) and make me unable to tolerate the cold Colorado winters. Practitioners of Oriental medicine cook almost all of their food in the belief that cooking predigests it, and because of the fear of food-borne parasites. Cooking food to make it more digestible sounds good in theory, but we might want to recognize that cooked food has not brought ultimate health to those who eat it. Now that I eat raw, I am amazed that it took me so long to overcome this prejudice. Coldness and dampness in the spleen are usually associated with impaired digestion—but I (like most raw foodists I know) am happy to say that, over time, the raw foods diet has made my digestive system work better than ever before.

People who do not practice Oriental medicine may nevertheless steer away from raw foods in the winter simply because it feels much nicer to have a hot bowl of soup warming up their insides. It's true that newcomers to a raw foods diet may feel cold more easily; one reason for this is that raw foods are less dense in calories, and calories produce heat as food is metabolized by the body. After some time, however, eating raw foods will cause your arteries and other blood vessels to become less congested, circulation will improve, and you will feel more comfortable in either cold or warm weather.

Rather than eating warm foods when the weather is cold, eat warming foods. "Warm" foods are heated and, as we've learned, have therefore lost some of their nutrients. "Warming" foods are those raw foods that offer concentrated nourishment, improve circulation and thereby increase body warmth, and otherwise help you tolerate the cold.

Try filling your diet with warming, concentrated, dark orange vegetables such as pumpkins, sweet potatoes, winter squash, and carrots. Eat more warming roots such as burdock, onions, rutabagas, and turnips, and warming greens such as arugula, mustard greens, and watercress. Consuming more nuts, nut butters, and dried fruit will help you develop better resistance to the cold. Getting adequate fats by consuming olive oil, avocados, durians, nuts, and seeds helps treat the dryness of skin and scalp that is so prevalent when heat is used in homes during the winter.

Use more of the warming culinary herbs to spice up your food and improve circulation. Good choices include:

- Black sesame seeds
- Cardamom
- Cayenne
- Cinnamon
- Curry (a combination of several warming spices)

- Garlic
- Ginger
- Horseradish

- Jalapeño
- Pepper, black or white

If you don't want to eat cold food, you can warm your raw meals up to 114°F without destroying any of the enzymes. You can also leave food out at room temperature, serve it on prewarmed plates, or place it in a glass jar with a secure lid and submerge the jar in some hot water to warm it up. Many raw foodists living in cold climates drink hot herbal teas in cold weather—just heat the water without boiling it.

People may ask, "Aren't you cold eating only raw food in the winter?" When they do, ask them right back, "Aren't you hot eating cooked food in the summer?"

How Do I Get Started?

Many people think that being raw will be difficult. It's not. It really does save time, money, and your health, and it's so very worth it.

As it can be a shock to the body to stop eating familiar fare abruptly, a gradual transition works best for some people. Begin by including a raw dish with each meal. Then, make one meal each day completely raw. Start having raw dishes for main entrées and relegate cooked foods to side dishes. Gradually increase the amount of raw food and decrease the amount of cooked food in your diet. Eliminate first those heavier, unhealthful foods you know you shouldn't be eating. Have baked or steamed rather than fried foods. Let go of prepackaged, instant, frozen, and other ready-to-eat, refined foods. Replace dairy, eggs, and meat with avocados, nuts, and seeds. Eventually, remove all the cooked, canned, and sugar- and flour-rich foods from your cupboards. Shop at natural foods stores or markets that sell organic produce, and avoid regular grocery stores. As much as possible, eat foods that are in season (see "Eating Seasonally" on page 136).

Some people take as long as a year to become totally raw. The hardest withdrawal period is at about two months. Salt cravings may indicate a need for more minerals: instead of potato chips, eat seaweeds. If you have cravings for sweet foods, eat celery to diminish them. If you strongly crave fats, eat avocados and nuts, and balance them with lots of greens, celery, and cucumbers. The one food you think you just can't give up—whether potato chips, coffee, chocolate, or any other—is very likely your greatest health impediment. To discourage cravings, drink green drinks, which are alkalinizing and calming to the emotions (where many cravings originate).

For motivation, take a "before" photo of yourself, and then take another photo after six months of being raw. Start a journal and write about your health history, keeping track of how your health improves or worsens (see The Detox Reaction on page 14) as you go raw. Make a list of five foods you would be better off without. Write down five limiting beliefs and replace them with affirmations: for example, "I am fat" can be replaced with "Every day, I am making healthier choices."

If you slip off the raw path, learn from the experience. Rather than feeling guilty, observe how you feel and get back on track as soon as possible. For best results, stick with the program and don't deviate.

It can be so helpful to have a raw buddy to share this process with you. Make a delicious raw meal for your friends; lend them books on the subject; and plan raw potlucks or raw theme dinners (Mexican, Indian, and the like; see "Theme Dinners" on page 258). To find other raw-interested folks in your area, offer to teach a class, or put up a sign in the local health foods store to connect with others for discussion, support, or meal sharing.

It may take up to three or four months on a raw foods diet before you are able to judge how it is working for you. Do your best to be at least 80 percent raw—and for ultimate health and healing, do it 100 percent!

3

Raw Foods Encyclopedia

*T*he foods that you eat maintain the health of your body, not only nutritionally but also therapeutically. Foods themselves do not technically heal the body, as only the body can heal itself. Eating the right foods, however, can help provide the right conditions for the body to heal itself. In this light, food can be seen as medicine. So in the case of illness or imbalance, instead of turning to pharmaceuticals, why not first try amending your diet? This chapter will help you understand the nutritional and healing properties of the fruits, vegetables, grains, nuts, and other foods that are commonly available to the Western consumer.

FRUITS AND VEGETABLES

Fruits and vegetables will form the vast majority of your raw foods diet. As much as possible, eat produce that is organic. Because no chemical pesticides or herbicides are used in its agriculture, organic produce supports not only your own health but also that of the soil and the planet. Although organic produce is still difficult to find in many areas, and tends to be more expensive than other produce, buying organic foods whenever you can puts pressure on the economic system to produce more of it. In effect, you'll be voting with your dollars for the continued development of organic agriculture.

Apple (*Malus* species)—Rosaceae (Rose) Family

Apples are sweet, sour, and alkaline, and have a cool energy. They are rich in flavonoids, beta-carotene, vitamin B, vitamin C, boron, calcium, phosphorus, potassium, and silicon. The more tart an apple, the higher its vitamin C content. Apples are also high in pectin, a soluble fiber that helps in

The Raw Facts

When not grown organically, the following plant foods receive high levels of pesticides and tend to carry the greatest amount of pesticide residue:

- Apples
- Cabbages
- Cantaloupe
- Carrots
- Celery
- Cucumbers
- Dates
- Grapes
- Lemons
- Nectarines

- Peaches
- Peanuts
- Pears
- Peppers (bell peppers and others)
- Spinach
- Strawberries
- String beans
- Sweet potatoes
- Tomatoes
- Winter squash

The following foods receive the least amount of pesticide treatment and tend to be relatively free of pesticide residue:

- Avocados
- Corn
- Figs
- Garlic

- Nuts*
- Papayas
- Watermelon

*Except peanuts, which may bear residue, and are really a legume; see "The Raw Facts" on page 83.

lowering blood pressure and cholesterol levels, especially of harmful low-density lipoprotein (LDL for short).

The old expression "An apple a day keeps the doctor away" has it right: apples are a superb, overall tonic for the body and especially for *yin* (see "Yin, Yang, and Chi" on page 27). This fruit has antibacterial, anti-inflammatory, antiviral, astringent, diuretic, tonic, and some estrogenic activity. Apples stabilize blood sugar levels, which is helpful in both hypoglycemia and diabetes. They promote good digestion, prevent intestinal fermentation, and reduce colon inflammation, thereby improving both diarrhea and constipation. They are of benefit in cases of arthritis pain, edema, gout, morning sickness, asthma, catarrh, hardening of the arteries, skin diseases, liver and gallbladder sluggishness, and rheumatism. Eating apples stimulates saliva flow, cleans the teeth, and stimulates gum tissue. It helps lubricate the lungs and cleanse the lymphatic system. Apples can also aid in weight loss, neutralize the effects of smoking, curb cravings for alcohol, and remove radiation from the body.

Apples taste best when they are in season and firm to the touch, as those yielding to the pressure of a fingertip will be mealy. Store them at 35°F. Apples can be enjoyed in pies, tarts, sauces, cakes, and salads, juiced alone or with other fruits or vegetables, or dried—but for maximum health benefits, eat them in their fresh, raw state! They are best eaten unpeeled, because their pectin is concentrated near the skin, and the peel also contains other dietary fiber. If you can't find organic apples, however, you should peel your apples before eating them, because commercial apples are often coated with wax and have pesticide residues on the skin.

Yin, Yang, and Chi

According to ancient Asian philosophy, *yin* and *yang* are the vital polarities that permeate the universe from the tiniest mote to the grandest star system. They are not warring opposites but different sides of a continuum, merging into one another. Neither can exist without the other, and the balance of the two affects the life force of every object and organism, including the human body.

In traditional Oriental medicine, ailments are often described in terms of a *yin-yang* imbalance. *Yin* embodies coldness and dampness, whereas *yang* embodies heat and dryness. A *yang* deficiency, for example, could result in a damp, cold condition such as lower back pain, lethargy, or edema. A *yin* deficiency, on the other hand, could result in a dry, warm condition such as insomnia, nervous exhaustion, or dizziness. Treatment is therefore focused on restoring *yin-yang* balance to the affected system or organ, and the root of that treatment is often the diet.

Chi (also spelled Qi) means life force or vital energy. It is a colorless, tasteless, odorless, formless substance that exists in the universe. We extract chi from food, which combines with the chi from the air we breathe, which contributes to health and vitality.

Apricot (*Prunus armeniaca*)—Rosaceae (Rose) Family

Apricots are sweet and sour, and neutral in energy. Apricots are rich in beta-carotene, vitamin C, copper, iron, magnesium, potassium, silicon, and cobalt. They are a natural laxative because of their high fiber and pectin content. They also contain a trace amount of lycopene, which is being researched as a cancer preventative.

Apricots are alkaline, nutritive, and antioxidant. They are an excellent fruit for midsummer, as they moisten the lungs and provide the body with *yin* fluids. They have been used to treat acne, anemia, asthma, bronchitis, catarrh, constipation, hypertension, toxemia, and tuberculosis. Apricot pulp can be used as a facial to soften the skin and reduce the appearance of wrinkles.

Apricots are most delicious when orange in color, without any green; otherwise, they are immature and will be sour. Enjoy them fresh as a snack or added to smoothies and fruit juices. Dried apricots can be soaked overnight and enjoyed in the morning as a breakfast of "stewed" fruit.

Note: Excess ingestion of apricots may cause diarrhea; therefore, during pregnancy, they should be eaten only in moderation. Also, most commercially dried apricots are treated with sulfur dioxide, a preservative that can cause allergic reactions in some people and should be avoided by all (see the Resources section for suppliers of untreated dried fruit).

Arugula (*Eruca vesicaria*)—Brassicaceae (Mustard) Family

Arugula, also known as rocket, roquette, Italian cress, and roka, is pungent and highly alkaline, with a warm energy. Arugula contains beta-carotene, vitamin C, calcium, iron, and sulfur. It also contains dithiolthiones (antioxidant and anticancer compounds) and is recommended as an anticancer food by the American Cancer Society. Arugula stimulates the liver and lungs and exhibits antibiotic and antiviral properties.

Eat arugula's young, green leaves, as the older leaves tend to be bitter and intensely flavored. Because of its strong flavor, arugula is best when mixed in a salad with other greens.

Asparagus (*Asparagus officinalis*)—Liliaceae (Lily) Family

Asparagus is alkaline, slightly warm, bitter, and pungent. Fresh, young asparagus shoots are rich in beta-carotene, vitamins B, C, and E, iodine, potassium, and zinc. They also contain the alkaloid asparagine, which is an effective diuretic and helps dissolve uric and oxalic acids as well, making asparagus a useful adjunct in the treatment of arthritis (the buildup of these acids contributes to arthritic symptoms).

Asparagus cools fever, increases production of mother's milk, boosts vitality, inhibits tumor growth, reduces the size and occurrence of kidney stones, and clears dark circles from under the eyes. Asparagus has long been used as an aphrodisiac, perhaps in part because of its phallic shape, but also because it increases circulatory activity in the genito-urinary system. So if you're wondering what to serve that special someone . . .

Look for bright, green asparagus spears with compact tops. Flat or thick stalks are likely to be woody and stringy. Asparagus is best eaten in spring, its natural ripening time. It is delightful added raw to salads, puréed in soups, or mixed with other vegetables.

Avocado (*Persea americana, P. gratissima*)—Lauraceae (Laurel) Family

Avocado is sweet and is considered to have a cooling energy. Avocados are rich in vitamin E, B-complex vitamins, beta-carotene, potassium (two to three times that of bananas), fluorine, copper, and lecithin. A single avocado has about 300 calories, in part because it is about 20 percent monounsaturated fat. This is the type of fat that helps maintain levels of good cholesterol (high-density lipoprotein, or HDL) in the body. People who have difficulty digesting fats will usually find avocado easy to assimilate.

Avocado nourishes the blood, lubricates the lungs and large intestines, balances liver function, and, in cases of cystitis, soothes the bladder. A traditional remedy for erectile dysfunction, constipation, nervousness, and insomnia, it is also recommended for convalescence, ulcers, and colitis. Mashed avocado applied to the face or scalp is nourishing and conditioning, and is especially beneficial for dry skin and hair.

Look for avocado fruits that yield slightly when pressed. If an avocado is very firm and not yet ripe, you can place it in a paper bag in a warm location to speed the ripening process. Once ripe, avocados should be refrigerated to keep them from becoming rancid (avoid rancid or overripe fruits). Avocado is excellent as a garnish, in fruit or vegetable salad, as a sandwich filler, and, of course, in guacamole. Many suprising uses for avocado will be found in the Raw Recipes chapter.

Banana (*Musa acuminata, M. sapientum*)—Muscaeae (Banana) Family

Bananas are considered cold and have a tendency to move energy inward in the body. They are sweet, being rich in carbohydrates (mostly the sugars glucose and fructose), as well as in folic acid, vitamins B_6 and C, potassium, and pectin. They also contain an enzyme that aids in the production of sex hormones. As bananas are high in calories but low in fat, they are an excellent food for pregnant mothers, babies, and children.

Bananas provide long-term energy and improve stamina. They moisten the *yin* fluids of the body, including the lungs and large intestines, and have some antiseptic activity. They support the friendly intestinal flora (helpful bacteria within our bowels) and stimulate the proliferation of cells that provide a protective coating between the stomach and harsh digestive acids. Bananas also stimulate the production of serotonin, a neurotransmitter that can improve sleep and elevate mood.

Bananas have been used to treat alcoholism, arteriosclerosis, celiac disease, colitis, constipation, depression, diarrhea, dyspepsia, exhaustion, hemorrhoids, hypertension, weak muscles, and ulcers. They have also been used to help treat insulin shock in diabetics. Ripe bananas are very easy to digest—even easier when mashed—and are recommended for those suffering from weak digestion, vomiting, or emaciation.

Bananas are ripe when they are solid yellow without any green, and are overripe once they develop large brown spots. Unripe bananas contain enzyme inhibitors and are therefore constipating and difficult to digest, whereas ripe bananas do not have the inhibitors and are considered laxative. Avoid commercial bananas, which are picked unripe and then treated with ethylene gas to hasten ripening during shipment; instead, purchase organic bananas and place them in a paper bag to encourage natural ripening. To preserve bananas at the peak of ripeness, store them in the refrigerator, which will turn the skin brown but not adversely affect the flavor, or keep them in a dark, plastic bag sealed with a twist tie.

Use bananas in puddings, pies, fruit salads, and smoothies. Bananas blended with water make nourishing banana milk. Snack on them fresh, or try a sandwich of banana and raw almond butter. Freeze peeled bananas and run them through a juicer to make dairy-free "ice cream." Dried banana chips make a tasty, sweet treat.

Note: People who are exceedingly cold, frail, or lethargic should only consume bananas in moderation, as eating them may exacerbate those conditions.

Beet (*Beta vulgaris*)—Chenopodiaceae (Goosefoot) Family

Beets are sweet. They abound with nutrients including beta-carotene, B-complex vitamins, vitamin C, iron, calcium, phosphorus, sodium, and manganese. Betaine, the red pigment that gives beets their color, helps increase oxygen intake. Being round roots, beets are considered to have a downward energy, affecting the lower organs and especially benefiting the colon, kidneys, bladder, spleen, and liver.

Said to be both blood cleansing and blood building, beets help build red corpuscles and have long been used therapeutically to treat anemia. They have also been used to treat constipation, infectious hepatitis, irregular menses, acne, lumbago, and low blood sugar.

Try beets grated raw into a salad. They are also lovely when seasoned with a bit of honey and lemon. Other seasonings that bring out the best in beets include dill, basil, parsley, and tarragon. Carrot-beet juice is a bona fide *energizing elixir*. The root is not the only edible part of the beet plant: beet greens are delicious when finely chopped and added to salads.

Note: Beet greens are even richer in iron than spinach is, but they do contain high levels of oxalic acid, which makes them suitable for occasional use only. Also, be aware that eating lots of beets may add a red color to your urine or stools, and remember that you have been eating beets before you rush off to the emergency ward!

Bell Pepper (*Capsicum annum*)—Solanaceae (Nightshade) Family

Bell peppers are sweet, pungent, alkaline, and warm. Rich in beta-carotene, vitamin C, silicon, and bioflavonoids, they contain some vitamin B_6, E, and folic acid as well. Peppers also contain lycopene, a carotenoid believed to help reduce the risk of prostate, cervical, bladder, and pancreatic cancers.

Bell peppers have antioxidant and circulatory-stimulant properties, and are considered useful in warding off angina, atherosclerosis, cataracts, constipation, colds, high blood pressure, macular degeneration, obesity, and respiratory ailments (asthma, bronchitis, catarrh, sinus congestion). Their high silicon content makes them an excellent "beauty food" for skin, hair, teeth, and nails.

Look for firm, unwrinkled, brightly colored peppers that are heavy for their size. Red bell peppers are more ripe, sweet, and nutritious than green ones. The refinement of their shape does not matter, as being crooked will not adversely affect their quality or taste. Store peppers in a cool place. Eat them stuffed, as a garnish, or in salads, sauces, crudités, and soups.

Note: People who suffer from arthritis may benefit from avoiding peppers and other members of the nightshade family (eggplant, potatoes, and tomatoes), as these foods contain solanine, an alkaloid that can inhibit calcium absorption if overconsumed.

Blackberry (*Rubus* species)—Rosaceae (Rose) Family

Blackberries are sweet, sour, and cooling. They contain vitamin C, niacin, pectin, sugars, anthocyanins, and flavonoids (especially kaempferol and quercitin).

Blackberries have alterative, astringent, blood-tonic, diuretic, hemostatic, nutritive, refrigerant, uterine-tonic, and *yin*-tonic properties. They have been used in the treatment of anemia, cholera, diarrhea, dysentery, fever, hemorrhoids, and infertility. They help dispel heat, reduce inflammation, cool fever, and dry excess dampness in the body.

Blackberries are a tasty treat all by themselves. Of course, they also can be enjoyed in raw pies, tarts, jams, and soups, and can even be used as food coloring.

Blueberry (*Vaccinium myrtillus, V. corymbosum, V. ashei, V. angustifolium*)—Ericaceae (Heath) Family

Blueberries are sour, astringent, and moist, with a cold energy. They contain beta-carotene, vitamin C, iron, and potassium, and are rich in silicon, which is believed to help regenerate the pancreas. They also contain pectin, which binds with cholesterol, lowering its levels and helping prevent the buildup of plaque in the blood. It is believed that anthocyanadin, a flavonoid and antioxidant found in blueberries, makes the walls of blood vessels stronger by interacting with their collagen, helping deter capillary fragility and the development of varicose veins. Myrtillin, another compound in blueberries, lowers blood sugar levels, and for that reason this fruit is considered beneficial in preventing and treating diabetes.

Blueberries are considered alterative, anti-emetic, antifungal, anti-inflammatory, antioxidant, antiseptic, antiviral, astringent, and diuretic. A *yin* tonic, they cool and cleanse the kidneys and liver. A urinary antiseptic, they help prevent bacteria from adhering to the bladder wall and are used to prevent and treat urinary tract infections. These berries have long been used in treatments for anemia, arthritis, dry skin, dysentery, *E. coli* infection, hemorrhoids, dysmenorrhea (menstrual cramps), fevers, gout, intestinal flu, joint inflammation, mouth sores, obesity, ulcers, and worms. They reduce platelet aggregation, thereby helping to prevent clumps or clots from forming in the blood. Large amounts of blueberries are laxative, though small amounts can be used to treat diarrhea.

Because blueberries improve circulation to the brain and extremities, and particularly increase circulation to the eyes, they are recommended against a wide range of eye diseases and have been used in treatments for eye weakness, cataracts, glaucoma, diabetic retinopathy, macular degeneration, myopia, and night blindness. They are especially helpful for people whose work can lead to strained eyesight, such as computer workers, drivers, pilots, and air traffic controllers.

Look for firm, plump, organic blueberries. They are wonderful eaten plain or added to pies, tarts, jams, cobblers, muffins, breads, ice creams, and yogurt.

Broccoli (*Brassica oleracea italica*)—Brassicaceae (Mustard) Family

Broccoli is pungent and slightly bitter, and is considered cooling. It is rich in fiber, beta-carotene, vitamins B_2, C, and K, pantothenic and folic acid, boron, calcium, chromium, iron, potassium, selenium, and sulfur. It contains many antioxidants including dithiolthiones, quercitin, lutein, zeaxanthin, and glutathione, as well as monoterpene carotenoids that have antioxidant properties and protect against breast, cervical, colon, esophageal, lung, and stomach cancers. Broccoli also contains indoles and sulforaphanes, which are believed to activate enzymes that, in turn, deactivate estrogens that can contribute to tumor growth.

Broccoli has immune-stimulating, antiviral, diuretic, and anti-ulcer activity. It aids in the digestion of fats, moves blockage and stuck energy from the liver, and helps regulate insulin and blood sugar levels. Broccoli also helps prevent constipation, high blood pressure, nearsightedness, neuritis, obesity, and toxemia.

This vegetable is most nutritious when consumed raw, because cooking destroys many of its valuable anticancer compounds. Look for dark-colored broccoli featuring compact clusters of buds. Use it in salads and soups, or as a crudité for dips. Broccoli sprouts (an excellent anticancer food and a rich source of calcium and folic acid) are also delicious.

Note: As eating raw broccoli can inhibit iodine absorption, people with low thyroid function should ensure adequate iodine intake.

Brussels Sprout (*Brassica oleracea gemmifera*)—Brassicaceae (Mustard) Family

Brussels sprouts are pungent, sweet, slightly bitter, and warming. These vegetables are alkalinizing and antioxidant, and their high sulfur content makes them warming. They are a good source of beta-carotene, vitamins B_6 and C, folic acid, flavonoids, calcium, iron, and phosphorus.

Brussels sprouts contain indoles, which are believed to prevent breast cancer by blocking the activity of estrogens that contribute to tumor growth, and sulforaphanes, which block carcinogens from damaging healthy cells. Brussels sprouts are also considered a preventative to colon cancer, and their high fiber content promotes bowel health. They stimulate the liver and have an affinity for the pancreas. They have been used to remedy acidosis, arteriosclerosis, catarrh, constipation, bleeding gums, and high cholesterol.

Select firm, compact, bright green Brussels sprouts. Puffy sprouts tend to taste bland, and smaller ones (less than $1\frac{1}{2}$ inches in diameter) tend to taste better. Their flavor improves after they have been through a frost, so they are most popular as a fall and winter vegetable. Young, tender Brussels sprouts can be enjoyed raw, sliced into salads, or used as crudités.

Note: For some people, especially for those prone to constipation, Brussels sprouts may induce gas and bloating; remember, however, that this reaction is caused by the vegetable's cleansing activity.

Cabbage (*Brassica oleracea*)—Brassicaceae (Mustard) Family

Cabbage is sweet and pungent in flavor, neutral to warming in energy, and alkaline. It is a good source of fiber, protein, histamine, beta-carotene, folic acid, vitamins B_1, B_6, C, K, and U, bioflavonoids, calcium, fluorine, iodine, iron, potassium, and sulfur. Cabbage also contains indoles, which help prevent breast cancer by inhibiting estrogens from stimulating tumor growth; monoterpenes, which are antioxidants that give protection against heart disease and cancer; and various other compounds shown to have anticancer properties.

This vegetable has alterative, anti-inflammatory, antiseptic, and diuretic properties. Esteemed as a circulatory stimulant, vermifuge, and muscle builder, it also strengthens the eyes, gums, teeth, bones, hair, liver, and nails. Cabbage is believed to lower the risk of heart disease, strokes, cataracts, and cancer of the colon, esophagus, lungs, skin, and stomach. It has been used to treat a wide range of conditions: asthma, high cholesterol, colds, colic, constipation, cough, depression, diabetes, eye infections, fibrocystic breast disease, gout, headaches, hearing loss, insomnia, irritability, kidney and bladder disorders, lumbago, lung congestion, radiation exposure, skin ailments, tuberculosis, ulcers, and yeast infections.

Chopped cabbage leaves are used as a topical treatment on painful joints, bug bites or stings, burns, eczema, rashes, varicose veins, and wounds, including gangrene. In fact, they are a soothing poultice for just about any skin irritation. Try them on hemorrhoids!

Many varieties of cabbage exist: Savoy (crinkly), bok choy, Napa (or Chinese), red, and white (sometimes called green). Look for firm, crisp heads with no evidence of decay or worm infestation. It is an inexpensive vegetable and stores well over the winter, especially if kept in a cool location.

Cabbage can be stuffed, used in slaws, salads, and soups, or juiced. Fermenting it, with or without the addition of salt, makes sauerkraut (rinse before serving to lower the sodium content). Unpasteurized sauerkraut contains microorganisms that promote healthy intestinal flora.

Note: Cabbage contains goitergens, which can interfere with normal thyroid function when iodine levels are low. Regular consumption of sea vegetables will prevent iodine deficiencies. Some people complain that cabbage causes gas, but this is probably the result of cabbage's action in loosening old bowel pockets, such as those that occur in diverticulitis. This action vanishes after being on a raw diet for several months.

Cantaloupe (*Cucumis melo*)—Curcurbitaceae (Gourd) Family

Cantaloupe is sweet and cooling. Cantaloupe is delightfully low in calories, and it is ideal for breaking a fast, being one of the easiest foods to digest. Ninety-four percent of a cantaloupe is highly mineralized water. In addition to those minerals, this fruit is rich in fiber, pectin, beta-carotene, vitamins B_6 and C, flavonoids, potassium, carbohydrates, and protein. The part of the melon close to the rind is rich in silicon. Cantaloupe also contains adenosine, a compound used in modern medicine as a blood-thinning agent.

Cantaloupes are alkalinizing, anticoagulant, antioxidant, cleansing, diuretic, hydrating, laxative, rejuvenative, and *yin* tonic. They cool heat in the body and can benefit lung ailments. These melons have been used therapeutically to treat arthritis, poor blood quality and quantity, constipation, fever, high blood pressure, kidney and bladder disorders, obesity, rheumatism, and skin diseases. In China, cantaloupe is used to treat hepatitis.

Look for cantaloupe that is symmetrical in shape and heavy for its size, with an even color and a warm, floral aroma. They are best when a hollow remains at the end where the stem was attached; melons that have a wet or soft stem end, or make a watery sound when shaken, are overripe. Search out organic cantaloupe whenever possible, as the nonorganic ones generally have high levels of pesticide residue. Cantaloupe is best eaten on its own or combined with other melons in a fruit salad. Peeled, seeded, and frozen melon run through a juicer makes an instant sorbet, and you can freeze melon juice in Popsicle holders for kids of all ages.

Note: People who have diarrhea or feel chilled are better off saving melon for another time.

Carob (*Ceratonia siliqua*)—Fabaceae (Pea) Family

Carob is sweet and alkaline, with a warm energy. It contains natural sugars, pectin, calcium, and B-complex vitamins. It is best known as a substitute for chocolate, but unlike chocolate, carob does not contain caffeine.

As a therapeutic agent, carob calms nervousness and is mildly laxative. For a good snack, chew on a whole carob pod. Use powdered carob to give a chocolatey taste and appearance to smoothies and desserts. Look for *really* raw carob.

Carrot (*Daucus carota sativa*)—Apiaceae (Carrot) Family

Carrots are sweet, alkaline, and warming. They contain beta-carotene, vitamins B_6 and C, calcium, phosphorus, potassium, pectin, and fiber, and their leaves are rich in flavonoids and potassium.

Carrots have antibacterial, anti-inflammatory, antioxidant, astringent, diuretic, galactagogic, laxative, and liver-tonic properties. They strengthen the stomach, spleen, liver, and lungs—if we all ate one carrot a day, lung cancer rates in our population could be cut in half. This root vegetable has been used as a urinary antiseptic to treat cystitis as well as bladder and kidney stones. Carrots have also been used in treating acne, asthma, cancer, catarrh, colitis, constipation, cough, diarrhea, dry skin, eczema, gallstones, gastritis, gout, high cholesterol, indigestion, irritable bowel, jaundice, obesity, parasites, pyorrhea, sore throat, tonsillitis, toxemia, ulcers, and vision problems such as dry eyes, Bitot's spots, and night blindness.

Choose whole, unwilted, colorful carrots. Most commercially grown carrots are subject to a wide variety of chemical sprays and need to be peeled before being eaten, but organic carrots can be eaten with the peel still on, which is beneficial for our skin. Carrots are delicious in salads, soups, cakes, pies, and crudités. Young, fresh carrot tops can be used in salads too. Carrot juice is an excellent remedy to cleanse the liver but should be diluted with water, as it is very sweet.

Cauliflower (*Brassica oleracea botrytis*)—Brassicaceae (Mustard) Family

Cauliflower is pungent and sweet with a cooling energy. This vegetable is high in fiber and low in calories. Its white color denotes that it lacks the chlorophyll and carotenes of many of its more nutritious relatives. Cauliflower is rich, however, in vitamins B_6 and C, bioflavonoids, folic acid, biotin, boron, calcium, iron, phosphorus, potassium, and sulfur. It also contains anticancer compounds, including indoles and sulforaphane.

Cauliflower is antioxidant and alterative. It helps move blockages in the body, such as stuck chi, lumps, fibroids, and constipation, and dispel heat in the lungs. Because its anticancer compounds enhance enzyme activity that neutralizes carcinogens so they are unable to attack and transform cells, cauliflower is believed to reduce the risk of colon and stomach cancer in particular. It also aids in the body's metabolism of excess estrogen, helping curb breast cancer and fibrocystic breast disease. Cauliflower has been used to treat acne, asthma, bladder and kidney disorders, constipation, high blood pressure, gout, and obesity. Consumed raw, it helps remedy bleeding gums. According to folklore, cauliflower is said to be beneficial for mental function because it resembles the brain.

Look for firm, compact heads without brown spots. If the leaves (which are edible) are still attached, they should be fresh and green. Refrigerate cauliflower with the stem upward to prevent moisture from collecting on its top and hastening deterioration. Cauliflower can be chopped into salads, used as crudités, or made into soups or pâtés. It is best eaten raw, as cooking deactivates its indole activity.

Note: Eating large quantities of cauliflower may cause indigestion or flatulence in some people, especially if new to a raw diet.

Celery (*Apium graveolens*)—Apiaceae (Carrot) Family

Celery is cool in energy and its flavor is both sweet and bitter. It is about 95 percent water by volume but is rich in beta-carotene, folic acid, vitamin C, calcium, magnesium, potassium, silica, sodium, chlorophyll, and fiber. The seeds and stalks contain a calming compound called phthalide, which can soothe a sensation of heat in the stomach when ingested. Celery also contains coumarins, compounds believed beneficial in cancer prevention.

One of the most alkaline of foods, celery helps neutralize acids in the body. It is considered blood purifying, diuretic, and tonic. It is used to cool and detoxify the liver and has a special affinity for the stomach and kidneys as well. Celery helps dry overly damp conditions including yeast over-growth and excess phlegm. It is a traditional remedy for acne, arthritis, asthma, canker sores, constipation, diabetes, edema, eye inflammation, gallstones, gout, headache, hypertension, insomnia, cracking joints, nerv-ousness, obesity, pyorrhea, rheumatism, burning or bloody urination, ure-thritis, and wounds. After exercising, drinking celery juice helps replace lost electrolytes.

The commercial celery crop is subject to intensive chemical "support": the plants are often grown in nitrate fertilizers and sometimes the leaves are blanched. For this reason, eat organic celery. Look for varieties that are darker green (more nutritious) and select stalks that are not cracked, dam-aged, or wilted. Celery can be enjoyed in salads and soups and as an alter-native to chips for dips. Spread raw almond butter into celery stalks for an afternoon treat. Celery makes an excellent vegetable juice, especially com-bined with carrot and apple.

Note: During pregnancy, eat celery only in moderation, as it can pro-mote the onset of menses.

Chayote (*Sechium edule*)—Curcurbitaceae (Gourd) Family

Chayote (pronounced "chy-O-tay") is the pear-shaped fruit of a West Indi-an vine in the gourd family. Chayote is cooling and its flavor is similar to a blend of apple and cucumber. The smooth-skinned female fruit is lumpy with small ridges and is considered more delectable than the male fruit, which is covered with wartlike spines. Chayote was a staple food of the Aztecs and is high in vitamin C. In Central America, a tea made from the leaves is used to treat hypertension and arteriosclerosis.

Look for chayote with unblemished skin and an ivory to dark green color. Avoid wet, bruised, or soft fruits. Store the fruit in a dry, cool place; in the refrigerator, it keeps for several days. Chayote can be substituted for summer squash in most recipes. It can also be enjoyed whole, sliced, grat-ed into salads, puréed, or added to soups. If the fruit is large, it should be peeled and seeded, but if the fruit is young and tender, the peel can be eaten. Young root tubers of chayote can be eaten as well.

Cherimoya (*Annona cherimola*)—Annonaceae (Custard Apple) Family

Inside the spiky, yellow-green skin of a cherimoya is a lush, white meat with a cooling energy and a delicious flavor similar to a combination of banana, blueberry, and pineapple. Related to soursop, it is rich in vitamin

C, calcium, and iron. Cherimoyas have been used to remedy acidosis, bad breath, constipation, and kidney and bladder inflammation.

Cherimoya fruits are harvested while they are still firm and will ripen at room temperature on a sunny window. When ripe, they yield to the gentle pressure of a fingertip, much like an avocado. Avoid brown, bruised, or squishy fruits. Ripe cherimoyas will keep in the refrigerator for up to five days. Enjoy them plain or in fruit salads, sherbets, and smoothies. The seeds can be spit out.

Cherry (*Prunus avium, P. cerasus*)—Rosaceae (Rose) Family

Cherries are alkaline and sweet and considered to be warm—in the Orient, they are known as the "fruit of fire." Cherries are rich in beta-carotene, vitamins B_1 and C, calcium, copper, iron, manganese, phosphorus, potassium, silicon, flavonoids, and pectin. They also contain ellagic acid, an anticancer compound.

Cherries are a circulatory stimulant that dispel stagnation in the bloodstream and impart a rosy glow to the complexion. They make an excellent detoxifying food, helping the body eliminate uric acid and cleanse the kidneys. They also function as a laxative, a stomach and spleen tonic, a stimulant, and a cavity preventative. Cherries are a traditional remedy for anemia, arthritis, asthma, catarrh, constipation, cramps, fatigue, gallstones and kidney stones, gout, high blood pressure, hypochondria, lumbago, measles, numbness, obesity, rheumatism, stunted growth, paralysis, and frequent urination.

Cherries are one of the most chemically contaminated fruits, so it is always best to buy organic whenever possible. Select fully colored, plump, glossy-skinned cherries with fresh, green stems. The darker the cherry, the more minerals it contains. Avoid any that are soft, leaking, brown, or moldy. Cherries can be enjoyed plain or in fruit salads, pies, jams, puddings, smoothies, and juices. They can also be dried for year-round consumption.

Note: Because cherries increase circulation and warmth in the body, avoid eating them in cases of extreme heat, such as fever.

Chive (*Allium schoenoprasum*)—Liliaceae (Lily) Family

Chives are pungent with a warm energy. They are rich in beta-carotene, B-complex vitamins, vitamin C, calcium, iron, and sulfur.

Chives promote the circulation of energy and blood and help dry excess dampness in the body. Considered to be an antiseptic and a digestive aid, they have a special affinity for the liver, kidneys, and stomach. They help clean the circulatory system, lower blood pressure, and inhibit the growth of viruses, fungi, and unfriendly yeasts. Chives are used to treat stomachache and arthritis due to internal coldness, to strengthen the kidneys, and to increase sex drive.

Chives complement the flavor of many other vegetables including carrots, onions, and potatoes, and are often added as a garnish. The hollow stalks can be used fresh or dried. The edible, purple flowers have a peppery taste and make an attractive garnish as well.

Collard

See Kale and Collard (page 47).

Cranberry (*Vaccinium oxycoccus, V. macrocarpon*)—Ericaceae (Heath) Family

Cranberries are acidic and sour, with cool energy. They contain vitamin C, bioflavonoids, ellagic acid (an anticancer compound), and fiber. Their high flavonoid content is believed to be beneficial in the formation of visual purple, a pigment in the eyes that is essential to night vision.

Cranberries have antiscorbutic (scurvy-preventing), bronchodilating, antifungal, antiviral, and vasodilating properties. They have been used to treat asthma, burning urination, cancer, cystitis, diabetes, fever, hemorrhoids, kidney stones, poor appetite, skin disorders, and urinary tract infections. A urinary antiseptic, cranberries inhibit the adhesion of bacteria (including *E. coli*) to the urinary tract, perhaps through the action of a polymer contained in the fruit.

Look for plump, bright red, shiny, hard cranberries, and avoid those that are soft, leaky, or shriveled. Good cranberries actually tend to bounce. They keep for up to a couple of months in the refrigerator. Cranberries are tart but can be sweetened with honey or dates and used in jams, relishes, sauces, breads, cakes, and stuffing, as well as being juiced. Dried cranberries can also replace raisins in any recipe.

Note: Cranberries contain tannic and oxalic acids, which, if overingested, can contribute to the formation of kidney stones and inhibit the body's absorption of iron and calcium. For this reason, cranberries should be consumed only in moderation.

Cucumber (*Curcumis sativus, C. melo, C. citrullus*)—Curcurbitaceae (Gourd) Family

Cucumber is slightly bitter, alkaline, and cool in energy. Eating it can truly help relieve summer heat, helping one feel "cool as a cucumber." Although not regarded as highly nutritive (being 96 percent water), cucumbers contain erepsin, an enzyme that helps digest proteins and kill tapeworm. In addition, they contain phosphorus, potassium, vitamin E, beta-carotene, and folic acid, and the peel is rich in silicon and chlorophyll.

Cucumbers are both diuretic and laxative. They help moisten the lungs and are considered therapeutic for people suffering from acne, conjunctivitis, depression, diabetes, high blood pressure, obesity, pyorrhea, skin and stomach inflammation, sore throat, sunburn, and tapeworm. By reducing uric acid levels, cucumbers aid in dissolving kidney stones. In addition, the peel's high silicon content is believed to encourage healthy growth of skin, nails, and hair.

Cucumber can also help heal from the outside. Mashed cucumber applied topically cools burns, wasp stings, and tired, swollen feet. As a facial, it clears up acne and encourages wrinkle-free skin. Cucumber slices placed on puffy, tired eyes reduce redness and inflammation.

Look for young, small to medium-sized cucumbers with deep green skins. Overly large cucumbers are overgrown and bitter. Avoid cucumbers with yellowish skin or puffy, withered ends. Commercial cucumbers are often waxed and should be peeled before being eaten, but the peels from organically cultivated cucumbers can be consumed.

Enjoy cucumbers sliced, juiced, or chopped and added to yogurt dishes, salads, dressings, and relish. Try stuffing cucumbers by scooping out the seeds and pulp and filling with a mixture of sun-cured olives, chopped celery, and red bell pepper tossed with a bit of dressing.

Note: People who are excessively cold or weak or who have a health condition (such as diarrhea) involving excess dampness should avoid eating large amounts of cucumber.

Date (*Phoenix dactylifera*)—Palmaceae (Palm) Family

Dates are sweet, moistening, and easy to digest, with a warm energy. They are high in carbohydrates, glutamic acid, tyramine, niacin, boron, copper, iron, magnesium, potassium, and fiber.

Dates have strengthening, spleen-tonic, blood-tonic, energy-tonic, *yang*-tonic, and laxative properties. They have been used to treat anemia, bronchitis, catarrh, colitis, dry cough, low blood pressure, erectile dysfunction, hysteria, nervousness, palpitations, weak stomach, sore throat, and stomach ulcers. Dates are also recommended as a galactagogue for encouraging milk production in nursing mothers.

Although good dates are somewhat moist, they are naturally low in water and do not usually require drying after being harvested; however, they are sometimes fumigated with chemicals, pasteurized, frozen, or preserved with glucose to discourage mold, so investigate their source. Keep them in the refrigerator, as they can ferment at room temperature. Dates are delightfully delicious on their own, as a sweetener in raw desserts such as ice cream, puddings, cakes, cookies, and pies, or used to make chutneys and jams. They are also a great transition food for people who are trying to give up sugar and junk food. (I like to stuff a date with raw almond butter: with this trick, I was able to give up chocolate easily!)

Note: People prone to migraines, obesity, diabetes, and hypoglycemia should limit their intake of dates. Be sure to brush your teeth or rinse your mouth after eating dates, as their stickiness clings to the teeth.

Durian (*Durio zibethinus*)—Bombaceae (Durian) Family

Durians are the large, tasty fruit of one of the world's largest fruit trees, and a preferred food of wild elephants, orangutans, and tigers. Durians are high in oleic fats, vitamin E, and sulfur, and contain more protein than any other fruits. Despite their prickly rind and what many deem to be a foul, sulfurous smell, they are considered an aphrodisiac, as well as a longevity food, a vermifuge (worm-dispelling agent), and a strong blood cleanser.

Select durians with a brown or yellowish color, rather than green. (Although yellowish fruits tend to be overripe, this is an exception.) Avoid fruits with soft spots or holes, which can indicate mold or worms. A durian's ripeness can be determined by a sweet, pungent aroma, flattened spines, and a hollow sound when the fruit is tapped on the bottom with a heavy knife. If it is not quite ripe, it will continue to ripen if left out at room temperature. Durians can be frozen for long-term storage and thawed for eight to twenty-four hours before consumption. To eat a durian, simply split it open and scoop out the cream-colored meat. The seeds should be picked out and discarded.

Eggplant (*Solanum melongena*)—Solanaceae (Nightshade) Family

Eggplant is cooling with a sweet flavor. It contains potassium, bioflavonoids, and antioxidant compounds called monoterpenes that are believed to offer protection against cancer and heart disease. Eggplant also contains glycoalkaloids, substances that are used topically to treat skin cancers, including basal cell carcinoma. (However, there is conflicting evidence on eggplant's cancer-protective qualities, as a Japanese study showed it to be somewhat mutagenic.)

Eggplant has antiseptic, diuretic, and hemostatic properties. It helps dispel toxic heat from the body and improves blood circulation. It is used to relieve colitis, constipation, bleeding hemorrhoids, pain, hypertension, stomach ulcers, swelling, and tumors. A study at the University of Texas showed that eating eggplant impedes the rise in blood cholesterol levels that normally follows the consumption of fatty foods.

The purple variety of eggplant is most common, though it also comes in red, white, and yellow. Look for firm eggplant that is heavy for its size. Eggplant's meatlike flavor is excellent in many vegetarian dishes. Try marinating raw eggplant in a bit of tamari, lemon juice, and olive oil, and purée it into a dip. It can even be sliced thinly into noodles. To get rid of any bitterness and excess moisture in eggplant, many people slice it, cover it with a sprinkling of salt, place a weighted plate on top, wait thirty minutes, and then rinse it. This process is optional, however, because good eggplants are not bitter.

Note: Eggplant contains solanine, which in large amounts inhibits calcium absorption. Some individuals with arthritis find that abstaining from eggplant and other foods in the nightshade family (peppers, potatoes, and tomatoes) reduces their symptoms. During pregnancy, eat eggplant only in small amounts.

Endive and Escarole (*Cichorium* species)—Asteraceae (Daisy) Family

Escarole and endive are close relatives of chicory. All of these greens are fairly bitter, cool in energy, and moist. Endive has narrow, curled, finely divided leaves, whereas escarole, in general, has broader, flatter leaves. Both are rich in beta-carotene, vitamin C, calcium, iron, magnesium, phosphorus, and potassium.

The bitter flavor of endive and escarole stimulates the secretion of digestive juices including bile. These greens help rid the body of infection, increase the appetite, and have diuretic, laxative, and tonic properties. They are therapeutic for the heart, gallbladder, and liver, and are considered nourishing to the eyes and exciting to the central nervous system. Endive and escarole have been used in traditional medicine to remedy acidosis, arthritis, asthma, candida overgrowth, constipation, diabetes, edema, gas, gout, hypertension, hypoglycemia, jaundice, liver enlargement, obesity, rheumatism, and inflammatory skin conditions such as acne, boils, and eczema.

Endive and escarole are traditionally eaten in the spring as blood puri-fiers. Look for green unwilted leaves. Both the inner and outer leaves are edible, though the mellower inner leaves are used more often. They are best when mixed in salads with milder greens.

Fig (*Ficus carica*)—Moraceae (Mulberry) Family

Figs are sweet and alkaline, with a warming energy. They are rich in vita-min B_6, folic acid, calcium, copper, iron, magnesium, manganese, phos-phorus, and potassium. They have a high content of mucin, a soothing laxative. Figs also contain the compound benzaldehyde, which has been shown in Japanese studies to shrink tumors, as well as a sulfur compound called ficin, which helps reduce joint and tissue inflammation and is used to treat injuries.

This fruit is antibacterial, antiparasitic, and restorative. Considered a neutralizer of toxins, figs are suggested for consumption during times of cleansing. They have a special affinity for the stomach, spleen, and pan-creas, help moisten the lungs and large intestines, and improve liver func-tion, which can result in improved eyesight. Figs are used to treat anemia, arthritis, asthma, low blood pressure, cancer, catarrh, colitis, cough, dysen-tery, emaciation, exhaustion, gout, hemorrhoids, pleurisy, rheumatism, sore throat, tuberculosis, and ulcers. They are also used to deter cravings for sugar, alcohol, and drugs.

Look for figs that are free of mold. Enjoy fresh or dried figs as a snack or for dessert. Try them stuffed with raw almond butter. Use them like dates to sweeten cookies, pies, and puddings. Soak dried figs overnight in water for a breakfast compote. As they are very sweet, figs should be eaten only sparingly by people desiring to lose weight; however, they are an excel-lent food for body builders and people wanting to gain weight.

Note: Excess consumption of figs may cause diarrhea. Of all the dried fruits, dried figs are considered the healthiest, but be sure to avoid those treated with the preservative potassium sorbate. Remember to brush your teeth after eating dried figs, because their stickiness clings to the teeth and can contribute to tooth decay.

Grapefruit (*Citrus paradisi, C. decumana*)—Rutaceae (Citrus) Family

Grapefruit is classified as alkaline, cold, sweet, and sour. Grapefruit con-tains vitamin C, folic acid, calcium, iron, and potassium, as well as many anticancer compounds including flavonoids (found especially in the white inner rind and peel), terpenes, limonoids, and coumarins. Its phenolic compounds help the body produce substances that help detoxify carcinogens such as nitrosamines, and its pectin content helps in lowering blood cholesterol levels and dissolving arterial plaque. Grapefruit also contains naringin, an anti-inflammatory, antispasmodic flavonoid that helps eliminate old red blood cells from the body. Pink grapefruit contains lycopene, which is an antioxidant carotene.

Grapefruit has antimutagenic, antiseptic, antiviral, detoxifying, diuretic, and liver-cleansing properties. It helps promote the circulation of energy and clears heat and toxins from the body. It also helps remove inorganic calcium deposits and prevent heart attacks, stroke, and cancers, especially cancers of the pancreas and stomach. Grapefruit is used in treatments for numerous conditions including alcohol intoxication, atherosclerosis, bad breath, belching, broken capillaries, catarrh, constipation, cough, fever, gallstones, indigestion, jaundice, lupus, pneumonia, rheumatism, skin inflammation, and obesity.

Look for grapefruits that are firm but springy to the touch and heavy for their size. Thin-skinned fruits tend to be juicier. Grapefruits are best stored in a cool room rather than the refrigerator, and placing them in a closed bag encourages ripening. Enjoy grapefruit on its own or in fruit salads. It can also be juiced, although it's best to eat the whole fruit, because many of the important compounds, such as pectin, are in the pulp.

Grapes (*Vitis vinifera*)—Vitaceae (Grape) Family

Grapes are sweet, sour, and cooling. They contain beta-carotene, B-complex vitamins, vitamin C, boron, calcium, magnesium, potassium, and pectin. In addition to malic, citric, and oxalic acids, grapes also contain ellagic acid, a compound that scavenges carcinogenic factors and moves them out of the body.

Grape skins contain resveratrol, which prevents platelet aggregation and elevates levels of high-density lipoprotein (HDL) in the bloodstream. Red- and purple-skinned varieties are more strengthening, more blood building, and richer in iron than white or green varieties, and also contain the antioxidant quercitin. Grapes containing seeds are rich in procyanolic oligomers and leukocyanidins, which are both types of antioxidant flavonoids that are used to treat varicose veins and other vein disorders as well as atherosclerosis. The outer layers of grape seeds contain tartaric acid, which helps cleanse catarrh from the body.

Grapes are easy to digest and are considered therapeutic for the lungs, liver, kidneys, and spleen. They have antibacterial, antiviral, and diuretic properties. Being highly alkaline, they help the body eliminate uric acid. They are a blood and *chi* tonic and nourish the *yin* fluids of the body. Grapes have been used therapeutically to strengthen the sinews and bones and to treat cancer, constipation, cough, digestive disorders, edema, gout, hepatitis, jaundice, and rheumatism, and strengthen immunity. They also help improve mental focus.

Purchase fresh grapes with a powdery blush that look firm, rather than soggy, where the fruits attach to the stem. A bunch with lots of small, green berries is likely to have been picked unripe and will be sour. Grapes are among the most pesticide-laden of all fruits in a grocery store, so go for organic ones or avoid them altogether. Pick off any bad grapes after purchase and store the bunch in the refrigerator, where it should keep for a couple of weeks. Grapes are excellent by themselves or in fruit salads, jellies, or juices.

Note: Raisins, of course, are dried grapes with many of the same properties as fresh grapes; they have an even higher concentration of sugar, however, so people with diabetes or hypoglycemia should ingest them with caution. Like other dried fruits, raisins can stick to the teeth and promote dental decay, so rinse your mouth or brush your teeth after eating them. Because grapes (and raisins) contain salicylates, people with aspirin sensitivity may react adversely to them.

Jalapeño
See Cayenne and Jalapeño Pepper (page 106).

Jicama (*Pachyrhizus erosus, P. tuberosus*)—Fabaceae (Pea) Family
The root vegetable jicama (pronounced "HEE-ka-ma") has a flavor similar to that of water chestnut, and many restaurants use it as a less-expensive substitute. Jicama is rich in beta-carotene, B-complex vitamins, vitamin C, calcium, iron, and potassium.

Select jicama that is firm and heavy for its size. Overly large or shriveled jicama is likely to be woody and tough. Jicama can be stored whole and unwrapped in the refrigerator for several weeks, but storing it in plastic accelerates mold growth. Once jicama is cut, it is best to use it within a day or two. Peel it, slice it like potato chips, and serve it with dips. In Latin America, it is common to serve sliced jicama with a squeeze of lemon or lime and a dash of salt. Jicama can be juiced, grated into a salad, or grated to the size of rice grains and used as a rice replacement.

Kale and Collard (*Brassica oleracea acephala*)—Brassicaceae (Mustard) Family

Kale and collard greens are very similar, but kale often has curly leaves, and while collards thrive in a warmer climate, kale grows best in a cooler one. Both are considered warming, with a sweet, slightly bitter-pungent flavor similar to that of cabbage. Kale and collards are rich in iron, potassium, sulfur, beta-carotene, vitamin C, folic acid, chlorophyll, and calcium—in fact, 1 cup of kale or collard greens has more calcium than 1 cup of milk. They also contain indoles that protect against colon, breast, and lung cancer.

Kale and collards have antibiotic and antiviral properties. They benefit the stomach, dispel lung congestion, rejuvenate the liver, and have been used to treat arthritis, constipation, dental problems, gout, obesity, pyorrhea, skin disorders, and ulcers.

Select tender, dark green, or even bluish-green leaves, avoiding those that are yellowed. Kale and collard greens can be finely chopped and added to salads, steamed, stir-fried, made into soup, or included in vegetable juices.

Note: People with an overly acidic condition may find that kale and collards are intestinally cleansing and may therefore cause flatulence when initially "going raw." This can be prevented by adding a bit of ginger, cumin, or caraway to the greens.

Kiwi (*Actinida chinensis*)—Actinidiaceae (Kiwi) Family

Kiwis are cool, sweet, and sour. They are rich in fiber, vitamin C (having twice that of oranges), and potassium. Like papaya and pineapple, kiwi contains enzymes that aid the digestion of proteins and speed the healing of sores, wounds, and inflammation. Because of these enzymes, kiwi cannot be used in gelatin or agar dishes, as they will inhibit the jelling effect.

Kiwi improves blood circulation and has been used to remove excess sodium from the body, as well as to treat high blood pressure, heartburn, and indigestion. In Oriental medicine, this fruit is recommended to treat breast and stomach cancer, and as a tonic for developing children and postpartum women.

The commercial kiwi crop tends to be heavily sprayed, so look for an organic source. Kiwis should be firm but not too hard, yielding just slightly to the pressure of a fingertip. They will ripen at room temperature and can then be kept in the refrigerator for up to nine months. Most people peel kiwi before eating them. Enjoy kiwi plain, in fruit salads, in desserts, as a garnish, in marinades, or juiced (along with the seeds and peel).

Kumquat (*Fortunella margarita*)—Rutaceae (Citrus) Family

Kumquats are pungent, sweet, and sour, with a warm energy. They are high in vitamin C, most of which is in the peel, as well as vitamin E. Kumquats promote *chi* circulation and are mucolytic (help break up phlegm). They have been used to treat fevers, gallstones, indigestion, hernial pain, stomachache, hepatitis, high blood pressure, prolapse of the uterus and anus, asthma, catarrh, cough, pneumonia, respiratory congestion, and whooping cough.

Look for firm, plump, golden fruits that are heavy for their size. Kumquats can be eaten whole (peel and seeds included), made into jams, used as a garnish, added to desserts, dried, or preserved in honey.

Lemon (*Citrus limon*)—Rutaceae (Citrus) Family

Lemons are sour and alkaline, and are considered cooling. Compared to oranges, they are more acidic and less sweet. Lemons are high in vitamin C and potassium. They also contain limonene, which is used to dissolve gallstones and is being studied for its anticancer properties. Limonene is most prevalent in the white, inner portion of the rind.

Lemons have antiparasitic, antiseptic, astringent, phlegm-resolving, refrigerant, and antiseptic properties: lemon juice poured experimentally into shellfish destroyed 92 percent of the bacteria in the shellfish within 15 minutes. Lemon improves the assimilation of minerals by the body. It also stimulates bile production, which helps cleanse the liver and lower cholesterol. Lemons are used medicinally to treat asthma, bronchitis, colds, fever, gallstones, headache, indigestion, obesity, and neuritis.

Lemon juice can be applied topically to calm itchy insect bites, pimples, corns, warts, boils, and poison ivy. A cotton ball saturated with lemon juice and applied inside the nostril can be used to stop a nosebleed. After shampooing, the juice of a lemon added to the final rinse water refreshes the scalp and promotes shiny hair. The juice of half a lemon in a cup of warm water can be used as a gargle for sore throats. Although it might sting, lemon juice can also be used as an antiseptic agent on cuts.

Look for thin-skinned, bright yellow lemons. Lemons tinged with green are likely to be more acidic, and thick-skinned lemons will have less juice.

Citrus versus Scurvy

In 1753, the Scottish naval surgeon James Lind demonstrated in a controlled experiment that citrus fruits cured scurvy, which at the time was a common, life-threatening ailment for seafarers, who went months without any fresh produce. Still, it took 45 years and the death of 200,000 more British sailors before Lind's finding was taken seriously. In 1795, the British Admiralty ordered members of the Royal Navy to take daily rations of lemon or lime juice (with a ration of rum) to prevent scurvy: hence the nickname "limeys" now applied to British sailors.

Add lemon juice to fruits and vegetables to preserve their color. Substitute lemon juice for vinegar in salad dressings. The juice of half a lemon in a glass of warm water is a great way to start the day, as opposed to coffee. Grated lemon rind gives food a zesty flavor, but if you're going to use the rind, make sure it's organic, because nonorganic lemons are often coated in wax.

Note: Lemons should not be sucked on, as their acid content can damage dental enamel. They help thin the blood and so should be used cautiously by people who are overly thin, weak, or irritable. Also, lemons contain psoralens, compounds that can make one photosensitive.

Lettuce (*Lactuca sativa*)—Asteraceae (Daisy) Family

Lettuce is alkaline, bitter, sweet, and cool. It can be 92 to 95 percent water, but also contains chlorophyll, lactucin (a calming alkaloid), beta-carotene, folic acid, vitamins B_1, B_6, C, E, and K, and the minerals calcium, iron, potassium, and silicon. Although about 75 percent of the lettuce consumed in the United States is the iceberg variety, this is the least nutritious of all lettuces. Darker varieties like bibb, Boston, and romaine are more nutritious.

Lettuce has anodyne, anti-inflammatory, antioxidant, antispasmodic, diuretic, expectorant, galactagogic, and sedative properties. It helps dry excess dampness in the body, including yeast overgrowth and phlegm, and is considered beneficial in helping prevent stomach and endometrial cancers, cataracts, heart disease, and stroke. Lettuce has a slowing effect upon digestion and has been used to treat acid indigestion, anemia, arthritis, catarrh, colitis, constipation, cough, gastritis, gout, insomnia, irritable bowel, obesity, sexual addiction, stress, and ulcers.

Look for fresh, crisp greens without signs of decay. Buy organic lettuces whenever possible, as nonorganic lettuces are generally laden with pesticides. Lettuce keeps best in its own sealed container. Storing it with apples, pears, and tomatoes, all of which naturally emit ethylene gas, will cause lettuce to turn brown more quickly. In the raw diet, lettuce can be used in salads, sandwiches, and *hors d'oeuvres,* and to make "wraps" stuffed with tasty fillings.

Lime (*Citrus hystrix, C. aurantifolius, C. latifolia*)—Rutaceae (Citrus) Family

Limes are sour, cooling in energy, and rich in vitamin C, bioflavonoids, and potassium.

Considered antioxidant, antiseptic, and astringent, limes improve energy circulation and stimulate bile production. They are also used in treatments for arthritis, colds, constipation, edema, fever, flu, gallstones, high blood pressure, liver dysfunction, obesity, phlegm, and uterine and anal prolapse. And if you're in the tropics and happen to have a run-in with fire coral, squeeze lime juice over the affected area to cool the burn.

Select firm limes that are heavy for their size. They should be solid green, but yellow mottling is also acceptable, as limes left on the tree to ripen fully can turn yellow and be even more flavorful. Limes have a shorter shelf life than lemons do; refrigerated limes keep longer and do not develop mold, but give less juice. If you're going to use the rind, make sure the fruit is organic, because nonorganic limes are often coated in wax.

Limes can be substituted for lemons in most recipes. Use lime juice to make limeade, salad dressings, margaritas, sorbets, and pies. A squeeze of lime juice also helps prevent the discoloration of cut fruits such as apples and avocados.

Note: Like lemons, limes (especially the peels) contain psoralens, which can make one photosensitive.

Litchee (*Litchi chinensis*)—Sapindaceae (Lychee) Family

Litchee (also spelled lychee or lichi) is a sweet fruit just a bit smaller than a walnut, with a flavor reminiscent of grapes and an aroma like a rose. Fresh litchee fruits have a cool energy, but when dried, they are called litchee nuts and have a warm energy. Litchee contains vitamins B_1 and B_2, niacin, and vitamin C.

Litchee is considered a blood and *yin* tonic that improves the circulation of energy. The fruits are used to relieve asthma, cough, diarrhea, hernial pain, tumors, and glandular enlargements. The nuts are used in Oriental medicine to enhance intelligence and make one's complexion more beautiful.

Look for plump, uncracked litchee fruits. Enjoy them alone as a snack or in fruit salads and sherbets. In the Orient, litchees are often eaten at the end of a meal or served in syrup. The inner seed is not edible.

Lycium Berry (*Lycium chinense*)—Solanaceae (Nightshade) Family

Lycium berries, also known as wolfberries or goji berries (the more popular term in the raw food community), are sweet and considered neutral. They are highly nutritive, containing beta-carotene, vitamins B_1, B_2, and C, and linoleic acid. These berries are said to "brighten the spirit," and prolonged use promotes cheerfulness.

Lycium berries have many virtues, including being an aphrodisiac, a rejuvenative, and a tonic for the blood, energy, liver, and *yin* (fluids) of the body. They help remove toxins from the blood by strengthening the kidneys and liver, and protect the liver against damage from toxin exposure. They are also a supreme eye food, helping with night blindness and blurred or poor vision. Lycium berries have been used to treat anemia, asthma, bronchial inflammation, diabetes mellitus, erectile dysfunction, pneumonia, tuberculosis, vertigo, and weak knees and back.

Look for bright red lycium berries that have not been treated with sulfur. Eat them plain like raisins, added to trail mix, or mixed into a smoothie (soaked first to facilitate blending).

Mango (*Mangifera indica*)—Anacardiaceae (Cashew) Family

Mango is sweet and sour, with a cooling energy. It is rich in amino acids, beta-carotene, niacin, vitamins C and E, flavonoids, calcium, iron, magnesium, and potassium. Mango also contains pectin, which is useful in lowering blood cholesterol levels.

This fruit is considered a *yin* tonic, providing moistening fluids for the body and quenching thirst. It has alterative (blood purifying), antiseptic, diuretic, and laxative properties. Mangoes have been used to treat anemia, bleeding gums, clogged pores, constipation, cough, cysts, fever, hypertension, indigestion, nausea, nephritis (kidney inflammation), nausea, respiratory ailments, seasickness, and weak digestion. They calm the emotions, benefit the brain, strengthen the heart, and provide energy.

Some mango species do not turn red, yellow, or orange, which means that with some varieties you are likely to buy them green and must look for other signs of ripeness. A ripe mango yields to the pressure of a fingertip and has a sweet fragrance. Putting a mango in a paper bag in a warm place helps the ripening process. Avoid shriveled fruits with large, dark areas on their skin, as these are overripe.

Eat mango by itself—enjoy a mango in the bathtub so you don't have to worry about the mess! Share one with your beloved. Add mango to fruit salads or use it in pies, ice creams and sorbets, smoothies, juices, and salsas.

Note: Some people are allergic to mangoes, especially to the juice under the peel. It's not surprising—after all, this fruit is in the plant family Anacardiaceae, along with poison ivy.

Okra (*Hibiscus esculentus*)—Malvaceae (Mallow) Family

Okra is commonly used in Creole cooking. It has a sweet bland flavor and cooling energy. Okra is a rich source of beta-carotene, B-complex vitamins, vitamin C, calcium, iron, phosphorus, potassium, and sodium. Its rich electrolyte content helps preserve the body's balance of fluids, which is necessary for nerve impulse transmission. Okra also contains pectin, which helps lower blood cholesterol levels.

Being very alkaline, okra helps neutralize acids and provides a temporary, protective coating for the digestive tract. As a bulk laxative, it helps lubricate the large intestine. Okra is a supreme vegetable for people who feel weak, exhausted, or depressed. It has been used to treat lung inflammation, irritable bowel, sore throat, and ulcers, and to keep joints limber. Topically, an okra poultice can be applied to heal burns or to soothe poison ivy or psoriasis, and okra juice can be used as a gargle for sore throats.

Select okra that are small (less than 4 inches long), firm, and resilient for maximum tenderness. Wheel-like slices of okra can be added to salads or used in soups as a thickener. Try it in dips or added to vegetable juices. Okra combines well with tomatoes, which minimize its gelatinous consistency. Dried okra pods can be ground into high-protein flour, and okra seeds can be pressed for their edible oil.

Olive (*Oleum europea, O. olviva*)—Oleaceae (Olive) Family

Olives have been cultivated for more than 4,000 years. The fruits of the olive tree are sweet, pungent, hot, and moist in nature. In addition to containing linoleic, linolenic, and oleic acids and lecithin, olives are an excellent, vegan source of protein.

Olives have antioxidant, antiseptic, demulcent, emollient, laxative, nutritive, and tonic properties. They have been used in treatments for gallstones and gout and as preventatives for heart disease and ulcers.

Before they can be eaten, olives must be cured in salt, oil, or vinegar. Green olives are harvested and cured unripe, and therefore are more acidic in flavor. Black olives are collected and cured when ripe. Look for olives that have been sun-cured rather than pasteurized, canned, or otherwise heated.

Onion (*Allium cepa*)—Liliaceae (Lily) Family

Onions are pungent with a hot energy. They are a good source of beta-carotene, vitamins B and C, potassium, selenium, and sulfur. Because of their anticancer phytochemicals, including cepaene, disulfides, trisulfides, and quercitin, they are considered a supreme food in preventing stomach and skin cancer and tumor growth. Onions also contain small amounts of prostaglandins A1 and E, which help in lowering high blood pressure.

These bulbs are antibiotic, antiseptic, anti-inflammatory, antioxidant, antiviral, diuretic, expectorant, laxative, sedative, and tonic. Onions help prevent blood platelet aggregation, have a cleansing effect upon the lymphs, warm the kidney's *yang*, stimulate the liver, dispel phlegm and respiratory congestion, and help prevent heart attack and stroke. They are used to treat anxiety, flu, atherosclerosis, asthma, blood clots, bronchitis, catarrh, colds, cough, diabetes, hay fever, hypoglycemia, high cholesterol, high blood pressure, hoarseness, insomnia, obesity, parasitic invasion, pneumonia, rheumatism, sinus congestion, tuberculosis, and urinary infections.

Onions can be strong or mild, with white being the mildest. Red and yellow onions have more antioxidants than other varieties. Look for firm onions with dry skins that are free of soft spots, and store them in a cool, dry place. Scallions, along with chives and leeks, are milder relatives of onion.

Many people become teary when cutting into onions, as a result of the volatile, sulfurous oil found in the bulb. Peeling and chopping onions under cold, running water prevents the vapors from rising to the eyes. Enjoy onions in salads, dressings, vegetable dishes, and soups. Banish onion breath by eating some parsley sprigs.

Note: Onions cause flatulence or bowel irritation in some people.

Orange (*Citrus sinensis, C. aurantium*)—Rutaceae (Citrus) Family

Oranges are alkaline, cooling, sweet, sour, moistening, and cleansing. In addition to vitamin C, oranges contain beta-carotene, vitamin B_1, folic acid, calcium, potassium, glutathione, and pectin. Orange essential oil contains limonene, which has been found to shrink tumors. When eating oranges, be sure to consume some of the inner membrane, where the flavonoids, including rutin and hesperidin, are located.

Oranges are a circulatory stimulant and a cardiac and immune tonic with alterative, antioxidant, antifungal, antiseptic, antiviral, and carminative properties. Their high vitamin C content helps counteract carcinogens called nitrosamines, and the fruit has been used to help prevent bladder, breast, cervical, esophageal, lung, pancreatic, rectal, and stomach cancer. Oranges are also used to treat arthritis, rheumatism, asthma, bronchitis, catarrh, colds, fever, flu, pneumonia, tuberculosis, arteriosclerosis, thrombosis, broken capillaries, high blood pressure, high cholesterol, and constipation. Some alcoholics find that drinking fresh-squeezed orange juice reduces cravings for alcohol.

Look for firm oranges that are heavy for their size, and avoid those that are puffy or spongy or have soft spots. Store them in a cool place (but they do not need to be kept refrigerated). If an orange develops mold, remove it from the others so they don't quickly follow suit. Oranges are best eaten fresh, juiced, tossed with mixed greens, or made into fruit salads, pies, sherbets, sauces, or other desserts. Orange peel, also known as orange zest, is a digestive aid and a popular garnish; nonorganic oranges are often waxed, however, so if you're going to use the peel, be sure to get organic fruit.

Note: Some people find that eating oranges causes them to break out in a rash. In many cases, the rash is the result of an increased discharge of toxins that is stimulated by the oranges, and will clear up when the cleansing is complete. Avoid excess consumption of oranges in cases of stomach ulcers or stomach or intestinal inflammation.

Papaya (*Carica papaya*)—Caricaceae (Pawpaw) Family

Papaya is sweet and bitter, with a neutral to cooling energy. Papaya is high in beta-carotene, vitamins C and E, calcium, magnesium, and potassium. It also contains the protease (protein-digesting enzyme) papain, which is an anticancer agent, and carpaine, an anti-tumorigenic compound.

This fruit is a digestive aid and tonifies the stomach. It has anti-inflammatory, antiparasitic, anti-tumorigenic, emmenagogic, and emollient properties; although it helps dry excess dampness in the body, it moistens the lungs. Papaya has traditionally been used to treat allergies, arteriosclerosis, cancer, catarrh, colds, cough, diarrhea, diverticulitis, dysentery, flatulence, gastritis, menstrual irregularities, rheumatism, stomachache, and ulcers. It can also help reduce the risk of stroke and heart attack. When consumed regularly, papaya improves the health of the skin, hair, nails, and eyes. The unripe fruit can be mashed and used in facial masks to nourish the skin and lighten freckles, or applied as a poultice for tumors.

The enzyme papain is found in highest concentrations in the milky juice of the unripe papaya—little of it occurs in the ripe fruit. Papain is used to treat allergies, asthma, indigestion, chronic diarrhea, digestive disorders, gluten intolerance, hay fever, sports injuries, and weak lungs, and is dabbed topically on warts. Papain powder is applied to bee stings to reduce pain and inflammation, and is also used as a tooth and gum cleanser.

Select smooth, unblemished papayas that are heavy for their size, and avoid those that are entirely green, shriveled, or marked with dark spots. A ripe papaya will yield slightly when pressed, and at least half of its skin will be a deep yellow, orange, or red. If you buy one that is slightly underripe, leave it out at room temperature to ripen. Enjoy papaya plain or in fruit salads, pies, puddings, ice creams and sorbets, salsas, and smoothies.

Note: The latex exuded by an unripe papaya may cause contact dermatitis in some people.

Parsnip (*Pastinaca sativa*)–Apiaceae (Carrot) Family

The sweet, warming parsnip looks like a pale version of its relative, the carrot (both are members of the Apiaceae, the carrot family). Parsnip contains beta-carotene, folic acid, vitamin C, calcium, potassium, silicon, pectin, and fiber. It is also rich in carbohydrates, making parsnip a good substitute when you have a craving for processed sugars and starches.

This root vegetable has analgesic, diaphoretic, diuretic, and laxative properties. Parsnip is considered therapeutic for the liver, spleen, pancreas, and stomach, and has been used to rid the body of kidney, bladder, and gallstones. It has also been used in treatments for colds, colitis, cough, gout, headache, hemorrhoids, ulcers, and shortness of breath. Because parsnip builds strength and corrects states of deficiency, it is considered strengthening for people with hypoglycemia or tuberculosis, and for people recovering from serious illness or surgery.

Look for smooth, firm, well-shaped roots of small to medium size. Nonorganic parsnips are often treated with wax as a preservative and should be peeled before being eaten. Parsnips are at their sweetest once they have been exposed to cold temperatures (such as those preceding a frost) for a couple of weeks. Mash them as an alternative to mashed potatoes, grate a small amount onto salads, or use them in vegetable juice combinations.

Note: Avoid consuming parsnip leaves, which are considered toxic.

Pea (*Pisum sativum*)—Fabaceae (Pea) Family

Peas are sweet, alkaline, and moistening, and are considered neutral in temperature. They contain protein, fiber, chlorophyll, carbohydrates, beta-carotene, B-complex vitamins, vitamin C, iron, manganese, phosphorus, potassium, and zinc. Due to their content of an anti-fertility substance called m-mylohydroquinone, peas have been investigated as a potential contraceptive agent for both men and women. Peas also contain protease inhibitors and isoflavones, which inhibit the activation of carcinogens.

Peas are anti-inflammatory, galactagogic, and laxative. They are tonifying to the liver, spleen, pancreas, and stomach, and may also help stabilize blood sugar levels and reduce the risk of heart disease. Peas have been used to remedy anemia, boils, high cholesterol, constipation, cough, diabetes, edema, hiccoughs, hypoglycemia, and spasms, and to relieve ulcer pain.

Look for crisp, fresh peas with shiny pods that squeak when rubbed together. If they are young and tender, peas can even be eaten in the pod. (Snow peas are a variety with pods that remain tender and edible through maturation.) They can be enjoyed as a snack, added to salads, pâtés, casseroles, juices, or soups. Fresh peas are easier to digest than dried peas.

Note: If peas are consumed in excess, they can be thyroid inhibiting. They also contain compounds called purines, which can aggravate gout in people prone to the disorder.

Peach (*Prunus persica, P. vulgaris*)—Rosaceae (Rose) Family

Peaches are sweet and sour, with a cool energy. They are rich in beta-carotene, vitamin C, calcium, boron, magnesium, phosphorus, potassium, and flavonoids.

This fruit has antioxidant, digestive, diuretic, expectorant, and laxative properties. Peaches have been used to treat acidosis, anemia, asthma, atherosclerosis, constipation, cough, gastritis, high blood pressure, high cholesterol, indigestion, kidney stones, nephritis (kidney inflammation), obesity, and ulcers, and to rid the body of intestinal worms. They help improve skin tone, lubricate the intestines, strengthen the lungs, promote circulation, and reduce excess perspiration. Mashed peach can be applied as a facial for radiant skin.

Look for unblemished fruits. Unripe peaches will ripen faster if placed in a paper bag and sealed for a day or two. When ripe, they will yield to the pressure of your fingers, and should be stored unwashed in the refrigerator. Enjoy them alone or in fruit salads, cold soups, ice creams, jams, pies, and cobblers.

Pear (*Pyrus communis*)—Rosaceae (Rose) Family

Pears are sweet, alkaline, mildly sour, and cool. They are a good source of beta-carotene, folic acid, vitamin C, boron, calcium, iodine, iron, phosphorus, and potassium, and they contain even more pectin than apples do. Most of a pear's nutrients are concentrated in the skin.

A *yin* tonic, this fruit lubricates dryness, tonifies the intestines, and dissolves uric acid, helping reduce swollen joints. Pears have been used to treat acidosis, alcoholism, diabetes, high cholesterol, dizziness, gallstones, hypertension, phlegm conditions, nephritis, colitis, constipation, diverticulitis, gastritis, indigestion, irritable bowel, obesity, and difficulty in urination, as well as blurred vision, lost voice, and tinnitus.

Pears are usually harvested and sold unripe, but will ripen at home if left at room temperature or placed in a paper bag. Look for fruit that is firm and unblemished. Pears are ripe when they yield to the pressure of your fingers, and should then be stored in the refrigerator. Enjoy them plain, juiced, or in fruit salads, pies, puddings, sorbets, and smoothies—they add a natural sweetness to any dish.

Note: Pears are very sweet, so remember to brush your teeth or rinse your mouth after eating them to deter dental problems. Practitioners of Oriental medicine recommend consuming this fruit only in moderation during pregnancy, as it is cooling and can increase the risk of miscarriage. Dried pears, unless from a health foods store, should be avoided, because they are likely to contain sulfites.

Persimmon (*Diospyros virginiana, D. kaki*)—Ebenaceae (Ebony) Family

Persimmons are sweet, astringent, and cooling. Their astringent flavor comes in part from the tannins they contain, which break down as the fruit ripens until practically none are left. Persimmons are a good source of beta-carotene, vitamin C, calcium, magnesium, phosphorus, and potassium.

Persimmons help tonify the *yin* (moistening fluids) of the body and have a special affinity for the large intestine and the heart. They lubricate the lungs, strengthen the spleen and pancreas, improve energy, and contain enzymes that help break down damaged cells and foreign microbes. This fruit has been used to treat bronchitis, catarrh, cough, diarrhea, dysentery, goiter, hangover, hemorrhoids, hiccoughs, hypertension, mouth sores, pleurisy, stomachache, and ulcers.

Persimmons are best when harvested after a frost. Look for plump fruits with an intact green cap. Allow persimmons to ripen at room temperature; ripening can be hastened by placing them in a paper bag along with some ripening bananas. Light-colored persimmons taste sweet only when mushy, but darker persimmons can be eaten before becoming overly soft. Enjoy persimmons by themselves, added to salads, or used in jams, chutneys, puddings, and pies.

Pineapple (*Ananas comosus*)—Bromeliaceae (Pineapple) Family

Pineapple is sweet, sour, cooling, and moist. It is rich in beta-carotene, B-complex vitamins, vitamin C, magnesium, manganese, potassium, carbohydrates, and fiber. Pineapple also contains the protein-digesting enzyme bromelain, a powerful anti-inflammatory agent that is believed to block inflammatory prostaglandins and inhibit blood platelet aggregation.

Pineapple has antibacterial, antiviral, demulcent, diuretic, and mild phytoestrogenic properties. It cools the blood, helps the skin retain youthfulness, promotes bone density, and speeds healing after an injury. It has been used to treat angina, arthritis, blood clots, bronchitis, catarrh, constipation, diphtheria, dyspepsia, edema, goiter, hypertension, indigestion, excessive menses, multiple sclerosis, obesity, sinusitis, sore throat, sunstroke, and tumors, and to expel intestinal worms. Pineapple is very helpful in cases of fever with sweating and much body heat. Topically, it can be used to to relieve swellings and speed tissue healing, and a small amount can be used instead of soap to wash the face.

When selecting a pineapple, look for a fragrant aroma, light yellow or white meat, and heaviness for its size. Another sign of ripeness is when the topmost center leaf pulls out easily. This fruit is delicious simply peeled and sliced. It can also be used in salads, marinades, juices, breads, cakes, cookies, pies, and gelatin-free puddings. Cut a pineapple into a "basket" to hold other fruits. In order to be effective therapeutically, pineapple must be eaten raw, as many of its helpful constituents are destroyed by heat.

Note: Underripe pineapple is too acidic for the teeth and stomach. Pineapple is not suggested for people with over-acidic digestion, eczema, or health conditions involving excessive dampness.

Plum (*Prunus domestica*)—Rosaceae (Rose) Family

Plums are sour, sweet, and mildly cooling. They can be eaten fresh or dried; when dried, they are called prunes. Plums and prunes are rich in vitamins B_1 and C, calcium, iron, phosphorus, and potassium.

Plums have antibacterial, antiviral, diuretic, and laxative properties. They provide energy, stimulate the liver, and are considered a tonic for the brain, nerves, and blood. They have been used to treat liver disease, bronchitis, constipation, diabetes, flatulence, hemorrhoids, obesity, skin eruptions, and tumors. Eating two plums daily improves digestion and helps curb bleeding gums.

Look for plums that are slightly soft. Add plums or soaked prunes to fruit salad, puddings, pies, jams and sauces, or eat them by themselves as a tangy snack.

Note: Plums contain some oxalic acid, which can inhibit the body's absorption of iron and calcium. People with ulcers or acute gastroenteritis should limit their intake of plums and prunes.

Pomegranate (*Punica granatum*)—Lythraceae (Henna) Family

Pomegranate is sweet, sour, and cooling. It is a rich source of vitamin C and potassium. The seeds also contain phytoestrogenic compounds, and eating half a pomegrate daily is said to improve fertility.

This fruit has alterative and antiseptic properties and is considered a *yin* tonic that builds the kidneys, liver, blood, and bladder. Studies in Israel have shown pomegranate to have anti-aging properties and to prevent cancer and hardening of the arteries. Pomegranate is used therapeutically to treat arthritis, bladder infection, diarrhea, intestinal worms (especially tapeworm), weak gums, liver congestion, and mouth sores. It helps encourage creativity.

Look for pink- to red-colored fruits that are heavy for their size. Pomegranates keep very well, sometimes until spring from their autumn harvest, even if not refrigerated. Try rolling the whole fruit on a hard surface to crush the succulent seeds, then making a hole in one end to suck out their rich juice. You can also slice open the fruit and scoop out the seeds, which are great in fruit salad or a pomegranate sorbet. Best of all is to eat a pomegranate with your lover.

Pumpkin (*Curcurbita pepo*)—Curcurbitaceae (Gourd) Family

Pumpkins are sweet, slightly bitter, and neutral to cooling in nature. They are high in beta-carotene, and also contain vitamins B and C, potassium, sodium, and carbohydrates. Pumpkin seeds are rich in zinc and are especially strengthening to the adrenal glands and prostate gland.

Pumpkins are considered antioxidant, diuretic, laxative, and immune tonic. They are believed to lower the risk of cancer, especially of the lungs, skin, and bladder. Being rich in beta-carotene, they improve respiratory health, including asthma and coughs. Pumpkins have been used to remedy acidosis, colitis, gastritis, indigestion, cataracts, edema, flu, and heart disease. Their alkalinity enables them to dry excess dampness in the body, thus benefiting people with conditions such as edema, eczema, and dysentery. Pumpkins also support the spleen, stomach, and pancreas, thus benefiting people with hypoglycemia and diabetes. Many cultures use pumpkin seeds as a vermifuge to help eliminate tapeworm and roundworm.

The heart-shaped leaves of the pumpkin vine can be used as a tea for diarrhea or as a plaster for chills and fevers. The beautiful, delicate flowers can be administered as a tea for jaundice, measles, and smallpox. Native Americans applied mashed pumpkin topically to soothe abscesses, boils, bruises, burns, carbuncles, headaches, and sprains. Filipinos used the sap of the pumpkin stem as an application for earaches.

Look for pumpkins with bright orange skin that are firm to the touch and heavy for their size. Smaller, "pie" pumpkins are good for eating, whereas the larger varieties are better for jack o'lanterns. Open yourself to the delectable possibilities of pumpkin soup, muffins, pies, cookies, and puddings. You can also try grating pumpkin meat into salads.

Radish (*Raphanus sativus*)—Brassicaceae (Mustard) Family

Radishes are pungent and sweet. They are neutral in temperature with the potential to be warm: they taste hot initially and then leave a feeling of coolness. Radishes are high in vitamin B_1, C, E, iron, potassium, and silicon. Their high sulfur content makes them a useful part of a cancer prevention program. They also contain raphanin, which helps balance the thyroid gland, and the enzyme diatase, which aids in the digestion of starches (this may be why it is common in Europe to eat radishes with bread and cereals).

Radishes are considered diuretic, expectorant, and stimulant. Thought to be a beautifying food, radishes are especially beneficial for the hair, nails, skin, teeth, and gums. Radishes cleanse the liver, prevent constipation, dispel phlegm, clear congested sinuses, remedy laryngitis and sore throat, and prevent viral infections such as flu. They are also used against gall and kidney stones. In Japanese folk medicine, a drink made of carrots and daikon radishes is used to reduce and eliminate deposits of hardened fats in the body.

Radish juice can be applied topically as an underarm deodorant or to heal bruises, insect bites, frostbite, and minor burns.

Look for firm radishes of moderate size, as those that are overly large tend to be pithy. Removing the leaves (which can be added to salad) will help radishes keep longer. Add sliced or shredded radishes to salads, eat them with dips as an alternative to chips, and add them in small amounts to vegetable juices.

Note: Minimize consumption of radishes in cases of excess digestive heat or inflammation, such as gastritis or ulcer.

Raspberry (*Rubus* species)—Rosaceae (Rose) Family

These delectable, warming, sweet-and-sour berries are known for their high content of vitamin C and potassium. Raspberries also contain pectin, which is useful in the "setting up" of jams and jellies. Flavonoids give the fruit its rich color.

In Chinese medicine, raspberries are regarded as a tonic for the kidneys and liver. They are cleansing and have been shown to have antiviral properties. Because they help build the blood, they are a good food for people with anemia. Raspberries are very alkaline and help improve phlegmy conditions such as catarrh. They have been used as a traditional remedy for diarrhea, frequent urination, erectile dysfunction, high blood pressure, parasites, excess menstrual bleeding, and rheumatism. The leaves of the plant are also edible and rich in minerals, and have a flavor similar to that of black tea.

They are available in early summer to autumn. Avoid mushy or moldy fruits. Raspberries are lovely when eaten plain or in fruit salads, and as a garnish for green salads and desserts. Mashed and mixed with honey, they make a delicious syrup for pancakes (raw or otherwise).

Rhubarb (*Rheum rhabaarbarum, R. rhaponticum*)—Polygonaceae (Buckwheat) Family

Rhubarb is sour and cooling. It is rich in vitamin C, calcium, and potassium.

Rhubarb increases the production of saliva and gastric juices, including bile, and is considered detoxifying to the liver. Being somewhat laxative, it improves peristalsis. Rhubarb is recommended for bronchitis, constipation, neuritis, obesity, and tumors. In folk medicine, brushing teeth with fresh rhubarb juice is thought to protect dental enamel from decay.

Rhubarb stalks are best eaten fresh and in season. You can simply peel the stalks, dip them in a bit of salt, and enjoy them raw. Rhubarb is also wonderful in jams, pies, puddings, sauces, and homemade wines. It is very tart, so the addition of apples, honey, and raisins make a sweeter treat.

Note: Rhubarb leaves are toxic and should never be consumed. Do not confuse garden rhubarb with Chinese rhubarb, which is used as a potent purgative. Consume rhubarb in moderation. Due to its high content of oxalic acid, which can inhibit the absorption of calcium and iron, rhubarb is best avoided altogether by people suffering from arthritis, gout, kidney stones, and rheumatism.

Rutabaga (*Brassica napus*)—Brassicaceae (Mustard) Family

Rutabagas are sweet and warming They are a good source of beta-carotene and also contain some vitamin C, B-complex vitamins, calcium, potassium, fiber, and carbohydrates. Like other members of the mustard family, rutabagas are rich in antioxidant dithiolthiones, sulfur, and indoles, which have anticancer activity. Rutabaga stimulates the liver and is recommended in treatments for constipation, digestive disorders, and intestinal worms.

Look for firm vegetables that are heavy for their size, as lightweight ones are likely to be withered inside. Rutabagas grow well in cold climates and last long into the winter if stored in a cool place (not necessarily the refrigerator). They can be puréed to make soup, mashed as a substitute for potatoes, grated raw into salads, or sliced for crudités. Nonorganic rutabagas are likely to be waxed, so be sure to peel them before use.

Shiitake Mushroom (*Lentinus edodes*)—Polyporaceae (Mushroom) Family

Mushrooms are fungi: primitive plantlike organisms that derive energy not from photosynthesis but from decomposed vegetation. The name "shiitake" is derived from that of the shii tree (*Pasania* species) upon which these mushrooms grow. Shiitake mushrooms are sweet and neutral. They are rich in niacin, vitamins B_2, B_{12}, C, and D, glutamic acid, germanium, potassium, selenium, and zinc, as well as the polysaccharide lentinan, which boosts macrophage (white blood cell) activity. They are also believed to be a source of interferon, a protein that interferes with the viral takeover of cells.

Shiitakes are considered to have antitumor, antiviral, aphrodisiac, immune-tonic, and rejuvenative properties. They encourage stem cells in the bone marrow to create more B and T cells (important in boosting the body's immunity). Shiitakes have been used to treat AIDS, cancer, chronic cough, fatigue, high blood pressure, and high cholesterol. They also help the body get rid of excess salt.

Shiitake mushrooms are available fresh or dried; dried mushrooms should be soaked for two hours before use. Shiitakes are great marinated, dehydrated, or used in soups.

The Raw Facts

The common white mushroom (*Agaricus bispora*) that is most widely available in grocery stores is not typically recommended in the raw foods diet. White button mushrooms contain hydrazide, a suspected carcinogen, and have not been found to provide therapeutic benefits.

Soursop (*Annona muricata*)—Annonaceae (Custard Apple) Family

The fruits of the soursop tree can be as heavy as 10 pounds. Their flavor can be likened to musky pineapple and their aroma to that of black currants. Soursop contains almost all of the known vitamins and minerals as well as protein and carbohydrates. It is an excellent source of calcium, iron, and phosphorus.

Soursop is considered aphrodisiac and diuretic. It has been used to treat hemorrhoids, obesity, heart and kidney ailments, urethritis, and, in some parts of the world, leprosy and liver ailments.

Soursop fruit is harvested when its thin, leathery skin has turned a yellowish green but the fruit itself is still firm to the touch. It can then be ripened at home at room temperature, and yields to the gentle pressure of a finger when ripe. Soursop is delicious plain or added to fruit salads, sherbets, preserves, and juices.

Note: Soursop seeds are toxic and should not be consumed.

Spinach (*Spinacia oleracea*)—Chenopodiaceae (Goosefoot) Family

Spinach is sweet, cool, and moistening. It is rich in beta-carotene, vitamins B_6, C, and K, folic acid, calcium, iron, potassium, sulfur, and chlorophyll, and contains more protein than most vegetables. Its high lutein content makes spinach an excellent, medicinal food in cases of vision weakness and night blindness and as protection against macular degeneration.

Spinach has antioxidant, digestive, diuretic, laxative, lymph-cleansing, nutritive, and tonic properties. It is considered a cancer preventative with a

64   *Rawsome!*

special affinity for the lungs and large intestines. It soothes intestinal inflammation, detoxifies the digestive tract, and promotes peristalsis. Traditionally, spinach is used to restore energy and treat acne, alcoholism, anemia, constipation, hemorrhoids, neuritis, obesity, and scurvy.

Look for unwilted, dark green leaves. Spinach grows best in sandy soil, so give it several rinsings before serving to avoid getting grit in your food. Spinach makes an excellent addition to salads, soups, dips, and fillings for wraps and sandwiches.

Note: Spinach contains oxalic acid, which can bind to iron and calcium and inhibit their absorption by the body. Cooking or canning converts the oxalic acid into an inorganic form that is deposited in the kidneys and can thus lead to a calcium deficiency, so eating spinach raw is considered most healthful.

Star Fruit (*Averrhoa carambola*)—Oxalidaceae (Wood Sorrel) Family

Star fruit, also known as carambola, is named for its shape: when sliced horizontally, each piece looks like a golden star. These fruits are cooling and range in taste from sweet to sour. Star fruit is a good source of beta-carotene, vitamin C, and potassium.

They help dispel excess heat from the body and are a *yin* tonic, detoxifier, and diuretic. They are used to treat arthritis pain, cough, diarrhea, fever, hangover, hemorrhoids, hiccough, indigestion, kidney and bladder stones, mouth sores, and toothache.

Look for even-colored, firm fruits without brown spots. Allow star fruit to ripen at room temperature; when a fruity aroma and golden yellow color are evident, the ripe fruit can be refrigerated for up to a week. Eat them by themselves, add them to salads, desserts, sherbets, jams, puddings, and chutneys, or juice them. Float slices of star fruit in punch bowls and use them as a garnish.

Strawberry (*Fragaria* species)—Rosaceae (Rose) Family

Strawberries are sweet, sour, cool, and moist. They are rich in flavonoids, vitamins B, C, and E, and iron. They also contain ellagic acid, which is a potent, anticancer compound.

Strawberries have blood-purifying, astringent, diuretic, liver-tonic, and wound-healing properties. This fruit is a medicinal food in cases of anemia, constipation, fevers, hangover, high blood pressure, and jaundice. Because strawberry helps the body eliminate uric acid, it is used for gout, arthritis, and rheumatism. Because it moistens the lungs, it has been helpful for dry cough, sore throat, and tuberculosis. Cut strawberries can be rubbed over the teeth to whiten them and remove dental plaque without damaging enamel.

Strawberries are among the most hybridized and pesticide- and herbicide-contaminated produce items on the market. It is worth your time and your money to search out organic varieties. Berries that are overly large often lack flavor, and berries with whitish tips were collected too soon before proper ripening. Store strawberries in an open container in the refrigerator, removing any spoiled ones first. Leave the green caps on while rinsing, to prevent water from entering the berry and diluting the flavor.

Strawberries are a heavenly snack and can also be added to jams, pies, tarts, yogurts, and smoothies, to name but a few possibilities. They are sweet enough to satisfy a dessert craving and make wonderful culinary decorations. The leaves of the strawberry plant are also edible; like raspberry leaves, they are rich in minerals and have a flavor similar to that of black tea.

Note: Strawberries, especially when they are not vine ripened, can be allergenic for some people, causing skin eruptions or indigestion, which may simply be a result of clearing toxins from the body.

String Bean (*Phaseolus vulgaris*)—Fabaceae (Pea) Family

String beans, also known as snap beans, are neutral in energy and sweet in flavor. They are very alkaline and are rich in beta-carotene, B-complex vitamins, calcium, and potassium. Green string beans contain more nutrients than yellow ones.

String beans are considered a spleen, kidney, and *yin* tonic. They nourish the pancreas and increase the fluids of the body. String beans also help in eliminating uric acid and are thus useful in relieving the inflammation of arthritis and gout. They have traditionally been used in treatments for acne, diabetes, diarrhea, leucorrhoea, night sweats, thirst, and frequent urination.

Good-quality string beans have a bright color and snap easily when broken. Look for beans with immature seeds. Large, swollen seeds foretell a tough string bean, but a bean with enough fuzz on its skin that it clings to your shirt is most likely to be tender. Use string beans in salad, soups, and vegetable juices, for dipping, and to add crispness to other vegetable dishes.

Summer Squash (*Cucurbita* species)—Curcurbitaceae (Gourd) Family

A sweet, cooling food, summer squash is ideal for the hot season. Summer squash varieties include the popular zucchini (*Cucurbita pepo*), yellow squash, yellow crookneck squash, and pattypan squash. Although they are less dense in nutrients than the harder, deeper-colored winter squash varieties, summer squash are a good source of beta-carotene, folic acid, vitamin C, calcium, and potassium.

Summer squash is alkaline, alterative, anti-inflammatory, antispasmodic, and diuretic. It is a wonderful, medicinal food in treatments for colitis, constipation, hypertension, indigestion, kidney and bladder disorders, obesity, and ulcers.

Summer squash is ideally harvested when it is immature, or less than 6–9 inches long. If left on the vine, it will grow as big as a baseball bat and be about as tasty. Look for young, tender squash that is heavy for its size and blemish free. Refrigerate, but do not store squash in plastic bags, as this will encourage spoilage. Scoop out the insides of summer squash and stuff with celery, chopped spinach, and nuts. Use slices for dipping or as crudités. Try summer squash chopped or grated into salads, made into pickles, or puréed into soups and sauces. Use a spiral slicer (see Chapter 4) to shred it into noodlelike threads for a low-carbohydrate "pasta" dish. Just about any type of summer squash can be substituted for another in recipes. The flowers of all summer squash are also edible and can be stuffed with guacamole or other fillings.

Sweet Potato (*Ipomoea batatas*)—Convolvulaceae (Bindweed) Family

Sweet potatoes are alkalinizing, warming, and, of course, sweet. They are rich in beta-carotene, vitamins B_1, B_6, C, and E, niacin, calcium, iron, potassium, and carbohydrates. Sweet potatoes also contain protease inhibitors, which have been shown to inhibit the formation of cancer cells, as well as a substance called phytochelatin, which binds with heavy metals such as mercury, lead, cadmium, and copper and carries them out of the body.

In a Japanese study of twenty-eight fruits and vegetables, sweet potato was best able to bind with cholesterol and thereby lower cholesterol levels in the body. It increases milk production in nursing mothers and is an excellent food for people who undergo heavy muscular activity, as it enhances strength. And because sweet potato is naturally very sweet and nutritionally dense, eating it can help curb the desire for refined sugar.

Sweet potatoes are considered an energy, lung, stomach, spleen, and kidney *yin* tonic. They are easy to digest and are used for treating ulcers and inflamed colon conditions. Because of their high beta-carotene content, they can help prevent cataracts and promote healthy night vision; beta-carotene is also helpful in preventing heart disease, strokes, and cancer, especially cancers of the bladder, lung, breast, cervix, and ovary. Sweet potatoes have long been used in treatments for anemia, constipation, diarrhea, dysentery, poor circulation, hemorrhoids, high blood pressure, mastitis, and premature ejaculation.

Look for firm, smooth-skinned sweet potatoes. The skin is generally thin and can be eaten; nonorganic sweet potatoes, however, are often waxed and should be peeled. The brighter and darker the color of the meat, the higher the beta-carotene content. Store sweet potatoes in a cool, dark, dry environment, where they will keep for weeks. Remove any that develop bruises, as a bruise can cause the entire potato to taste unpleasant. Raw sweet potatoes can be sliced into chips, grated into salads, puréed, or mashed into pies, puddings, and soups.

The Raw Facts

Sweet potatoes are sometimes mislabeled as yams. True yams are native to West Africa and are rarely grown or available in the United States. The orange tubers sold in North America as "yams" are usually sweet potatoes.

Swiss Chard (*Beta vulgaris cicla*)—Chenopodiaceae (Goosefoot) Family

Swiss chard is salty, cooling, and alkaline in nature. This wonderful green is a good source of calcium, beta-carotene, vitamin C, phosphorus, sodium, potassium, and iron. It is considered a digestive aid and is beneficial for people suffering from a cold. Look for brightly colored firm leaves.

Note: Swiss chard contains oxalic acid, which can inhibit the absorption of calcium and iron, and so should be consumed only in moderation, especially if cooked.

Tomato (*Lycopersicum esculentum*)—Solanaceae (Nightshade) Family

Tomatoes are cool in energy and sweet and sour in flavor. Although they are acidic, they have an alkalinizing effect on the blood. Tomatoes contain beta-carotene, B-complex vitamins, vitamins C and E, phosphorus, potassium, sulfur, quercitin, histamine, and lycopene. Lycopene, a potent antioxidant, protects against stroke, heart disease, and cataracts, and is being studied as a preventative for cancers of the lungs, prostate, pancreas, stomach, and cervix.

Tomatoes have antiseptic, antiscorbutic (scurvy-preventing), and laxative properties. They aid digestion in cases of inadequate stomach acid secretions. They are considered beneficial to the liver and help the body eliminate uric acid. Tomatoes have been used in treatments for headache, tuberculosis, high cholesterol, hypertension, and constipation.

Avoid tomatoes that are bruised or mushy. Ripe ones should have a smooth, firm skin but yield slightly to the pressure of a finger. Vine-ripened tomatoes are best, because nonorganic, commercial tomatoes are sometimes picked green and then ripened with ethylene gas. Grocery stores will usually advertise vine-ripened tomatoes as such. They can be kept unrefrigerated for several days. Serve sliced tomatoes at room temperature, or add them to salads, soup, sauces, or vegetable juices.

Note: Some people find that tomatoes cause irritable bowel, heartburn, migraines, and/or skin irritation. Like other members of the nightshade family (eggplant, peppers, and potatoes), tomatoes contain the alkaloid solanine, and also oxalic acid, which can inhibit absorption of iron and calcium. People with arthritis should therefore eat tomatoes only in moderation, especially if they are cooked.

Turnip (*Brassica rapa, B. campestris*)—Brassicaceae (Mustard) Family

Turnips, a white version of rutabagas, can grow in poor soil and were thus historically associated with poverty, so potatoes quickly became more popular than the lowly turnip upon their introduction to Europe. Turnips, however, yield both roots and greens that are edible, whereas potato greens are toxic. Also, turnips have one-third the calorie content of potatoes.

Turnips are sweet, bitter, and pungent, and considered warming and alkalinizing. They are believed to reduce the risk of cancer due to their indole content, and because they speed the metabolism of estrogen. Turnips are high in vitamin C, calcium, potassium, sulfur, and carbohydrates. Turnip greens are even more nutritious than the root, being rich in beta-carotene, vitamin B_2, vitamin B_{12} (when soil is well composted), and folic acid.

Turnips are a digestive aid, a lung tonic, and an energizer for the stomach and intestines. They help dry excess dampness in the body, clear up phlegm, neutralize toxins, move stagnation, and build the blood. Turnips have been used to treat asthma, bronchitis, high cholesterol, constipation, diabetes, hoarseness, insomnia, jaundice, nervousness, skin diseases, sinus disorders, and tuberculosis. When eaten raw, they clean the teeth and gums.

Turnip greens are considered excellent for anemia, asthma, bladder disorders, bronchitis, coughs, high blood pressure, gout, liver ailments, and tuberculosis. In folk medicine, a few turnip leaves are applied to the back of the neck to stop a nosebleed.

Even turnip flowers and seeds are edible. In Oriental medicine, the flowers are considered a liver tonic and an aid to visual acuity. The seeds are diuretic and used to dispel excess, damp heat from the body, improve vision, and remedy jaundice and dysentery.

Turnips must be in their prime to be flavorful. Old ones are bitter and pithy. The best roots are small to medium-sized, smooth, and firm. The root and stem will ideally be intact, and if the greens are still attached, they should not be wilted. Nonorganic turnips are often waxed. In general, turnips should be peeled before consumption. Store turnips in a paper bag in the refrigerator, where they will keep for several weeks. Turnip roots can be grated into salads or puréed in soups. Turnip greens can be substituted for kale or collard greens in most recipes. Raw turnip greens are considered bitter, but this is remedied by marinating them in lemon juice, olive oil, and salt.

Note: People with low thyroid function should be sure they are getting enough iodine (from kelp and dulse, for example), as eating turnips on a regular basis can inhibit thyroid activity. People who often experience constipation may find that turnips induce flatulence (especially when first "going raw"), because they help detoxify the bowels.

Watercress (*Nasturtium officinale*)—Brassicaceae (Mustard) Family

Watercress is pungent, bitter, sweet, and alkaline, with a warm energy. Cooking decreases this green's pungency but also decreases its nutritional value. It is rich in beta-carotene, chlorophyll, folic acid, vitamins C and E, bioflavonoids, calcium, iodine, iron, manganese, potassium, sulfur, zinc, and, sulfur.

As a medicinal food, watercress is considered an alterative, antioxidant, antipyretic, antiseptic, aphrodisiac, diuretic, expectorant, hypoglycemic, laxative, metabolic-stimulant, and nutritive agent. It stimulates bile production, detoxifies the liver, and builds *chi*. Watercress has been used in treatments for anemia, asthma, bronchitis, cancer, canker sores, dermatitis, diabetes, eczema, edema, eye disorders, flatulence, goiter, gout, hair loss, headaches due to nerves, infection, jaundice, yellow phlegm, obesity, scurvy, urinary stones, poor teeth, and tuberculosis.

Choose crisp, unwilted bright green leaves and store them in the refrigerator. The leaves can be mixed with milder greens, used in salads, sandwiches, dips, soups, and as a garnish, and added to vegetable juices. Watercress combines well with a bit of citrus flavor.

Note: Watercress can harbor parasites such as liver flukes if collected from contaminated water, so thoroughly washing and soaking watercress in a natural cleansing solution is advisable.

Watermelon (*Citrullus lannatus, C. vulgaris*)—Curcurbitaceae (Gourd) Family

Watermelon is cold, sweet, and alkalinizing. It has only half as much sugar as an apple does, yet tastes sweeter, because it is mostly (92 percent) water. Watermelon is a good source of beta-carotene, vitamin C, potassium, and silicon. It also contains the pigment lycopene, which is being investigated as a cancer preventative, and glutathione, which guards against cataract formation. The inner, pale green rind of watermelon contains chlorophyll and can be eaten along with the pink meat. The fruit's black seeds contain curcurbocitrin, which dilates the capillaries, and are a traditional remedy for strengthening the kidneys.

Watermelon has antibacterial, antioxidant, anticoagulant, diuretic, and laxative properties. It lubricates the intestines, has an affinity for the bladder, kidney, stomach, and heart, and is considered a rejuvenating tonic for the blood. Watermelon can help lift the spirits from depression and has been used in treatments for halitosis, hangover, mouth sores, sore throat, and urethral pain. It is a digestive aid and makes an ideal food during a cleanse.

When on the vine, the melon develops a white spot where it touches the ground; when this white spot turns yellow or cream colored, it indicates ripeness. A ripe melon will also be heavy for its size, have a sweet fragrance, have skin that can be scraped off easily with a fingernail, and make a dull, hollow sound when thumped. Avoid melons with a green or white belly. Watermelon is best enjoyed on its own, but you can add it to other melons in a fruit salad, juice it, or freeze the purée for a cool watermelon sorbet. For a truly invigorating watermelon tonic that will help build the blood and strengthen the glands, try juicing the seeds, rind, and pink meat all together.

Winter Squash (*Curcurbita maxima*)—Curcurbitaceae (Gourd) Family

Winter squash are warm, alkaline, and sweet. The varieties of winter squash include acorn, banana, buttercup, delicata, Hubbard, spaghetti, and turban. They are very nourishing, being rich in beta-carotene, vitamin C, folic acid, magnesium, potassium, sodium, carbohydrates, and fiber. In general, darker winter squash are more nutritious than paler ones. The flowers and large seeds of all winter squash varieties are also edible. The seeds are high in protein, beta-carotene, and B-complex vitamins.

Winter squash have anti-inflammatory, antioxidant, energy-tonic, and immune-tonic properties. They clear toxins from the body and nourish the stomach and spleen. Their high antioxidant content helps prevent stroke, heart disease, and cancers of the bladder, lung, skin, and stomach. Winter squash have been used to improve vision, reduce cataracts, treat bladder infections, lower cholesterol, improve dry skin, and promote weight gain. Their seeds are used to protect the prostate gland and eliminate worms from the body.

Winter squash are generally harvested in the fall and have hard shells. Look for firm, smooth squash that are heavy for their size. Those with the stem still attached will keep longer. They generally do not need to be stored in the refrigerator—a cool, dry location will suffice. They must be peeled before they can be eaten, which is easiest if they are first cut into segments. Use the meat of winter squash like you would use pumpkin: cubed or puréed, or in soups, puddings, and pies.

GRAINS

A grain is the fusion of seed and fruit that is the reproductive mechanism of cereal grasses and a few other types of plants. Although grains are a major element of the typical Western diet, they have only limited use in the raw foods diet. What's more, grains such as rice, oats, wheat, and barley have a tough, outer husk that needs to be removed before they can be eaten, making them labor-intensive to produce.

Grains are heavy in starches, which are difficult to digest, taking from thirty-six to seventy-two hours. Overeating grains can cause you to feel groggy and "hungover" the next day. The sharp fiber in grains, often referred to as nonsoluble fiber, can irritate the intestinal mucosa, contributing to irritable bowel, spastic colon, diverticulosis, Crohn's disease, and a host of other maladies. Grains also tend to be low in calcium, and contain acid-forming compounds of chlorine, iodine, sodium, and sulfur, which can contribute to cancer, obesity, urinary (kidney and bladder) stones, and hemorrhoids.

Grains also contain antinutrients such as phytates, which must be cooked, sprouted, soaked, or fermented in order to be neutralized or inactivated. Although cooking grains inactivates much of their phytate content, cooked starches are difficult to digest. Sprouting, however, inactivates phytates in grains while converting their starch to an easier-to-digest fructose and their proteins to amino acids. In addition, gluten, which is found in wheat, rye, oats, and barley, is a common allergen. Fortunately, people who are allergic to a particular grain are rarely allergic to that grain in its sprouted form.

With these above concerns in mind, I recommend that a raw diet include only a minimal amount of grains if at all, and that they always be sprouted. I also encourage you to seek varieties that are as close to their "heirloom" or "native" state as possible, with minimal hybridizing. Grains tend to be sweet and acid forming (except millet, which is alkalinizing). The following grains can be useful and beneficial in the raw foods diet.

Amaranth (*Amaranthus* species)—Amaranthaceae (Cockscomb) Family

Amaranth was an important food crop for the Aztecs and Incas. It contains higher levels of calcium, phosphorus, and amino acids, including lysine, than most other grains, and is gluten free. The tiny grains are considered astringent, diuretic, and hemostatic. Amaranth is generally used in small amounts, mixed with other grains.

Barley (*Hordeum vulgare*)—Poaceae (Grass) Family

Barley, which originated in western Asia, is believed to be one of the first grains to be cultivated. It thrives in areas where most other grains refuse to flourish, such as arid or saline soils and even in the arctic climate. It is lower in gluten than wheat is, and is therefore less likely to be allergenic. Barley is esteemed for its high content of protein, carbohydrates, B-complex vitamins, calcium, germanium, iron, phosphorus, potassium, and sulfur. It also contains hordenine, a substance that helps relieve the bronchial spasms associated with asthma.

Barley is considered one of the easiest grains to digest. It can help soothe ulcers and colon or bladder irritations, prevent gallstones, and lubricate dry lungs. It stimulates the liver and lymphatic system, aiding the body in discharging toxins. Barley is good for people who live in cold climates, are frail, or have low self-esteem, because it imparts warmth and vitality to the body.

Buckwheat (*Fagopyrum esculentum*)—Polygonaceae (Buckwheat) Family

Although buckwheat is used as a grain, it is technically a fruit or an achene (seed). It originated in Siberia and Manchuria and, being a warming food, is favored by peoples living in cold, damp climates.

Buckwheat has up to twice the amount of calcium found in other grains. It is rich in vitamins B and E and the amino acid lysine. It also contains rutin, which strengthens the capillaries and is an excellent tonic for the cardiovascular system. Rutin helps people with varicosities and people who bruise easily. Buckwheat has a tradition of use by people wishing to strengthen their kidneys, relieve constipation, and reduce high blood pressure.

To be edible, hulled buckwheat should be soaked overnight (or for at least four hours) and then rinsed. If you buy unhulled buckwheat, sprout it in a shallow tray of dirt, and within a few days you can harvest the delightful "buckwheat lettuce."

Corn (*Zea mays*)—Poaceae (Grass) Family

Corn was cultivated in the Americas long before European settlers arrived. It was originally hybridized from a native wild grass, and is North America's only native grain. Today, corn is highly hybridized, and it is the only grain that can't reproduce without human help, as it needs to be shucked and then planted. Corn is sweet and neutral. It is rich in beta-carotene, vitamins B, C, and E, folic acid, iron, magnesium, phosphorus, potassium, and zinc. It is an excellent source of fiber and essential fatty acids.

Corn is appropriately eaten in summer, as it is more cooling than other grains. It has antiviral, diuretic, and mildly stimulating properties. It helps remedy conditions involving phlegm and dampness in the body. Corn is a tonic food that is easy to digest, relieves constipation, and benefits the stomach, heart, and large intestines. It increases estrogen levels and stabilizes blood sugar levels. It helps build the bones, blood, and muscles and is also considered a sexual tonic.

Corn tastes best if left in the husk until right before use. Look for fresh, green husks and plump, milky kernels in nongenetically modified (non-GM) varieties. Yellow corn is more nutritious than white corn.

Kamut (*Triticum durum*)—Poaceae (Grass) Family

Kamut, believed to have originated in Egypt, is an ancient, nonhybridized ancestor of wheat. The genus name *triticum* is Latin for "grain" and the species name *durum* means "hard." It can be used in much the same way as wheat, whether sprouted, grown as grass, or fermented into Rejuvelac (see page 152). The International Food Allergy Association deems kamut to be an acceptable alternative for most people who are sensitive to wheat. Try growing kamut grass for juicing, or sprouting the grain to make raw breads.

Millet (*Panicum miliaceum*)—Poaceae (Grass) Family

Millet is an important staple in its native northern Africa and Asia. Its common name is derived from the Latin *mille,* meaning "thousand," in reference to the multitudes of tiny seeds produced on a stalk. Millet is high in protein, iron, and silicon. It is easily digested and is very alkaline, unlike most other grains, which are more acid producing. Millet is considered beneficial for the stomach and spleen. It helps balance blood sugar levels and helps overcome candida infection.

Oat (*Avena sativa*)—Poaceae (Grass) Family

Oats are sweet, warm, and moist. They are rich in protein, B-complex vitamins, and calcium.

Oats are considered antidepressant, antispasmodic, brain tonic, nutritive, and rejuvenative. They benefit people who are weak and have difficulty gaining weight. Oats have been used to treat attention deficit disorder, broken bones, depression, drug addiction, exhaustion, multiple sclerosis, nervous breakdown, osteoporosis, paralysis, and posttraumatic stress, among other maladies.

Note: Eating too many oats gives the skin a pasty complexion. Be sure to buy oats from a supplier of raw foods (see the Resources section), because most commercially available oats have been cooked. As a rule, if your oats won't sprout, don't eat them!

Quinoa (*Chenopodium quinoa*)—Chenopodiaceae (Goosefoot) Family

Quinoa, a close relative of spinach and beets, is native to the Andes and was a staple food of the Incans. It contains high levels of protein, the amino acid lysine, and calcium. Easy to digest, quinoa is is considered an energy food. It is also a galactagogue, increasing the milk production of nursing mothers. I like to use sprouted quinoa in place of my former, cooked staples, like bulgur wheat.

Rice (*Oryza sativa*)—Poaceae (Grass) Family

Rice grows in water and requires lots of oxygen. Because rice sucks air in through its pores, the Chinese associate it with the lungs. Rice contains less protein than most other grains, though it is rich in lysine. It is reputed to calm the nerves and lift the spirits. Most rice varieties available in grocery stores are heavily hybridized. Freshly harvested brown rice, which can be sprouted, is available from raw foods suppliers.

Rye (*Secale cereale*)—Poaceae (Grass) Family

Rye was developed from a wild grass of northeastern European origin. It has a nutritional portfolio similar to that of wheat and can be used in similar ways, but rye has less gluten. It contains B-complex vitamins, vitamin E, iron, and lysine. Rye is traditionally consumed to strengthen fingernails, hair, bones, teeth, and muscles, and to promote endurance and stamina.

Spelt (*Triticum aestivum*)—Poaceae (Grass) Family

Spelt is believed to be the oldest cultivated variety of wheat. It is not hybridized and is easy to digest. Spelt can be used in place of wheat and, although it contains some gluten, is usually tolerated by those with gluten sensitivities.

Teff (*Eragrostis tef*)—Poaceae (Grass) Family

Native to the region of the Nile, teff was a wild grass that eventually became cultivated. It is rich in iron, calcium, copper, and zinc. Teff also contains intrinsic (naturally occurring) yeast, which aids in the digestion of this grain. Teff has a low potential for being allergenic.

Wheat (*Triticum* species)—Poaceae (Grass) Family

Like barley, wheat was among the first grains to be cultivated. Throughout the world, wheat has now replaced many traditional grains such as barley, teff, and millet; for some Americans, wheat composes up to one-third of the diet. It is the most acidic of grains, and, of course, one of the most common sources of the allergen gluten. Whole wheat is high in B-complex vitamins, vitamin E, iron, magnesium, and zinc.

Wheat tends to build fat and cause weight gain. It also stimulates the liver; however, the ingestion of wheat causes a cleansing reaction that results in skin breakout, lethargy, and excess phlegm. This is one reason why overconsumption of wheat can become such a health detriment.

Wild Rice (*Zizania aquatica*)—Poaceae (grass) Family

Wild rice is technically not a grain but the seed of an aquatic grass. Wild rice is almost always parched after harvesting and so is not usually available as a bona fide *raw food*.

NUTS AND SEEDS

Nuts and seeds contain the genetic potential for starting a new life, and are endowed with sufficient nutrition to sustain their offspring. This, in turn, makes nuts and seeds a powerhouse of nutrition for us, providing beneficial fats, vitamins, minerals, proteins, and carbohydrates.

Nuts have a higher fat content than seeds do, whereas seeds tend to be higher in iron. Both contain beta-carotene, B-complex vitamins, vitamins D and E, and calcium, and are excellent sources of vegetarian protein; in fact, by volume, nuts and seeds provide more protein than meat or milk. They contain phytosterols, or plant hormones, that have a structure similar to that of human hormones and support the endocrine system and all its functions, including reproductive health. Raw nuts and seeds also contain lipase, an enzyme that helps the body digest fats.

Nuts and seeds can help regulate blood sugar levels, and also help clean and strengthen teeth and gums. They relieve constipation, have a "grounding" effect, calm nervousness, and strengthen weakness. Nuts and seeds are excellent for bodybuilders, for those who work with their muscles, and for increasing sexual desire in both men and women.

The Raw Facts

"Nut" is a term used loosely for any dry, hard-shelled fruit. Technically, however, all nuts are actually seeds.

Many people avoid nuts and seeds because of their high fat content. However, when consumed in moderation, nuts and seeds (and the lipase they contain) can actually help control fat and cholesterol levels in the body. They are themselves cholesterol free and can help lower levels of LDL (low-density lipoprotein, the undesirable type of cholesterol). For example, eating 3 ounces of almonds daily, along with a low-fat diet, can lower levels of LDL within three weeks.

Most nuts and seeds are warm and damp in energy, so eating too much of them can build up warmth and dampness in the body, contributing to pimples, digestive disorders, and gas. People with health conditions involving excess dampness (as evidenced by acne, candida infection, tumors, cysts, obesity, or phlegm) should therefore minimize their consumption of nuts and seeds, with the exception of pumpkin, sesame, and sunflower seeds, which are warm and dry.

With the exception of almonds, nuts are acidifying. They should be eaten only in small amounts, preferably with alkalinizing, leafy green vegetables. They can be a bit hard to digest, so people with sensitive digestion will find that nuts are best eaten alone or combined with green or non-starchy vegetables. New raw foodists tend to over-eat nuts and seeds, but they are a heavy, fatty food, so some raw foodists eat them only occasionally. If you do make them a regular part of your diet, eat no more than 6 ounces of nuts and seeds a day, and every couple of months, take a week or so off from eating them.

Nuts and seeds are best when bought in the shell and cracked as needed. The shells prevent free radical damage from light and air, and nuts and seeds in the shell will keep for about a year. The next best option is to buy them shelled and whole; if stored in glass jars in the refrigerator, they will keep for several months. Slivered, cracked, blanched, or broken nut pieces are likely to be rancid (rancidity is caused by the oxidation of oils). Nuts that are rubbery, moldy, rancid, or acrid should be composted. Rancid nut or seed products irritate the lining of the stomach and intestines, cannot be assimilated, weaken the immune system, can damage the health of the liver and gallbladder, and have had their vitamins A, D, and E destroyed. Almonds are less prone to rancidity. Brazil nuts, macadamias, pecans, sunflower seeds, and walnuts tend to turn rancid more quickly than other nuts and seeds.

Oils pressed from nuts and seeds are not typically included in a raw foods diet. Once pressed, these oils are subjected to chemical solvents or heat in order to preserve them, and as a result they are often denatured or contain traces of the solvents. Exceptions in this category are cold-pressed coconut oil and, in some cases, flaxseed oil and hemp seed oil, which are not treated with heat or solvents. (Olive oil, which is also beneficial in a raw foods diet, is technically not a seed oil but a fruit oil; see page 103.) These oils should always be stored in the refrigerator, where they'll keep for several months. Most nut butters (including tahini) are subjected to high enough temperatures to destroy the enzymes (even those labeled "raw"). A brand we use is from Rejuvenative Foods (see the Resources section). Look for nut butters made by manufacturers who avoid subjecting the nuts to heat in the grinding process.

By endowing nuts and seeds with enzyme inhibitors, nature curbs their ability to sprout until conditions are favorable, thereby preventing them from germinating at the wrong time (such as during the winter, or in the grocery store's bulk bins). Soaking nuts and seeds activates protease, a compound that neutralizes the enzyme inhibitors and thus initiates the sprouting process. Even if you don't allow the nuts and seeds to carry the germination process all the way through to sprouting, soaking activates the life force that they contain and improves their digestibility.

Nuts and seeds can be soaked in or out of the refrigerator, but in hot climates it's a good idea to refrigerate those that require long soaking times. Use twice as much water as the volume of nuts or seeds you are soaking. It's best to soak nuts and seeds for eight to twelve hours. If you soak them for longer than twelve hours, rinse them after the first twelve hours and replace the soaking water with fresh water. If you are in a hurry, even soaking them for twenty minutes can improve their digestibility. After soaking nuts or seeds, rinse and drain them. If you're not going to use them immediately, store them in the refrigerator. When blended, soaked nuts or seeds have a creamy texture; blended, unsoaked nuts are oilier and grainier.

The following nuts and seeds can be healthful components of a raw foods diet. Use them for garnishing recipes, as snacks, in trail mixes, or to give crunch to cookies. One nut can be substituted for any other in most recipes.

Almond (*Prunus amygdalsu, P. dulcis*)

Almonds are members of the Rosaceae (rose family) along with peaches, apples, and other relatives. Sweet and neutral in temperature, almonds contain about 18 percent protein and are a good source of vitamin E, calcium, iron, magnesium, potassium, and zinc. They also contain amygdalin, otherwise known as laetrile (vitamin B_{17}), which is a proposed anticancer nutrient. Because almond skins contain lots of tannins (acidic pigments), some people advise not eating the skins.

Almonds have anti-inflammatory, antispasmodic, demulcent, emollient, and tonic properties. They are known as a brain and bone food. They help alkalinize the blood and relieve *chi* stagnation (energy blockages) in the liver. Almonds are used to lubricate the lungs, relieve asthma and coughing, dispel phlegm, strengthen the nervous system, improve energy, and increase strength and sexual vitality. In Ayurvedic medicine, they are used to strengthen *ojas,* the essence that exemplifies intellect and spiritual receptivity. Yogananda, an Indian yogi and author of *Autobiography of a Yogi,* said almonds foster "self control and calmness of the mind and nerves."

Brazil Nut (*Bertholletia excelia*)

Brazil nuts are members of the Lecythidaceae (Brazil nut family). They are harvested in the wilds of the Amazon River Valley, where they fall from their trees in pear-shaped fruits that weigh from 2 to 4 pounds. (Watch your head if you're walking through the jungle!) Brazil nuts are sweet and warming and highly acidic. They are a good source of the amino acids cysteine and methionine, making them beneficial in a vegetarian diet. They are a good source of selenium as well, and rich enough in calcium to be beneficial for teeth and bones. They are also 67 percent fat—finding once that we had no birthday candles for a cake, we stuck fresh raw Brazil nuts in the cake and lit them, and they burned like candles!

In order to remove their shells, unshelled Brazil nuts are boiled for five minutes. This might render them not raw, but most people feel that the thick, hard shell protects the nut inside from becoming too hot.

Cashew (*Anacardium occidentale*)

Cashews are members of the Anacardiaceae (cashew family) and related to mangoes, pistachios, and poison ivy. Their name is derived from the Brazilian Tupi-Indian word *acaju,* meaning "nut." The cashew nut grows attached to the bottom of a cashew apple, which is eaten fresh and made into jams. Because the fruit spoils quickly, it is rarely seen outside of its native regions. Sweet and warming, cashew nuts are composed of about 20 percent protein.

Between the inner and outer shell of the cashew nut is a toxic oil called cardol, which can irritate the skin. To release the cardol, the uncracked cashews are roasted at 350°F, and then the cracked nuts are roasted again to remove the inner shell. Very few cashews, even those labeled "raw," are packaged for sale without having undergone this roasting process. Try purchasing truly raw cashews from raw foods suppliers (see the Resources section).

Chia Seed (*Salvia columbariae, S. hispanica*)

Chia is a member of the Lamiaceae (mint family). *Salvia,* the genus name, is derived from the Latin *salvere,* meaning "to save." The common name comes from the Mayan *chiabaan,* meaning "strengthening." Sweet, bitter, and neutral, chia seeds are rich in omega-3 fatty acids. They are considered an energy tonic that moistens *yin* (fluids). Chia seeds have long been used by the native peoples of the American Southwest for endurance, and in Latin America, the seeds are used to treat constipation.

Coconut (*Cocus nucifera*)

Coconut, the largest known seed, is the fruit of the coconut palm, in the Palmaceae (palm family). Its name comes from the Spanish/Portuguese word *coco,* meaning "monkey face." In Sanskrit, the coconut palm is called *kalpa vriksha:* "the tree that supplies all that is needed to live." An ancient South Pacific saying is, "He who plants a coconut tree plants vessels and clothing, food and drink, a habitation for himself, and a heritage for his children."

Sweet and warming, coconuts are 70 percent fat, most of which is saturated (see Coconut Oil, page 104). They are also high in iodine, which is important for normal thyroid function, and are a good source of protein, beta-carotene, B-complex vitamins, and minerals. Coconut is considered an energy tonic, and is excellent fare for vegetarians.

Coconut milk (made by puréeing the meat and blending it with the water) compares favorably with mother's milk, as they both contain lauric acid, protein, fat, and minerals. Although infants are always better off with mother's milk, coconut milk can be used as a replacement for mother's milk for older children. Coconut milk can also be used to relieve sore throat and to treat stomach ulcers.

A coconut under six months of age has a gelatinous meat that is soft enough to be eaten with a spoon. Considered a delicacy, this "spoon coconut" is also used to feed babies and nourish the sick. Spoon coconut restores damaged body tissues, boosts male sexual fluids, and can be used to rid the body of tapeworm.

Young, green coconuts can contain up to a pint of rejuvenating coconut water, a supreme source of electrolytes and an excellent rehydration beverage. Coconut water cools the body, benefits the elderly and infirm, and helps treat kidney stones and intestinal worms. It can also be fed to infants suffering intestinal distress. This liquid is surprisingly similar in composition to human blood plasma, and was used in intravenous solutions by Japanese doctors during World War II. Coconut water can be applied topically to treat rashes, such as those caused by chicken pox and measles, and it has even been used as eyedrops to treat cataracts.

When shopping for coconuts, look for those that are light in color, indicating their freshness and immaturity. We have recently found out that many of the white coconuts available in this country are dipped in a bleach solution. It is unlikely that any chemicals would seep into the inner portions of the nut. Brown-shelled coconuts are more mature and contain tougher meat. A coconut should have a full, liquid sound when shaken. Avoid any with moldy spots or with moisture that has seeped under the plastic covering. In addition to a "mouth," a coconut has two "eyes," which are soft enough to puncture with a screwdriver so you can pour out the coconut water. Then, tap around the head of the shell with a hammer until it cracks and the coconut meat can be pried out.

It's best to eat fresh rather than dried coconut, because the dried, shredded coconut available in grocery stores is often sweetened, pasteurized, or preserved with propylene glycol. We like to remove fresh, young coconut meat from the shell carefully with a spoon and then slice it thinly into "noodles"; they are excellent in Asian dishes and can also be chopped fine for adding to raw puddings and ice creams.

Flaxseed (*Linum usitatissimum, L. lewisii*)

Flax is a member of the Linaceae (flax family). The genus name is derived from the Greek *linon,* meaning "cord," and the species name *usitatissimum* means "most useful." Flaxseed, sometimes known as linseed, is sweet, warm, and moist. Rich in omega-3 and omega-6 fatty acids, protein, and vitamins A and B, it contains more vitamin E by volume than any other known seed. Flaxseed is 60 percent linolenic acid, which helps maintain cell wall integrity and inhibits the production of tumor-producing acids. It is also high in phytoestrogenic lignans (plant hormones that can mimic some of the actions of human hormones like estrogen), which can help relieve some of the concerns of menopause, including hot flashes.

Flaxseed's healing properties are tremendous. It is considered analgesic, anti-inflammatory, antitussive, decongestant, demulcent, emollient, expectorant, and mucilaginous. It helps clean the arteries, soothes irritation in the intestinal tract, and benefits the cardiovascular system. Flaxseed is often recommended as a daily supplement to support bowel and skin health. It is a potent laxative: just eat 1–2 tablespoons of the seeds, which can be easily chewed as is, or grind or soak them beforehand—and be sure to consume plenty of fluids to aid their laxative action.

Flaxseed has been used to treat arthritis, asthma, breast cysts, bronchitis, constipation, cystitis, eczema, hemorrhoids, and sore throat. Topically, flaxseeds can be used as a poultice for boils, burns, inflammations, pleurisy, psoriasis, and shingles. Nutritionally speaking, golden flaxseeds are considered the best.

Note: Flaxseed contains a small amount of prussic acid, which in very large amounts can be toxic; however, you'd have to eat enormous quantities of the seeds to be at risk from prussic acid toxicity. Do avoid eating immature, unripe flaxseeds, which may be toxic. Also, flaxseed oil turns rancid rapidly, faster than other seed and vegetable oils, especially when exposed to light, heat, or oxygen.

The Raw Facts

In the eighth century, the French king Charlemagne passed a law requiring his people to consume flaxseed so that they would be healthier subjects. Centuries later, Mahatma Gandhi said, "Whenever flaxseeds become a regular food among the people, there will be better health."

Hazelnut/Filbert (*Corylus avellana, C. maxima*)

Hazelnuts are members of the Corylaceae (hazel family). The genus name *corylus* is derived from the Greek *korys,* meaning "helmet," in reference to the nut's helmet-shaped husk. The wild nut is known as a hazelnut, whereas the cultivated nut is called a filbert. Both are rich in calcium and minerals, are acid forming, and strengthen teeth and gums. Hazelnuts are sweet and warming.

Hemp Seed (*Cannabis sativa*)

The seeds of this member of the Cannabaceae (hemp family) contain more protein than any other plant food except for soy, yet hemp seed is easier to digest than soy and is less likely to cause allergic reactions. Hempseeds are sweet and warming. Like flaxseed, hemp seed is rich in omega-3 fatty acids, but it has a longer shelf life. Unlike many seeds, hemp seeds are free of trypsin inhibitors (enzymes) and do not need to be soaked before use. Hemp—both the seed and the plant—has many wonderful uses and is economically and environmentally a great agricultural product. For more information, consult one of the many books that have been written about hemp.

Macadamia Nut (*Macadamia tertrphylla, M. integrifolia*)

Macadamia nuts, also known as Queensland nuts, are members of the Proteaceae (protea family). The nuts are sweet and warming. Macadamia nuts are high in fat (70 percent) and low in protein (8 percent), but they also contain carbohydrates, calcium, iron, phosphorus, selenium, and zinc. They are said to rejuvenate the liver, discourage alcohol cravings, improve anemia, and aid in convalescence. Macadamias are also a phlegm-forming food.

The Raw Facts

Peanuts are not actually nuts but legumes. They are often contaminated, especially when raw, with a mold called aflatoxin that is considered a carcinogen. They are hard to digest, so excess consumption of peanuts can promote lethargy. Additionally, they can aggravate skin breakouts. Peanuts are often produced through crop rotation with cotton, which means they are grown in cotton's pesticide-laden fields. For all of these reasons, peanuts are not considered an optimal raw food.

Pecan (*Carya illinoensis*)

Pecans, in the Juglandaceae (walnut family), are a close relative of walnuts. Pecans are sweet and warming. Pecans are about 71 percent fat. They are also a rich source of protein, minerals, and B-complex vitamins, especially B_6 (pyridoxine). Pecans are considered especially nourishing for the nervous system and helpful in repairing damaged cells in cases of heart disease. The nuts are generally steamed to remove the shells, but the steaming is brief enough that most raw foods enthusiasts do not consider it detrimental.

Pine Nut (*Pinus* species)

Pine nuts, also called *pinons* or *pignoli,* come from those pine trees (members of the Pinaceae, or pine family) that have large, palatable seeds. Sweet and warming, pine nuts are 14 percent protein and known for lubricating the lungs and large intestines. They are delicious in pesto.

Pistachio (*Pistacia vera*)

Pistachio nuts are members of the Anacardiaceae (cashew family). They are neutral in energy, sweet, bitter, and slightly sour. Pistachios are similar in nutritional value to almonds, but higher in iron and vitamin B_1. They are also 55 percent fat and 20 percent protein. The green color of the nut is due to its chlorophyll content. Pistachios lubricate the intestines and tonify the kidneys and liver.

Poppy Seed (*Papaver rhoeas*)

The poppy is a member of the Papaveraceae (poppy family). The seeds are incredibly tiny; you'd need more than ten million of them to make 1 pound. Poppy seeds are sour and have a cool energy. Poppy seeds contain protein, calcium, and zinc.

These seeds are considered analgesic, anodyne, antispasmodic, diaphoretic, expectorant, and mildly narcotic and sedative. They have been used to treat anxiety, asthma, bronchitis, coughs, insomnia, pneumonia, pleurisy, and tonsillitis.

Poppy seeds are good sprinkled on vegetable dishes or blended into poppy seed butter in a food processor. They also make good bird food. They do not need to be soaked before using in raw recipes.

Pumpkin Seed (*Curcurbita maxima, C. pepo*)

Pumpkins are members of the Curcurbitaceae (gourd family). Pumpkin seeds, also known as *pepitos,* are 29 percent protein and rich in omega-3 fatty acids, B-complex vitamins, and calcium. They are also rich in zinc and have anti-inflammatory properties, which makes them useful in the treatment and prevention of prostate gland enlargement. The seeds are sweet, slightly bitter, and have a neutral energy.

Pumpkin seeds help reduce the formation of calcium oxalate crystals, which can contribute to bladder and kidney stones, and help relieve nausea and erectile dysfunction. They can be beneficial in expelling worms (tapeworm, pin worm, and roundworm).

Sesame Seed (*Sesamum indicum*)

Sesame is a member of the Pedaliaceae (sesame family). Sesame seeds are sweet and neutral in temperature. They are about 50 percent oil and 25 to 35 percent protein. They also contain vitamin E, calcium, iron, and sesamin, a lignin that is a powerful antioxidant and can inhibit cholesterol production. Sesame seeds are avaliable either hulled or unhulled. With the loss of their hull, seasame seeds also lose much of their fiber, calcium, potassium, vitamin B_1, and iron.

The seeds are considered demulcent, emollient, laxative, and a general tonic. They tonify the *yin,* relieve chronic wasting diseases, and strengthen the kidneys, liver, bones, hair, nails, and teeth. Black sesame seeds are especially good kidney tonics and are considered strengthening to the reproductive system. They are also used in Oriental medicine to prevent hair from graying. If you're buying them, make sure they're authentic black sesame seeds, and not regular sesame seeds that have simply been dyed black.

Grinding the seeds right before use makes them more digestible. Hulled sesame seeds are used to make tahini; unhulled seeds make sesame butter. Toasted sesame seed oil is indeed cooked, but if you're not a stickler for the rules, a tablespoon of it added to a large bowl of otherwise-raw food will make you reminisce about your favorite Asian dishes from the old days.

Note: Unhulled sesame seeds are high in oxalic acid, which can inhibit the body's absorption of iron and calcium, and should be consumed only in moderation. Hulled sesame seeds may be chemically treated, so it's best to soak them overnight and rinse them in the morning to remove any chemical residue.

Sunflower Seed (*Helianthus annuus*)

Sunflowers are members of the Asteraceae (daisy family). Sunflower seeds, like pumpkin seeds, are rich in zinc, which many regard as a remedy to protect the prostate. They are also rich in B-complex vitamins and linoleic acid.

As a medicinal food, sunflower seeds are antioxidant, diuretic, expectorant, and nutritive. Their high B-complex vitamin content makes them excellent for strengthening a debilitated nervous system and for building kidney strength. Their high linoleic acid content makes them useful in lowering cholesterol and preventing heart disease. Sunflower seeds are considered a tonic for the eyes because they decrease light sensitivity and prevent eye degeneration. They lubricate the intestines, benefit dry constipation, build energy, and increase sexual vigor in both men and women.

When you're trying to quit smoking, try eating sunflower seeds in the shell instead of lighting up; it is satisfying oral-manual work to crack open the shell and peel it off before enjoying the tender seed.

Walnut (*Juglans nigra, J. regia*)

Walnuts are members of the Juglandaceae (walnut family). The genus name *juglans* is derived from the Latin *Jovis glans,* or "nut of Jupiter," a reflection of the belief that gods dined on walnuts. The Chinese refer to walnuts as "longevity fruit" because a walnut tree lives for several hundred years.

Walnuts are sweet, bitter, and warming. They are about 60 percent fat and 20 percent protein; they also contain vitamin E, calcium, potassium, and zinc. They strengthen the lungs and kidneys and lubricate the large intestines. Because of the walnut's resemblance to the brain, in many cultures these nuts are considered a good brain tonic and used for treating head injuries.

WILD THINGS

Thirty-some years ago I lived on a farm in Reynolds, Missouri. Every Thursday, I would go help Mrs. Glore, a neighboring hill woman old enough to have outlived three husbands, and I'd work in her very large and wonderful garden in exchange for firewood. Mrs. Glore was an important teacher in my life. She taught me that most of the weeds we pulled were useful and edible plants. Rather than composting them, we would incorporate them into the evening's dinner and thus double or triple the yield of her garden. Mrs. Glore would declare "Why, you'ze can eat this. It's lamb's-quarter. It's wild spinach and its good fer ya! Even better than the store-bought kind!" Thus began my lessons in learning to love the weeds . . . lessons I would use in my own garden.

Wild plants are hardy, surviving without fertilizer or weekly waterings from the garden hose. Some, like dandelions, persist despite our best attempts to get rid of them. Their ability to overcome all sorts of adversity imparts to us a source of strength and vitality. Nourished by rain, sunlight, moonlight, and wind, they can furnish more nutrition than their cultivated progeny. Learn to enjoy the freshness of a salad that was collected five minutes before being eaten!

Use wild edibles in place of spinach, kale or collard greens in most recipes. Add wild greens to vegetable juices. Learn to love the weeds that heal and feed our needs!

Gathering Guidelines

- Make sure you are collecting the proper species, because many plants have poisonous lookalikes. Bring along a good guide, or at least a good guidebook.

- Be sure you are collecting the correct plant part. For example, blue elderberries are wonderful, but the leaves of the plant are toxic. Red elder is also toxic.

- Do not harvest any known endangered species.

- Ask permission before gathering on private land.

- If possible, water plants the day before collecting.

- When harvesting from a group of plants, identify the grandfather/grand-mother plant and leave it there to ensure the continuation of the strongest of the species.

- Never take more than 10 percent of a wild population of plants. Leave some for the wild animals.

- Vary the places from which you collect.

- Avoid collecting plants within 50 feet of a busy road, in areas that are polluted, or in areas that have been treated with pesticides or herbicides.

- Gather leaves and flowers in the morning, after the dew has evaporated and before the sun is too hot.

- Gather leaves not when the plant is already in full flowering but in the early stages of flowering, when its energy will still be in its leaves.

- It is kinder to take a whole leaf rather than to tear off part of a leaf.

- Replant seeds as often as possible.

- Collect plants in a way to ensure the continued survival of the species. For example, if all you need are the leaves and flowers, take only the tops. Cutting a plant back can actually help promote new growth. Leave the roots to continue their growing cycle. By gathering selectively, you can thin plants that are growing too close together, and give the other plants more room.

- Compost the plant parts you do not eat, or use them as mulch or in herbal preparations.

- Sing while collecting! Be joyful and thankful!

Amaranth (*Amaranthus* species)

Parts used: Leaf and seed

Amaranth, also known as pigweed or redroot, is so persistent that the Greeks considered it a symbol of immortality. Amaranth is bitter, sweet, and cooling in nature. The greens are high in calcium and magnesium.

Amaranth leaves are considered astringent and diuretic. Amaranth leaf tea has been utilized to treat diarrhea, dysentery, and excessive menstrual bleeding.

Amaranth leaves can be collected before flowering and eaten raw like spinach. The seeds can be collected in late summer or autumn, spread out on a paper bag, and allowed to dry for several days. Using your fingers or a colander, separate the seeds from the chaff. The seeds can then be ground or used as flour and added to dehyhdrated breads.

Note: Amaranth does contain some oxalates, which can inhibit calcium and iron absorption, so be sure your diet contains calcium if incorporating more than small amounts of amaranth.

Burdock (*Arctium lappa*)

Part used: Root

Burdock is bitter, sweet, and cooling. It contains vitamin C, calcium, magnesium, and iron. Burdock was used during the Industrial Revolution to help people cope with the health detriments of pollution. Unfortunately, the pollution hasn't gone away, but the good news is that burdock is still growing in our midst. Burdock root assists many of the body's organs of elimination including the colon, liver, kidneys, lymph nodes, and skin. It can be grated or sliced and added to salads.

Chickweed (*Stellaria media*)

Parts used: Leaf, flower, and stem

More than thirty bird species, including chickens, are known to eat this plant. It grows outward, instead of upward, and its very presence indicates a fertile soil: it helps the soil retain its nitrogen content. Chickweed is delicate and delicious, and is known for its high vitamin C content.

Traditionally, chickweed has been used to strengthen frail people. It has soothing and anti-inflammatory properties and can be prepared as a tea for bladder irritation, bronchial irritation, and ulcers. Chickweed is an excellent salve ingredient, helping to soothe everything from diaper rash to psoriasis. The leaves, flowers, and stems can be included in salads or made into soups. It keeps well in the refrigerator for up to a couple of weeks.

Dandelion (*Taraxacum officinale*)

Parts used: Leaf, flower, and root

Most people regard this plant as a nuisance, but dandelion has many uses.

Dandelion leaves are edible in the springtime, before the plant flowers, and are high in iron and beta-carotene. The leaves also have a diuretic effect, and although most chemical diuretics deplete the body of potassium, dandelion greens, by contrast, are rich in this mineral. Dandelion blossoms can be separated from the calyx and sprinkled on salads. They contain lutein, a nutrient that is beneficial for the eyes. Dandelion roots are also edible. We like to dig them up, scrub them, add a bit of olive oil and tamari, and then dehydrate them a bit—delicious! Dandelion-root tea has long been used to improve skin conditions such as acne and eczema, and also to improve liver function.

Knotweed (*Polygonum erectum, P. aviculare*)

Parts used: Aboveground plant and seed

The genus name for knotweed is derived from the Greek *polys,* meaning "many," and *gony,* meaning "knees," in reference to the plant's numerous, jointed stems. Perhaps this appearance led to its use as a tea remedy for swollen, arthritic joints and knees. Knotweed, also known as doormat grass, is considered an important kidney herb, as it is a valuable diuretic and can be used to eliminate kidney stones. Its high silica content makes it a good remedy for strengthening the lungs' connective tissue.

When knotweed stems are young and tender, between 6–8 inches in height, they can be collected, finely chopped, and added to salads. The seeds can also be used as a grain.

Lamb's-quarter (*Chenopodium album*)

Parts used: Leaf and seed

The goosefoot-shaped leaves of this abundant plant have long been used as a nourishing food during times of war and famine. Rich in iron, lamb's-quarter is considered a remedy for anemia. Lamb's-quarter, like spinach, contains oxalic acid, which can inhibit absorption of iron and calcium, but lamb's-quarter is also rich in calcium and magnesium. The leaves taste like spinach but are much easier to grow and even more nutritious. The seeds can also be used as a grain.

Malva (*Malva neglecta*)

Parts used: Leaf, flower, and seed

Malva leaves are soothing and anti-inflammatory. They are very rich in beta-carotene and have been included in teas and syrups for helping coughs and irritated lung conditions. As a tea, malva leaves are a traditional medicine for sore throats and ulcers. They also make a simple poultice for treating skin rashes, burns, and insect bites.

Malva leaves can be eaten by themselves or added to soups, where their high content of mucilage helps thicken the pot's contents. The seeds can be eaten raw or even pickled. Because the seeds have a high moisture content, they can be used to moisten the mouth when water is scarce. Malva's delicate, pink and white flowers are a lovely and edible addition to grace the dinner plate.

Mustard (*Alliaria petiolata, A. officinalis, Brassica juncea, B. sinapiodes, Cardaria draba, Descurania* species, *Lepidium perfoliatum, Sinapsis alba, Sisymbrium officinale*)

Parts used: Leaf, seed, seedpod, and flower
Mustard is an annual that grows 1–8 feet in height, depending on the species. Mustard flowers can be white, pink, yellow, or purple in color, but all have four petals in the shape of a cross with four sepals, six stamens, and one pistil. Mustard is pungent and hot, and its seeds and leaves are both used as food and medicine.

Mustard is considered antiseptic, expectorant, rubifacient, and stimulant. It stimulates appetite and secretion of gastric juices. Mustard has been used medicinally to treat chilblains, cough, and respiratory congestion.

Mustard leaves can be chopped and mixed in a salad with milder greens. The flowers and young seedpods are edible in salads and as a garnish. The seeds are used in pungent sauces.

Note: There are no poisonous mustards. However, eat mustards only in moderation, as they do contain some irritating oils that can cause intestinal irritation.

Nettle (*Urtica dioica*)

Part used: Young plant
Nettles are probably best known for their sting. The tiny hairs of the plant contain formic acid, the same substance that causes pain from ant bites. The hairs also contain choline acetyltransferase, acetylcholine, choline, and serotonin, all of which can improve brain function. There are actually health benefits to the stings, such as in relieving arthritis pain. Most people will want to wear gloves and use scissors when collecting nettles. However, people in the know have learned that getting stung by nettles is very therapeutic because the sting increases circulation to the area, relieving pain and inflammation. I have several friends who come over to "whack" their wrists in the nettle patch to relieve the soreness from playing guitar all night long.

Nettles are highly alkaline and very rich in iron, and are more effective than spinach in building the blood. Their abundant supply of beta-carotene and vitamin C strengthens the mucous membranes. In fact, nettles are so rich in nutrients that they help curb overeating. They are also considered anti-allergenic. Taking nettles in capsule, tea, or tincture form before the hay fever season even begins can minimize its annual discomfort.

Young nettle shoots can be finely chopped and marinated in a bit of olive oil, Celtic salt, and lemon juice. Nettles can also be puréed in a food processor to make a pesto (puréeing them deactivates the sting).

Note: Only young nettle plants should be consumed: once the plant starts to flower, it becomes irritating to the kidneys when ingested.

Purslane (*Portulaca oleracea*)

Part used: Leaf

Although its creeping, succulent leaves are tenacious invaders, purslane is truly a valuable plant. It is rich in omega-3 fatty acids and is therefore helpful in protecting the heart and lowering blood pressure and cholesterol levels. It is a cooling, summer vegetable with a high content of beta-carotene and vitamin C. Not only does purslane make a fine salad herb, but it is wonderful in raw soups like gazpacho.

Red Clover (*Trifolium pratense*)

Parts used: Leaf and flower

Red clover is a highly nutritive, blood-purifying herb. The flavor is salty and sweet. Red clover has a cooling quality. The young flowers and leaves are edible—try them in small amounts in salads. It contains protein, vitamin C, chromium, and iron.

Violet (*Viola odorata*)

Parts used: Leaf and flower

As we look deep into shady areas, heart-shaped leaves and brilliant purple flowers announce the everpresent violet. You might catch its beautiful aroma before you glimpse it. The flowers are at their prime in the spring. The leaves and flowers, both high in vitamin C, are an esteemed remedy for coughs, fevers, and lung complaints such as bronchitis. The smell and flavor of violets helps comfort those who are grief stricken. Violet leaves are wonderful in salads.

SEAWEEDS

Seaweeds, also known as sea vegetables, grow in the mineral-rich brine of the ocean and transform its fifty-six known minerals, including calcium, iodine, iron, potassium, and magnesium, into nutrients that we can assimilate. In fact, seaweeds contain ten to twenty times more minerals than land-grown plants do. Their abundant mineral content makes seaweeds an important element of the raw foods diet.

Seaweeds offer many benefits to human health. They increase metabolism, purify the blood, help break down fat, improve joint flexibility, and help heal mucous membranes. They are naturally alkalinizing, antibacterial, antifungal, and antiviral. They also strengthen the kidneys and beautify the skin and hair.

Energetically, seaweeds are cool and wet. They can help old "emotional programming" to resurface, allowing negative memories to come to light and have the opportunity to be resolved.

In addition, seaweeds contain alginic acid, a compound that binds in the body with heavy metals, environmental toxins, and other chemicals, and then carries them from the body through the stools.

The Raw Facts

In the warmth of tropical waters, sea vegetables are smaller, whereas in cold waters, they are larger and grow more abundantly.

Seaweeds are available commercially in dried form, often in small sheets. Crush and sprinkle them over salads, eat them plain as snacks, add them to soups as flavorings, or use them as wrappers to hold other raw delights. If you need to soften dried seaweed, soak it in room-temperature water for twenty minutes, then rinse and drain it. Use a bit of oil in preparing seaweeds to enhance your body's absorption of their minerals and vitamins A and D.

Agar (*Gelidiella acerosa*)

Agar grows in deep water and has a trunklike stem with thorny, tubular leaves. This seaweed is rich in calcium and phosphorus. It has a cooling effect on the digestive tract and contributes to the health of blood vessels and arteries. Agar can be used to replace gelatin in vegan recipes. (Usually, 3 tablespoons of agar are soaked in 3 cups of water for a few minutes. The water and agar are then brought to a boil for 1 minute, cooled slightly, and finally mixed with raw fruits, vegetables, or juices to thicken.)

Arame (*Eisenia bicyclis*)

Arame has a sweet, mild flavor and a relaxing nature. It is rich in beta-carotene and potassium, and supports the spleen, stomach, and pancreas.

Dulse (*Rhodymenia palmetta*)

Dulse is soft, flat, and delicate, resembling gloves or mittens. It is rich in iron, beta-carotene, and vitamin E, and it benefits the heart and spleen. Of all the sea vegetables, dulse is the easiest to digest.

Hiziki (*Hizikia fusiforme*)

Hiziki is rich in calcium, iron, and vitamins B_1, B_2, and C. It strengthens the intestines and enhances the assimilation of nutrients. Hiziki is often heated in its processing, so if you can't be sure that you're getting completely raw hiziki, you might consider using a different variety of seaweed.

Kelp (*Fucus versiculosis*)

Kelp is the most common type of seaweed. It contains mucopolysaccharides, protein, vitamin B_2, vitamin C, and minerals. Kelp is antibacterial, antibiotic, antioxidant, anticarcinogenic, diuretic, emollient, nutritive, and expectorant. It has a softening and draining effect on the body and can be used to help treat lymph node enlargement and tumors. When ingested, kelp combines with residues of drugs, chemicals, and radioactive strontium-90 and carries them from the body. It also stimulates a sluggish metabolism and can be helpful as part of a weight-loss program.

Kelp is often used in powdered form as a seasoning, as it imparts a salty flavor.

Kombu (*Laminaria* species)

With its long, flat fronds, kombu can grow up to 1,500 feet long. This seaweed is high in calcium, iron, potassium, sodium, and glutamic acid (a flavor-enhancing compound). Kombu is especially strengthening to the kidneys and reproductive system.

Nori (*Porphyra tenera*)

Nori is low-growing and fragile and makes its home in shallow water. It is high in protein, beta-carotene, and minerals. Nori stimulates circulation and gives short bursts of energy, relieving fatigue and loneliness. Buy only black nori sheets, as the green ones have been roasted.

Sea Palm (*Postelsia palmaeformis*)

Sea palm resembles a palm tree, grows on rocky shores, and is almost constantly pounded by the surf, enduring more hardship than most plants. It contributes greatly to stamina and supports glandular function.

Wakame (*Undaria pinnatifida*)

Wakame has serrated leaves and a strong spine. It is rich in protein, trace minerals, beta-carotene, and B-complex vitamins. Wakame helps support the liver and nervous system as well as mental flexibility.

GREEN SUPERFOODS

A "superfood" contains high concentrations of nutrients. The following three superfoods are packed with nutrients, including chlorophyll, and have energizing, detoxifying, rebuilding, and immune-strengthening properties. To feel more vibrant than ever before, make a habit of including at least one of these raw, green superfoods in your daily diet.

Blue-Green Algae (*Aphanizomenon flos-aquae*)

This species of algae is found in freshwater lakes, where it reproduces at a very fast rate (almost daily in the summer). Upper Klamath Lake in southern Oregon is the only place in the world where large quantities are available in the wild. Blue-green algae are said to be 65 percent assimilable protein, and the softness of the cell walls makes them easy to digest. The algae are also rich in neuropeptides, which can boost the activity of the brain's neurotransmitters. This superfood is a tremendous energizer and is available in both powder and tablet forms.

Spirulina (*Spirulina platensis*)

Spirulina, named for its spiral shape, is a multicelled algae that grows in warm, alkaline or salty waters. It is rich in gamma linoleic acid (GLA) and is 65 percent protein; in fact, 1 acre of spirulina yields 20 times more protein than an acre of soybeans. These algae are easy to digest due to their soft-walled cell structure. Popular with dieters, this superfood is loaded

The Benefits of Chlorophyll

All of the green superfoods contain bountiful supplies of chlorophyll, the green pigment that most plants require for photosynthesis. Chlorophyll could be considered the blood of the plant—in fact, there is but one atomic bond's difference between chlorophyll and hemoglobin.

Chlorophyll stimulates red blood cell production, strengthens the immune system, and minimizes the effects of pollution. It is an anti-inflammatory agent and relieves pain. Although it doesn't kill germs directly, chlorophyll fights internal and external infection by creating an environment that interferes with their growth; in helping the body to break down undesirable bacteria, it acts as a natural deodorizer and promotes better bowel function and digestion. Chlorophyll can help curb chronic skin conditions, sinusitis, pyorrhea, gastric ulcers, anemia, arteriosclerosis, and depression. It mitigates stress and calms the mind.

In 1943, *The American Journal of Surgery* reported that chlorophyll sped wound healing by 24.9 percent. It works in this way by reducing inflammation, reducing the synthesis of fibrin (a blood protein associated with platelet aggregation, or clotting), inhibiting bacteria, and promoting tissue repair by stimulating healthy granuloma tissue and fibroblasts (cell types that form a matrix to rebuild the damaged area). Chemical, heat, and radiation burns respond quickly to topical chlorophyll treatments. Before immune-suppressing drugs were available, chlorophyll was applied to skin grafts to encourage their acceptance by the body; there have even been cases of chlorophyll treatments saving limbs that were being considered for amputation.

Chlorophyll has also been shown to help neutralize and deactivate carcinogens. In 1986, the journal *Mutation Research* published research by Ong and colleagues on chlorophyll's potent antimutagenic effects against environmental and dietary substances. Tests showed that chlorophyllin (a water-soluble form of chlorophyll) neutralizes the cancer-causing activity of tobacco, fried beef, coal dust, and other compounds.

In contrast to the many pharmaceuticals that require increasingly larger doses to continue being effective, repeated use of chlorophyll does not cause the body to build up a tolerance to it. Chlorophyll also exhibits no toxicity whether ingested, injected, or applied topically, making it one of the most distinctive substances known to science.

with nutrients, including vitamin B_{12} and the amino acids phenylalanine and tyrosine, which suppress appetite and help one to feel satisfied. Spirulina is available in powder form, which can be sprinkled into salads, soups, or guacamole.

Wheatgrass (*Triticum* species)

Wheatgrass is the term for sprouted wheat berries that have been grown into a grass. The hard berries are usually sprouted outdoors or in trays of soil indoors and the wheatgrass appears, as the name implies, like small shoots of grass (see "The Raw Facts" on page 123 and Sprouting Guide on page 126). You can grow your own wheatgrass or buy it fresh at natural foods stores. It is usually consumed as juice but is also available in dried powder and tablet form.

Wheatgrass is an incredible superfood; though it is 95 percent water, the remaining 5 percent carries a host of nutrients, including 90 out of a possible 102 minerals. Wheatgrass is a rich source of beta-carotene, B-complex vitamins (including B_{12}), vitamins C, E, K, and U, calcium, cobalt, iron, magnesium, germanium, phosphorus, sodium, sulfur, zinc, seventeen amino acids (including the eight essential ones), and at least eighty enzymes. It also contains superoxide dismutase (SOD), which is a potent antioxidant that inhibits the activity of free radicals, and abscisic acid, which is a plant hormone believed to regulate growth and metabolism and to defeat cancer cells. According to some studies, dehydrated wheatgrass has a protein composition of 47.4 percent (three times higher than that of beef).

Wheatgrass is antibacterial, antiviral, and alkalinizing. It detoxifies, purifies, and builds the blood. It helps eliminate phlegm from the intestines, nourishes the brain and nervous system, and prevents degenerative disease. People who drink wheatgrass juice feel energized and clearheaded from their daily shots of "grass." Many health benefits are ascribed to wheatgrass and its juice, including:

- Relieving indigestion

- Improving body odor

- Relieving arthritis and rheumatism

- Reducing alcoholic tendencies

- Helping reduce obesity

- Cleansing the liver

- Helping alleviate depression

- Improving blood sugar levels

- Reducing high blood pressure

- Eliminating heavy metals (cadmium, copper, aluminum, lead, mercury) from the body

- Reducing inflammation of mucous membranes

- Reducing destructive effects of X-rays and other radiation

- Improving digestion

- Correcting anemia by increasing red blood cell count

- Stimulating growth of connective tissue

- Improving skin health

- Helping prevent hair graying

- Improving vision

- Slowing the harmful effects of carbon monoxide and other air pollutants

Applied topically to the affected area, wheatgrass juice or a poultice of the grass is said to:

- Accelerate healing of wounds and burns

- Eradicate moles and blemishes

- Reduce varicose veins

- Relieve scalp conditions such as dandruff

- Freshen breath

- Relieve toothache and sore throat

- Prevent tooth decay

- Treat canker sores and bleeding gums

- Restore gum tissue and control pyorrhea (infection and loosening of tooth sockets)

- Remedy athlete's foot

- Remedy yeast infection or vaginitis

When first added to one's diet, wheatgrass or its juice can cause nausea or stomachache, especially if too much is consumed. Start with 1 teaspoon of juice daily and gradually increase the amount to 2 ounces three times daily. Sip it slowly, mixing it well with your saliva. Do not eat for at least an hour after drinking more than 3 ounces of wheatgrass juice.

Juicing wheatgrass requires a special juicer, which can be obtained from any of the suppliers listed in the Resources section. Wheatgrass can be juiced in combination with other foods such as carrots, celery, parsley, spinach, kale, or dandelion greens. For those times when you can't juice your wheatgrass, its nutrients can be extracted very effectively by chewing it and then spitting out the pulp: 2 ounces of chewed wheatgrass is equal to 1 ounce of fresh juice. If the wheatgrass is very young, it can be eaten as is or mixed in with salads.

Note: People who are allergic to wheat are usually sensitive to gluten, a substance that is found in the grain but not in the grass. If you have a wheat allergy, start your wheatgrass regimen slowly, and discontinue it if you have an allergic reaction.

EDIBLE FLOWERS

Flowers, the sex organs of plants, add grace and beauty to any dish. The edible flowers on the following list are a wonderful addition to a raw foods diet. Be sure to use only organically grown or wild edible flowers, as many commercially grown ones are treated with chemicals.

- Acacia (*Acacia* species)
- Anchusa (*Anchusa officinalis, A. azurea*)
- Anise hyssop (*Agastache foeniculum*)
- Apple (*Malus* species)
- Arugula (*Eruca sativa*)
- Bachelor's buttons (*Centaurea cyanus*)
- Banana (*Musa* species)
- Basil (*Ocimum basilicum*)
- Beebalm (*Monarda* species)
- Begonia (*Hybrid tuberous begonia*)
- Borage (*Borago officinalis*)
- Broccoli (*Brassica oleracea*)

- Calendula (*Calendula officinalis*)
- Canary creeper (*Tropaeolum peregrinum*)
- Carnation (*Dianthus* species)
- Catnip (*Nepeta cataria*)
- Cattail (*Typha latifolia*)
- Chamomile (*Matricaria recutita, Chamaemelum nobile*)
- Chervil (*Anthriscus cerefolium*)
- Chickweed (*Stellaria media*)
- Chicory (*Cichorium intybus*)
- Chive (*Allium schoenoprasum*)
- Chrysanthemum (*Chrysanthemum morifolium, C. coronarium, Dendranthema grandiflora*)
- Clove dianthus (*Dianthus carophyllus*)
- Coriander/cilantro (*Coriandrum sativum*)
- Cowslip (*Primula veris*)—not American cowslip
- Dandelion (*Taraxacum officinale*)
- Day lily (*Hemerocallis* species)
- Dill (*Anethum graveolens*)
- Elder (*Sambucus canadensis, S. caerulea*)
- English daisy (*Bellis perennis*)—not American daisy
- Fennel (*Foeniculum vulgare*)
- Fuchsia (*Fuchsia* species)
- Garlic (*Tulbaghia violacea, Allium sativum*)
- Garlic chive (*Allium tuberosum*)
- Geranium (*Pelargonium* species)
- Gladiolus (*Gladiolus* species)
- Hawthorn (*Crataegus* species)
- Hibiscus (*Hibiscus* species)
- Hollyhock (*Alcea rosea*)
- Honeysuckle (*Lonicera japonica*)
- Hop (*Humulus lupulus*)

- Hyssop (*Hyssopus officinalis*)
- Jasmine (*Jasminum* species)
- Johnny-jump-up (*Viola tricolor*)
- Kale (*Brassica* species)
- Lavender (*Lavandula* species)
- Lemon (*Citrus limon*)
- Lemon balm (*Melissa officinalis*)
- Lemon geranium (*Pelargonium crispum*)
- Lemon verbena (*Aloysia triphylla*)
- Lilac (*Syringa* species)
- Linden (*Tilea* species)
- Lovage (*Levisticum officinale*)
- Magnolia (*Magnolia grandiflora, M. denudata*)
- Mallow (*Malva* species)
- Marigold (*Tagetes erecta, T. tenufolia*)
- Marjoram (*Origanum marjorana*)
- Meadowsweet (*Filipendula ulmaria*)
- Mint (*Mentha* species)
- Mullein (*Verbascum* species)
- Mustard (*Brassica* species)
- Nasturtium (*Tropaeolum majus*)
- Okra (*Abelmoschus esculentus*)
- Onion (*Allium* species)
- Orange blossom (*Citrus sinensis*)
- Oregano (*Origanum* species)
- Oxeye daisy (*Chrysanthemum leucanthemum*)
- Pansy (*Viola wittrockiana*)
- Passionflower (*Passiflora* species)
- Pea (*Pisum sativum*)
- Peony (*Paeonia* species)
- Peppermint (*Mentha piperita*)

- Peppermint geranium (*Pelargonium tomentosum*)
- Petunia (*Petunia hybrida*)
- Pineapple guava (*Feijoa sellowiana*)
- Pineapple sage (*Salvia ellegans*)
- Pinks (*Dianthus caryophyllus, D. plumarius*)
- Plum (*Prunus domestica*)
- Poppy (*Papaver* species)
- Primrose (*Primula vulgaris*)
- Purslane (*Portulaca oleracea*)
- Radish (*Raphanus sativus*)
- Red clover (*Trifolium pratense*)
- Redbud (*Cercis canadensis, C. siliquastrum*)
- Rocket (*Eruca vesicaria*)
- Rose (*Rosa* species)
- Rose geranium (*Pelargonium graveolens*)
- Rose of Sharon (*Hibiscus syriacus*)
- Roselle (*Hibiscus sabdarriffa*)
- Rosemary (*Rosmarinus officinalis*)
- Runner bean (*Phaseolus coccineus*)
- Safflower (*Carthamus tinctorius*)
- Saffron crocus (*Crocus sativa*)—not autumn crocus (*Colchicum autumnale*), which is poisonous
- Sage (*Salvia* species)
- Salad burnet (*Poterium sanguisorba*)
- Savory (*Satureja hortensis, S. montana*)
- Shungiku (*Chrysanthemum coronarium*)
- Snapdragon (*Antirrhinum majus*)
- Sorrel (*Rumex scutatus, R. acetosa*)
- Spearmint (*Mentha spicata*)
- Squash (*Cucurbita* species)—especially male zucchini blossoms
- Sunflower (*Helianthus annuus*)

- Sweet cicely (*Myrrhis odorata*)
- Sweet woodruff (*Galium odoratum*)
- Thistle (*Cirsium* species)
- Thyme (*Thymus* species)
- Tiger lily (*Lilium tigrinum*)
- Tulip (*Tulipa* species)
- Violet (*Viola cornuta, V. odorata*)
- Water lily (*Nymphaea odorata*)
- Watercress (*Nasturtium officinale*)
- Wild oregano (*Monarda* species)
- Yarrow (*Achillea millefolium*)
- Yucca (*Yucca* species)

Flower Sun Teas

*Many flowers (and some of their leaves) make
delicious sun teas. Choose your favorites from the list below,
and imbibe the beauty of a fresh-flower infusion!*

Beebalm leaf and flower (*Monarda* species)

Catnip leaf and flower (*Nepeta cataria*)

Lavender flower (*Lavandula* species)

Lilac flower (*Syringa* species)

Lemon balm leaf and flower (*Melissa officinalis*)

Lemon verbena leaf (*Aloysia triphylla*)

Anise hyssop leaf and flower (*Agastache foeniculum*)

Peppermint leaf and flower (*Mentha piperita*)

Rose flower (*Rosa* species)

Rosemary leaf and flower (*Rosmarinus officinalis*)

Spearmint leaf and flower (*Mentha spicata*)

Fill a glass pitcher with 1 cup of fresh flowers and leaves. Cover with a $1/2$ gallon of pure water. Allow to steep in the sun (or moonlight) for two hours. Strain the sun tea and serve. Garnish with a flower or mint sprig, if desired. Sun tea will keep for up to four days in the refrigerator.

FATS AND OILS

Fats are a necessary part of our diet. They are antioxidant, moisturize the skin, contribute to joint and muscle flexibility, and facilitate digestion by lubricating the body's digestive tract. In the body, they form a protective layer around the nervous system and insulate the nerves from shock. The linolenic acid and lineoleic acid found in raw fats can help the body metabolize stored deposits of cooked fats.

People deficient in fats tend to be irritable and unable to cope with stressful situations. A diet totally devoid of fats can cause previously accumulated fats to harden in the body, and can intensify cravings for fat. Too much fat, on the other hand, can cause acne, body odor, constipation, and a hot and hungover feeling.

The best fats are those found in whole, raw foods such as avocados, durians, nuts, sun-cured olives, soaked seeds, and young coconut. Oils, having been extracted from their source, are not exactly a whole food, but olive oil and coconut oil are two acceptable sources of raw fat. Hemp seed oil and flaxseed oil are also used to some degree, as both are rich in omega-3 fatty acids and benefit the skin, hair, and emotional balance. Flaxseed oil goes rancid quickly, whereas hemp seed oil is more stable.

Oils deteriorate quickly and are likely to become rancid in the presence of heat or light. All oils should be stored in dark, glass bottles and kept in the refrigerator, where they will solidify from the cold. Take them out of the refrigerator ten minutes before you need to use them, and they'll return to their liquid state readily.

Olive Oil

Olive trees can live for centuries, even as long as 2,000 years (though their average is 300–600 years). Although slow growing initially, the trees sprout new branches if cut, have deep taproots, and thrive in sunshine. Olives are rich in protein and polyphenols, which are water-soluble antioxidants with antifungal and antibacterial properties. Olives and olive oil soothe the stomach and help congested lymphatic system and lungs. Olive oil is digestible and nourishing; it penetrates, softens, and strengthens.

The first pressing of olive oil uses gentle pressure, with heat rising no higher than room temperature. The oil of the first pressing is marketed as "extra-virgin" olive oil. The next pressing's oil is marketed as "virgin." Subsequent pressings of olive pulp and seeds use solvents and high heat and are marketed as "pure" olive oil. The best olive oil is stone-pressed, extra-virgin.

Coconut Oil

Coconut oil, also known as coconut butter, is solid at room temperature but becomes a clear liquid at temperatures higher than 78°F. It is a primarily a saturated fat, but it is very digestible: so much so that it is often added to infant formulas, or fed to infants and children who cannot digest other fats. In the body, it is quickly metabolized for energy production. Raw coconut oil does not elevate cholesterol levels or promote blood platelet aggregation. To avoid harmful trans fats, use only cold-pressed or expeller-pressed coconut oil. Know your source. Some companies label their oils "cold pressed" even though the oil temperature may reach 200°F.

Coconut oil contains both short- and medium-chain fatty acids. In laboratory tests, the medium-chain fatty acids (MCFAs) have been shown effective against flu, measles, sinusitis, food poisoning, urinary tract infections, cavities, gonorrhea, toxic shock, fungal infections, hepatitis C, and candida. Coconut oil is antibacterial, antifungal, antiviral, and antiprotozoal. It helps stimulate thyroid function, normalize blood sugar levels, decrease seizures, and relieve chronic fatigue.

Coconut oil can be used in raw dishes such as Asian fare, cakes, candies, and salad dressings. A wonderful skin-care product with a long shelf life, it smells great and imparts beauty and radiance when rubbed on the skin. Coconut oil is used in massage, skin care, and first-aid creams to heal

Concerns about Oils

Most vegetable oils are extracted from their source with chemical solvents. The oils are then boiled to remove the solvents—but even after boiling, traces of the solvents remain. Even oils labeled "cold pressed" or "expellar pressed" are usually heated above 115°F; here, "cold" is a relative term, meaning that the pressing occurs at a temperature lower than normal but still hot enough to give you a good burn. Once the oil is extracted, preservatives are often added to extend the product's shelf life.

Heating fats, such as oils, produces carcinogenic free radicals. Heated fats impair the blood's ability to transport oxygen by clogging capillaries with fat globules, and can congest vascular walls, contributing to arteriosclerosis and other cardiovascular disorders. Heated fats can also cause acne, impaired liver function, and unpleasant body odor.

and prevent scarring. People suffering from psoriasis may benefit from topical applications of coconut oil. It can also be used as a sexual lubricant, though not with condoms or other latex forms of birth control.

SEASONINGS

Fresh, raw, organic food is delicious in itself. Seasonings simply complement that deliciousness, harmonizing with or providing a counterpoint to the food's flavor. Using herbs and spices with familiar flavors as condiments can help you make the transition to raw foods. Many seasonings offer many wonderful therapeutic benefits as well. Some have potent antimicrobial properties that aid in food preservation and prevent *E. coli* and salmonella contamination; and most culinary herbs and spices are rich in natural, volatile oils that improve circulation to our digestive systems and thus improve our ability to assimilate nutrients.

When seasoning your food with herbs, use fresh herbs whenever possible. If you have more fresh herbs than you'll need and they're still on the stalk, set them in a glass of water in the refrigerator. If you are using dried herbs, buy or harvest them whole and then grind or chop them only as needed. Store dried herbs in glass jars away from light and heat.

The following herbs, spices, and other seasonings are all wonderful accompaniments to a raw foods diet.

Fresh Herbs versus Dried Herbs

Most of the recipes in this book call for fresh herbs. Fresh herbs always contain more chi, or life force. However, organic herbs that are dried at low temperatures and are not irradiated are available yearround. Also, herbs that come from faraway places, such as cinnamon, will be available only in dried form. Dried herbs tend to have a stronger flavor and absorb moisture from the other ingredients. If you must substitute dried herb for fresh herb in a recipe, use half as much dried herb as the recipe specifies.

Allspice (*Pimenta dioica*)

Part used: Fruit

Allspice is a warming spice with antioxidant and antiseptic properties. It improves digestion and protein assimilation and mitigates flatulence. Allspice earns its name because it can take the place of cinnamon, cloves, or nutmeg in just about any recipe.

Anise (*Pimpinella anisum*)

Part used: Seed

Aniseed is a sweet, warming spice that is recommended to improve digestion and relieve colic, hiccough, and bloated bellies. It has long been used as a tea or in syrups for people with coughs and asthma to help expectorate phlegm. Chewing aniseeds after a meal will sweeten the breath.

Basil (*Ocimum basilicum*)

Part used: Entire herb

Basil is pungent, warm, and dry. It helps improve digestion and circulation. Using basil in food especially benefits the lungs, spleen, stomach, and large intestines. It is used to treat colds, coughs, headache, and nausea.

Caraway (*Carum carvi*)

Part used: Seed

Caraway is pungent and warm with antiseptic, expectorant, and galactagogic properties. It improves circulation and helps with many gastrointestinal problems such as nausea, Crohn's disease, colic, cramps, flatulence, and hiccoughs; in particular, it improves the digestion of starches. Chew a few caraway seeds when traveling at high elevations to help relieve shortness of breath.

Cardamom (*Elettaria cardamomum*)

Part used: Seed

Cardamom is pungent, slightly bitter, sweet, warming, and dry. It was favorite ingredient in ancient love potions, and to this day is considered an aphrodisiac. Cardamom helps relieve a wide range of digestive disorders including bloating, celiac disease, colic, flatulence, indigestion, nausea, and stomachache. When added to grains, it enhances their digestibility. Chew a few cardamom seeds removed from the pod after a meal to sweeten the breath.

Cayenne and Jalapeño Pepper (*Capsicum annuum*)

Part used: Fruit

Cayenne and jalapeño peppers are hot, pungent, and drying. They are rich in beta-carotene and vitamin C. Hot peppers like cayenne and jalapeño are consumed in large amounts in tropical climates because they induce perspiration, which helps a person to cool off. They have been used to improve circulation and in treatments for arthritis, chills, colds, coughs, dysentery, flu, and migraines. When ingested, cayenne and jalapeño also cause the brain to secrete more endorphins, which can block pain. Diluted and applied topically, powdered hot pepper inhibits the transmission of substance P, which would otherwise transport pain messages to the brain.

The Raw Facts

Hot peppers vary greatly in their amount of heat. Use them judiciously when preparing a recipe and taste-test as you go, so you don't end up creating something inedibly hot!

Celery (*Apium graveolens*)

Part used: Seed
When consumed with food, celery seed aids in the digestion of protein. The seeds are valued medicinally for their anti-inflammatory, antifungal, aphrodisiac, antirheumatic, antispasmodic, carminitive, deobstruent, diuretic, emmenagogic, galactagogic, hypotensive, nervine, sedative, sudorific, tonic, and urinary antiseptic properties. Celery seed reduces inflammation, dispels heat and toxins (including uric acid), cleanses the liver and kidneys, and softens deposits in the body.

Cinnamon (*Cinnamomum* species)

Part used: Bark
Cinnamon is warming, pungent, and sweet. It is a supreme digestive tonic and helps invigorate the abdominal area, relieving gas, nausea, and diarrhea. Cinnamon is regarded as an aphrodisiac and antifungal agent, and it also calms the nerves. When taken as a tea, cinnamon can help people whose rheumatism worsens from exposure to cold weather.

Clove (*Eugenia aromatica*)

Part used: Bud
Cloves are pungent and warm. They contain eugenol, a powerful anesthetic, and are often used in dentistry to numb the gums or tooth. Cloves are

used medicinally to treat indigestion, halitosis, parasites, nausea, and sexual debility. Clove essential oil exhibits activity against streptococcus, staphylococcus, and pneumonia bacteria. Sucking on a whole clove helps keep the breath fresh.

Coriander/Cilantro (*Coriandrum sativum*)

Part used: Seed

The seeds of *Coriandrum sativum* are known as coriander, and the plant that grows from the seeds is known as cilantro. Coriander is pungent and neutral in temperature. Coriander is used to improve digestion and break up mucus, and has antibacterial properties. Cilantro is considered a blood-purifying agent. Both are regarded as digestive aids that help treat bloating, colic, cramps, flatulence, and indigestion.

Cumin (*Cuminum cyminum*)

Part used: Seed

Cumin is slightly bitter, pungent, warm, and rich in flavonoids. An antispasmodic, it relieves coughs, diarrhea, indigestion, and headache, and is a galactagogue (increases milk production) in nursing mothers. Cumin is also used topically as a liniment for speeding the healing of bruises and sprains.

Dill (*Anethum graveolens*)

Part used: Seed

Dill seeds are pungent and warm. The name "dill" comes from the Old Norse word *dilla,* meaning "to lull," because these seeds were traditionally made into a tea that lulled colicky babies to sleep. Early American settlers referred to dill as "meetin' seed" because, during long sermons, it was given to small children to keep them calm and used by adults to quiet rumbling stomachs. Dill seeds aid digestion, freshen the breath, and relieve hiccoughs.

Fennel (*Foeniculum vulgare*)

Part used: Seed and leaf

Fennel is pungent, sweet, and warm. It aids digestion and is a galactagogue. Its expectorant properties make it helpful in calming a cough. Fennel leaves are a traditional eye, brain, and memory tonic and help disperse liver congestion.

Garlic (*Allium sativum*)

Part used: Bulb

Garlic is pungent, hot, and drying, and has a wide range of therapeutic benefits. It lowers blood pressure, and it prevents platelet aggregation (keeps blood from clumping together) so that circulation can flow better. Garlic exhibits broad-spectrum activity against disease-causing organisms including bacteria and viruses. It has some antiparasitic activity as well, and can make you a less-hospitable host to mosquitoes, ticks, and even giardia. Garlic improves lung capacity and is used for treating respiratory infections. To chase away garlic breath, eat parsley or a small piece of organic lemon peel.

Ginger (*Zingiber officinale*)

Part used: Root

Ginger is hot and pungent. It benefits digestion and improves circulation. Ginger helps increase the concentration of amylase in the saliva, thus improving carbohydrate digestion. It also increases intestinal muscle tone and aids digestion, particularly that of fatty foods. Ginger is beneficial in treatments for colds, menstrual cramps, and arthritis. In a double-blind study conducted at Brigham Young University, ginger outperformed Dramamine in preventing motion sickness. By the way, ginger does not have to be peeled before use.

Honey

Honey is sweet and has a neutral energy. It calms ulcers and lowers high blood pressure. Applied topically, it can soothe burns. Most commercial honeys have been pasteurized, causing them to lose their medicinal properties. Raw honey is available at natural foods stores and from raw foods suppliers. Darker honey tends to have a greater mineral content than lighter honey has. If you can't find raw honey, you can substitute six small, pitted dates for each tablespoon of honey called for in a recipe.

Horseradish (*Armoracia lapathifolia*)

Part used: Root

Horseradish is high in vitamin C and aids in the digestion of fatty foods. It has both antiseptic and decongestant properties, making it helpful for opening congested respiratory passages.

Buying Bee Products

For years, I avoided buying any bee products because of concern for the exploitation of the decreasing bee population, which was being traumatized by mites, urbanization, and pesticides. A beekeeper of a small local business reminded me that he and other beekeepers were doing all they could to sustain and protect the bees, and that in order for their efforts to be successful, they needed to be supported. So if you do buy honey, make sure it is from an environmentally conscious company that cares for the bees and does not allow them to be harmed. We depend upon viable bee populations to continue to pollinate so many of our vitally important plant foods.

Lemon Balm (*Melissa officinalis*)

Part used: Aboveground herb

Lemon balm improves digestion, strengthens the nervous system, and is mildly antiviral. The great Arab physician Avicenna wrote, "Lemon balm causeth the mind and heart to be merrie." The sourness of its lemony flavor helps stimulate the liver.

Miso

Miso is a purée of fermented soybeans, salt, and sometimes grain. It contains protein and enzymes. Miso helps neutralize environmental pollutants in the body. In the Orient, it is considered a longevity tonic. Look for unpasteurized miso. Lighter-colored miso has less enzymatic activity and tends to be less salty than darker miso. Lighter-colored misos are more cooling, while darker-colored misos are more warming.

Mustard (*Brassica nigra, B. juncea, Sinapis alba*)

Part used: Seed

Mustard seeds are pungent and hot, and rich in protein and sulfur. They have analgesic, antiseptic, and expectorant properties. Mustard seeds have been used to treat coughs and respiratory congestion.

Nutmeg (*Myristica fragrans*)

Part used: Kernel

Nutmeg is pungent, warm, and dry. Medicinally, it is an antiemetic, anti-inflammatory, antispasmodic, aphrodisiac, astringent, carminitive, circulatory stimulant, and stomachic. Nutmeg is used in treatments for bronchial irritations, colic, Crohn's disease, delirium tremens, diarrhea (especially diarrhea occuring first thing in the morning), digestive tract infections, insomnia, dysentary, eczema, flatulence, gastroenteritis, halitosis, indigestion, muscle spasm, nausea, rheumatism, and vomiting.

Nutritional Yeast

This type of yeast is generally grown on sugar beets or molasses and is available in the form of flakes. Nutritional yeast contains synthetic B-complex vitamins, as well as minerals (including phosphorus), and it imparts a cheesy flavor to raw dishes. Nutritional yeast is not a purely raw food itself, as it is heated to around 250°F during its processing, but some raw foods enthusiasts use it in small amounts; others choose to avoid it.

Oregano (*Origanum vulgare*) and Marjoram (*O. majorana*)

Part used: Leaf

Oregano and marjoram are pungent and warm. Both are valued as antioxidants, antiseptics, and cholagogues. Use these closely related herbs to treat lung problems such as bronchitis, cough, pleurisy, and tonsillitis. They can also help relieve headache, indigestion, measles, mumps, and nausea. Fresh oregano or marjoram leaves can be chewed at the site of a toothache.

Paprika (*Capsicum tetragonum*)

Part used: Fruit

Paprika, a mild relative of cayenne, is sweet and warm. It is high in beta-carotene, flavonoids, and vitamin C. Paprika has antibacterial properties and has been used to treat high blood pressure, scurvy, seasickness, and varicose veins. It improves the health of the circulatory system by promoting blood vessel elasticity. As a digestive aid, paprika improves the secretion of saliva and stomach acids as well as increasing peristaltic movements.

Parsley (*Petroselinum crispum*)

Part used: Herb

Parsley is neutral and sweet, and is rich in beta-carotene, vitamin C, and iron. It is also high in chlorophyll, which builds the blood. Parsley is a time-tested remedy for arthritis, edema, gout, halitosis, kidney inflammation, and kidney stones. The herb can also be used topically as a poultice to treat bruises.

Pepper (*Piper nigrum*)

Part used: Fruit

Pepper (black and white) is pungent and hot. It has antibacterial properties and helps dispel phlegm in the body. Pepper has been used to relieve arthritis, colic, diarrhea, flatulence, indigestion, and poor circulation. Black pepper comes from the unripe but fully grown berry, while white pepper comes from the peeled mature fruits.

Peppermint (*Mentha piperita*)

Part used: Leaf

Peppermint has a fresh, pungent, cooling flavor. Its antiviral properties make it beneficial in preventing illness. Peppermint has the added benefit of being a natural breath freshener.

Rosemary (*Rosmarinus officinalis*)

Part used: Leaf

Rosemary is warm, pungent, bitter, and drying. It is a natural antioxidant. Rosemary has been used to freshen the breath, aid digestion, ease anxiety, improve mental alertness, relieve headaches and coughs, and improve eyesight.

Rosewater

Rosewater is distilled from the petals of rose flowers (*Rosa* species). It is not truly a raw product and is rarely available in organic form. However, one teaspoon of rosewater added to a smoothie or dessert imparts a beautiful flavor. One drop of rosewater can be added to drinking water to improve digestion.

Saffron (*Crocus sativus*)

Part used: Stigma

Saffron is neutral and sweet. It is the most expensive spice in the world, as the stigmas (female organs) of about 100,000 saffron flowers are required to make a pound of saffron spice. Saffron relieves digestive and urinary problems. It is diaphoretic and helps the skin eliminate toxins from measles and chicken pox.

Sage (*Salvia officinalis*)

Part used: Leaf

Sage is pungent, warm, and drying. It is considered an anaphrodisiac (curbing sexual desire) and an antigalactagogue (inhibiting production of breast milk). It also reduces hot flashes and sweating and has antiseptic properties.

Consider sage a remedy for colds, diarrhea, and flatulence. A poultice of fresh sage leaves can be used to soothe insect bites and wounds.

Salt

The best type of salt for the raw diet is Celtic salt, which is harvested from a 9,000-acre ocean region of Brittany, France, and is not kiln dried. It contains over eighty trace minerals and has lower sodium content than other refined salts. Look for the coarsely ground variety, as finely ground Celtic salt is heated to 200°F during its processing. Celtic salt has a grayish color and appears damp compared to other commercially available salts.

Scallion (*Allium fistulosum*)

Scallions, also known as green onions, are pungent, bitter, and warm in energy, with a milder flavor than garlic or onion. Scallions are rich in sulfur and have antibacterial and antifungal properties. They are used in Oriental medicine to treat colds, flu, diarrhea, edema, and high blood pressure.

Spearmint (*Mentha spicata*)

Part used: Aboveground plant

Spearmint is pungent, cool, and drying. It has antibacterial and antiviral properties. Spearmint is an excellent digestive aid; it has been used to treat colic, fatigue, fever, flatulence, and nausea. Being a mild, less medicinally tasting mint, spearmint is often a better choice than peppermint for culinary recipes.

Tamari

Tamari is a type of fermented soy sauce made from soy, wheat, salt, and water. Raw foodists prefer the Nama Shoyu® brand, which is unpasteurized and contains active enzymes. Tamari is high in sodium (though lower than traditional soy sauces), so it should be used sparingly.

Tamarind (*Tamarindus indicus*)

Part used: Fruit pulp

Tamarind, the fruit pod of a tree native to India, is rich in beta-carotene, niacin, vitamin C, calcium, and phosphorus. In North America, the pulp that surrounds the pod is often sold in dry form; if it is tough, it may need to be soaked before use. This pulp is used as a sour condiment in Caribbean and Indian dishes. Tamarind pulp or paste is valued as a digestive aid, laxative, and refrigerant.

Tarragon (*Artemesia dracunulus*)

Part used: Aboveground plant

Tarragon is warm and moist. It improves digestion and has been used as an oral anesthetic to numb the mouth from toothache pain. Tarragon has carminative and galactagogic properties and is a traditional remedy for arthritis, flatulence, gout, halitosis, nausea, rheumatism, and worms.

Thyme (*Thymus vulgaris*)

Part used: Aboveground plant

Thyme is pungent, mildly bitter, warm, and drying. It is a powerful antiseptic with activity against bacteria, fungi, molds, and parasites. Thyme is excellent for treating respiratory infections, colds, and coughs.

Turmeric (*Curcuma longa*)

Part used: Rhizome

Turmeric is pungent, bitter, and warm. It contains the antioxidant curcumin, known for its anticancer and anti-inflammatory properties. It is an excellent herb for arthritis, asthma, candida infection, eczema, jaundice, and high cholesterol. Turmeric is an effective post-trauma remedy used both internally and topically to reduce inflammation in bruises, swellings, and wounds. It stimulates wound healing, works as an anticoagulant, and has antifungal properties. Turmeric helps beautify the skin, eliminating acne, boils, and other impurities by purifying the blood and imparting a healthy skin color and texture.

Vanilla (*Vanilla planifolia*)

Part used: Bean

Vanilla is sweet and warm, and best known as an aphrodisiac and digestive stimulant. It is also the second-most expensive spice in the world. The bees that once pollinated the orchids that produce vanilla beans are extinct as a result of pesticide use, and only a few species of hummingbirds and butterflies participate in the pollination process, so the plants generally must be hand-pollinated within a few hours of opening.

Be sure to use pure vanilla extract (not vanillin, which is artificial). Vanilla extract is available in vegetable glycerin or alcohol and is not truly raw. One-half inch of vanilla bean can be substituted for one teaspoon of vanilla extract, or the vanilla can be ommitted entirely, if desired.

Vinegar

Vinegar is a product of fermentation, and there are many different types. Fruit and grain vinegars, such as apple cider and balsamic, tend to be less acidic and milder in flavor than distilled white vinegar. Vinegars have a cool, drying effect on the body. Excess use can wrinkle the skin and weaken muscle tone. Interestingly, vinegars have a soothing and cleansing effect for people with a hot temperament. I tend to use lemon juice in place of vinegar, but if vinegar appeals to you, make sure it is raw and unpasteurized (mostly available as apple cider vinegar).

Spice Blends

You can buy premade, raw spice blends in bulk from natural foods stores (spice blends found in regular grocery stores tend to be irradiated or chemically treated), but making your own is fun and can be an opportunity for culinary creativity. For the best flavor, buy whole herbs (for example, the seed rather than the powder), which retain the aromatic and flavorful essential oils, and grind them yourself with a mortar and pestle or in a grinder.

Chili Powder

Add this blend to any dish that could use a south-of-the-border flair.

2 tablespoons cumin seeds

1 teaspoon coriander seeds

1 teaspoon turmeric

1 tablespoon dried oregano

Combine all of the ingredients and mix well. Use as needed.

Classic Herb Mix

This blend is similar to the stuff sold commercially as "poultry seasoning." Use it when you want to recreate dishes that remind you of all-American fare, such as raw burgers, stuffings, and nut loaves.

1 tablespoon dried sage

1 tablespoon dried thyme

1 tablespoon dried rosemary

1 tablespoon dried parsley

Combine all of the ingredients and mix well. Use as needed.

Curry Powder

*This blend offers the traditional, warming flavors of India
without the necessity of cooking.*

$\frac{1}{2}$ teaspoon mustard seeds

2 tablespoons cumin seeds

1 teaspoon coriander seeds

$\frac{1}{4}$ teaspoon cayenne powder

$\frac{1}{2}$ teaspoon turmeric

$\frac{1}{2}$ teaspoon ginger powder

Combine all of the ingredients and mix well. Use as needed.

Garam Masala

*This is a sweet and spicy Indian blend.
Try it on a side dish when Indian curry is the entrée.*

5 3-inch cinnamon sticks

$\frac{1}{2}$ cup whole cloves

$\frac{1}{2}$ cup cumin seeds

1 cup coriander seeds

$\frac{1}{8}$ cup ground black pepper

$\frac{1}{8}$ cup dried, medium-hot chilis

Combine all of the ingredients and mix well. Use as needed.

Tonic Gomashio

*This nutty blend contains milk thistle seeds, which help regenerate
and protect the liver against toxins, and black sesame seeds, which
make a wonderful kidney tonic. Sprinkle it on vegetables and salads.*

$\frac{1}{2}$ cup milk thistle seeds

$\frac{1}{2}$ cup black sesame seeds

3 tablespoons Celtic salt

Combine all of the ingredients and mix well. Use as needed.
(Store in the refrigerator in a glass jar.)

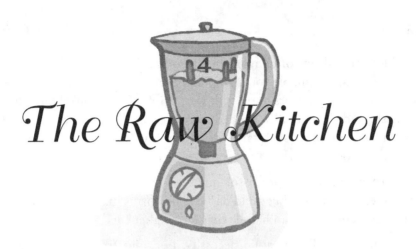

The Raw Kitchen

Raw food preparation is much easier with the following helpful kitchen tools. Although the initial cost of purchasing them all may seem steep, I highly recommend investing in setting up a fully equipped raw kitchen with these tools. You won't need much else, and then your first forays into a raw foods diet won't be met with the frustration of not being able to try a wide range of recipes. You can eventually get rid of your stove, pots, toaster, microwave, waffle iron, deep-fat fryer, and so forth. (Now that we don't use our oven, it makes a great place to store our juicer. We even grow trays of sunflower greens and buckwheat lettuce on the stovetop.) Talk to friends who own some of these tools and ask for their opinions and suggestions about the best types and brand names.

Blender. A sturdy blender works wonders for making smoothies, salad dressings, and purées. I prefer the Vita-Mix brand, which is multipurpose and super-powered. A regular two-speed (or more) blender also works fine for most recipes.

Citrus juicer. You'll be juicing lots of lemons and limes for salad dressings, and an electric model speeds up the process. A hand juicer will also do the job.

Colanders. Try to get one with "feet," as that enables excess water to drain away freely.

Food dehydrator. A dehydrator is the raw foodist's replacement for a stove. I highly recommend the Excalibur. Whatever the brand, you'll want a dehydrator with a temperature-control mechanism; most have one, but some don't. Without temperature control, temperatures might start at a level high enough to kill the precious enzymes. Be sure to get the solid, nonstick, reusable Teflex sheets or dehydrator sheets, as they are referred to in some recipes, that are available for many dehydrators. These sheets fit over the mesh trays in dehydrators to prevent wet, drippy food from sliding through the mesh, and they are also needed to make flax crackers, cakes, cookies, pizza crusts, and other such fare—don't think you can substitute with wax paper, as it doesn't work.

Food processor. A food processor quickly grates, chops, and purées, making it so easy to have a big salad daily. It performs many of the same functions as a blender but can handle bigger, tougher foods.

Ice cream maker. This is not a necessity, but your friends and family will love you for it.

Glass jars. Glass mason jars are great for storing dry goods such as nuts, grains, and dried food, and they also can contain drippier foods such as soups and salad dressings. They make cupboards neater than having bags everywhere. To prevent bug infestations, put a bay leaf in each jar.

Juicer. There are many varieties of juicers: centrifugal force juicers (a disk shreds the produce and the pulp is spun to the sides of the basket); masticators (the produce is grated and then pressed); single-gear juicers (a single auger crushes the produce against the sides of a strainer basket); and twin-gear juicers (the produce is shredded and the juice pressed from it by two gears). I prefer the twin-gear juicers, as they are the easiest to use, make excellent juice, and do not require you to extricate the mashed produce from the basket midway through juicing.

Knives. You'll need good kitchen knives, including a 10-inch paring knife. Ceramic knives are great, as they do not oxidize the edges of chopped food, but they are somewhat fragile and are not ideal for hard vegetables such as rutabagas.

Nutcracker. I recommend the Krakanut® brand.

Spiral slicer. You'll need the Saladacco Spiralizer®, the Spirooli®, or any other type of spiral slicer that allows you to make turn vegetables into angelhair-sized threads of "pasta."

Sprouting bags (also known as nut milk bags). Besides their uses in sprouting, these bags are great for straining nut milks and vegetable juices. They can also be used to strain excess liquid when making nut cheeses, for example.

Sprouting jars. Be sure to get sprouting jars with wide mesh lids.

Strainers. Having strainers of various sizes will make food preparation and clean-up easier.

Trays. Cafeteria-style trays or baking sheets of stainless steel or plastic can be used to grow wheatgrass and other sprouts (see Sprouting Guide on page 124).

Vegetable brush. With a sturdy vegetable brush, you can scrub roots clean without having to peel away their nutritious skins.

Water filter. If your water supply is anything but fresh, clean, unchlorinated, pure water, you'll want a water filter. Many raw foodists recommend the EcoWater® filter, as it's easy to use, effective, and economical.

Wheatgrass juicer. Fresh wheatgrass juice is an astonishing nutrifier, but a normal blender or juicer will not juice wheatgrass: you have to use one designed specifically for the purpose. Electric and hand-powered models are available. However, vegetable juicers such as Green Star, Green Power, Omega, and Samson can be used to make wheatgrass juice.

SPROUTING

Sprouts are truly a living food. Unlike fruits and vegetables, which stop growing when plucked from their mother plant, sprouts continue growing up until the moment they are digested, and impart a subtle life force to the body.

Germination, or the process of sprouting, releases the nutrients in a seed and makes them more available for absorption. It can also increase a seed's nutritional content by as much as 400 percent. Sprouting activates the seed's plant hormones (phytosterols) and increases its metabolic activity: the seed's starches are broken down into simpler sugars, proteins are predigested into easy-to-assimilate, free amino acids, and fats are converted into easily digestible and soluble fatty acids. Sprouts are considered excellent anti-aging foods due to their rich supply of enzymes. They also contain good amounts of vitamin C, B-complex vitamins (including B_{17}, also known as laetrile, which has been used in cancer treatment), and vitamin E, as well as chlorophyll.

Sprouts are especially beneficial in terms of their ability to provide enzymes to the body. Seeds—including beans and grains—are an important element of the human diet, but they contain enzyme inhibitors (factors that keep enzymes dormant until the right growing conditions—not those found in the bean bin at your local grocery—are present). Phytic acid, an enzyme inhibitor, inhibits the absorption of calcium, iron, and zinc. Ingesting enzyme inhibitors can lead to health problems, such as digestive difficulties, enlarged pancreas, or general poor health. Cooking destroys enzyme inhibitors, but it also destroys the enzymes. Sprouting gets rid of the enzyme inhibitors and preserves the healthful enzymes.

The most nutritious, easiest-to-grow sprouts are:

- Buckwheat
- Clover
- Fenugreek
- Mustard
- Radish
- Sunflower

The Raw Facts

Beans are best used in small quantities and not as a major part of a raw foods lifestyle. Even when sprouted, beans still contain lots of starches that are not completely transformed into simple sugars and can be difficult to digest. Personally, I find sprouted beans (with the exception of lentils and mung beans) hard to digest, and so I avoid them.

Jar Sprouting

For sprouting, it's best to use organic seeds, or at least seeds that have not been treated with chemicals. Weed seeds that can be sprouted using the jar method include amaranth, burdock, clover, dandelion, lamb's-quarter, mustard, plantain, sorrel, yellow dock, wild garlic, and onion.

You can sprout seeds in containers made of glass or ceramic, but not of metal, plastic, or wood. (Although plastic jars should be avoided, plastic lids are acceptable.) Glass is ideal, because it enables you to watch the amazing growth of new life. Removing the inner lid from a canning jar and replacing it with a piece of stainless-steel or plastic window-mesh can make an inexpensive sprouter. Health food stores carry different types of sprouters or sprouting lids that fit over canning jars. Make sure the container has a mouth that is wide enough to allow easy removal of the sprouts from the jar.

Pour the seeds into the sprout jar (discard any broken or chipped seeds, as they will not sprout). Small seeds should just cover the bottom of the sprouting jar. Bigger seeds should not fill the jar more than one-eighth full. Then, cover the seeds with two to three times their volume in room-temperature or cold water, and give the jar a little shake to get rid of air pockets between the seeds.

In general, soak small seeds for four to six hours and larger seeds for eight to twelve hours. (See Sprouting Guide on page 124 for more specific soaking times.) When you are soaking larger seeds, change the water twice during the soaking process. If seeds are left to soak for longer than twelve hours, they can ferment.

After the seeds have soaked, apply the sprouting lid and turn the jar upside down to drain out the water and let oxygen circulate into the jar. Place the jar upside down in a location where the temperature stays around 70°F. Most people sprout seeds in their kitchen or other moderately well-lit place, but sprouts will tolerate darkness for at least the first couple of days. After your sprouts have grown for a few days, increase their bounty of chlorophyll by placing them in indirect sunlight for at least six hours before harvesting. While the seeds are sprouting, rinse them two or three times a day, just enough to get rid of any foam, and after each rinsing, drain them and return the jar to the sprouting location. Be sure to keep the jar upside down, preferably at an angle so that oxygen can get into it. Excess moisture and inadequate ventilation are a sure way to grow mold as well as sprouts; however, do not allow the sprouts to dry out or they will die.

As a general guideline, when the "tail" of the sprout is one and a half times as long as the original seed, the sprout is ready for consumption. To harvest sprouts, soak them in a bowl of cool water, allowing the hulls to float to the top; scoop out and discard the hulls, and then drain and rinse the sprouts. If you rinse and drain the sprouts every three days after harvesting and store them in the refrigerator, they will keep for about a week.

Paper-Towel Sprouting

Small seeds like those of flax, chia, watercress, mustard, radish, and teff can be sprouted on paper towels (unbleached and undyed). First, soak the seeds as described for the jar method, above. Place two moistened paper towels in a glass pan. Sprinkle the soaked seeds evenly over the towels and cover with two more moistened paper towels. When the sprouts are about $\frac{1}{2}$ to $1\frac{1}{2}$ inches long, remove the paper towels on top and set the pan in sunlight for three to four hours to allow the sprouts to develop chlorophyll. They can be rinsed afterward and consumed immediately or placed in a covered container, stored in the refrigerator, and rinsed before use.

Tips for Troubled Sprouts

If your seeds don't sprout when you're using the jar or paper-towel method, the cause of the problem is likely to be one of the following:

- You soaked the seeds for too long or too short a period of time.

- The seeds were of poor quality, with a resulting low rate of germination.

- The seeds were old and they rotted rather than sprouted.

- The sprouts were crushed through rough handling.

- You left the seeds in a spot that became too hot and cooked them.

- The growing sprouts did not have adequate drainage and developed mold.

- You did not rinse the sprouts frequently enough and they dried out.

Tray Sprouting for Grains and Grasses

This method works best for barley, buckwheat, kamut, rye, spelt, sunflower, and wheat (when sprouting wheat, use the hard, red berries, not soft wheat). One pound of seeds will produce about 4 pounds of grass. Store the grain in a cool, dark location and in a sealed container to keep out bugs and rodents. It is best to procure seed in the fall, when it is freshly matured.

First, soak the seeds in at least twice their volume in water for twelve hours or overnight. Next, prepare a tray filled with about $5/8$ inch of growing medium. Black humus from the woods, including leaf mold and the black earth underneath, works well, and a bit of kelp can be added to the growing medium to enrich it with minerals. You can also use organic potting soil or a combination of equal parts of Canadian sphagnum or peat moss and organic, untreated soil. Whatever you choose, the soil should be light and airy.

Finally, spread the seeds out on the tray of dirt, without piling them on top of one another. The soil needs to be kept moist, so put the tray in the basement or cover it with plastic for the first few days to conserve moisture. In very dry climates, you may need to wet a paper bag and place it over the seeds. When the sprouts are about 2 inches high, remove any coverings and place the tray near a sunny window. Three hours of sunlight daily is adequate, although more light will speed the growing process. (If the grasses are pale, they are not receiving adequate sunlight.) Water the tray only once daily.

When the sprouts are 8 inches high (in about one week to twelve days), it's time to harvest them. Using scissors or a serrated knife, cut the sprouts as close to the soil surface as possible (many of the sprouts' nutrients are concentrated close to the soil). After the harvest, keep watering the tray to obtain a second harvest; the sprouts of the second harvest, however, will not be as nutritious as those of the first. When the second growth has been harvested, compost the contents of the tray, which will be filled with grass roots.

Sometimes mold forms on the seed of a sprouting grass. At first it looks like white cotton, but it becomes grayer as it matures (do not confuse mold with the young, ciliar hairs on the rootlets). Mold is most likely to form during hot, humid weather. It can also result from excess watering or from inadequate spacing between plantings. Mold does not make the grass unusable—simply wash it off the sprouts after harvest. If flies are attracted to the mold, just vacuum them up as best you can. If mold turns out to be a chronic problem for you, you can prevent it by soaking the seed for twenty-four hours in the refrigerator, draining and rinsing it well, and allowing it to sprout for twelve hours before placing it in the soil.

The Raw Facts

Strictly speaking, "wheatgrass" (one word) refers to trays of wheat that are sprouted indoors, whereas "wheat grass" (two words) refers to wheat sprouts grown outdoors. (For the purposes of this book, however, I have simply used the term "wheatgrass" to denote any sprouted wheat that has grown long enough to become a grass.) In mild climates, wheat can be sprouted outdoors in locations that are sunny but protected against direct sun from 11 A.M. to 3 P.M., when the sun's rays are most intense.

SPROUTING GUIDE

The following chart is a guide to sprouting. If you're a beginner, it will help you get started. If you're already familiar with sprouting, this chart will surely expand your repetoire.

SPROUTING NUTS, SEEDS, AND GRAINS				
Item	Soaking Time	Growing Time	Quantity	Yield
Alfalfa	4–6 hours	5–6 days	3 tablespoons	3–4 cups
Comments: Allow to grow two leaves in sunlight before harvesting; otherwise, these sprouts may contain canavanine, a toxin. Use the jar method.				
Almonds	8–10 hours	1–2 days	2 cups	4 cups
Comments: Sprouted almonds are easier to digest than unsprouted almonds. Use the jar method.				
Amaranth	4–6 hours	3 days	3 tablespoons	3 cups
Comments: The paper-towel method works best.				
Aniseed	4–6 hours	2 days	3 tablespoons	1 cup
Comments: These strong-flavored sprouts are best served mixed with other sprouts. Use the jar method.				
Azuki beans	12 hours	3 days	$\frac{1}{2}$ cup	4 cups
Comments: Allow to sprout in darkness. These sprouts are rich in calcium and iron. Use the jar method.				
Barley	10 hours	2–3 days	1 cup	$2\frac{1}{2}$ cups
Comments: It can be difficult to find viable barley that will sprout. It can be grown like wheatgrass, or use the jar method.				
Broccoli seeds	6 hours	3–4 days	3 tablespoons	3 cups
Comments: These sprouts are rich in protein, beta-carotene, and vitamins C and K. Use the jar method.				
Brown rice	8–10 hours	3 days	1 cup	$1\frac{1}{2}$ cups
Comments: These sprouts are rich in fiber and B-complex vitamins. Use the jar method.				
Buckwheat	8–14 hours	2–3 days	1 cup	2 cups
Comments: Use hulled seeds for jar sprouting. Unhulled seeds can be grown in soil.				
Cabbage seeds	6 hours	4–5 days	3 tablespoons	4 cups
Comments: These sprouts benefit digestion. They are a good source of minerals, beta-carotene, and vitamin C. Use the jar method.				
Chia	4–6 hours	2–3 days	1 tablespoon	$1\frac{1}{2}$ cups
Comments: Use the paper-towel method. Allow to grow two leaves before harvesting.				
Clover seeds	4–6 hours	4–5 days	1 tablespoon	$2\frac{1}{2}$ cups
Comments: Expose to sunlight on the last day to encourage the sprouts to develop chlorophyll. Clover can also be grown in a mix with alfalfa. Use the jar method.				
Corn	8–10 hours	3 days	1 cup	2 cups
Comments: These sprouts are sweet, but it can be difficult to find viable corn that will sprout. Use the jar method.				

Item	Soaking Time	Growing Time	Quantity	Yield
Fenugreek seeds	8 hours	3–5 days	$\frac{1}{4}$ cup	3 cups
Comments: These sprouts become bitter if allowed to grow taller than 1 inch. They help break up phlegm and purify the blood, lymphatic system, liver, and kidneys. Use the jar method.				
Flaxseed	6–8 hours	4 days	1 tablespoon	1 cup
Comments: Use the paper-towel method, but instead of rinsing, just remoisten the towel.				
Garbanzo beans	12–48 hours	3 days	1 cup	$3\frac{1}{2}$ cups
Comments: Rinse often. These sprouts are somewhat starchy. Use the jar method.				
Green peas	10–12 hours	2–3 days	1 cup	2 cups
Comments: These can be grown like wheatgrass, using the tray method. The sprouts taste like fresh peas.				
Kale seeds	4–6 hours	4–6 days	4 tablespoons	3–4 cups
Comments: Like broccoli sprouts, kale sprouts are rich in protein, beta-carotene, and vitamins C and K. Use the jar method.				
Kamut	8–14 hours	3 days	1 cup	3 cups
Comments: Use the jar method, or grow like wheatgrass.				
Lentils	6–8 hours	3–4 days	1 cup	4 cups
Comments: Lentils sprout easily. These sprouts are a good source of B-complex vitamins, iron, and easy-to-digest protein. Use the jar method.				
Millet	6–8 hours	2 days	1 cup	$1\frac{1}{2}$ cups
Comments: Use the paper-towel method. These crunchy sprouts are best used in small amounts in salads.				
Mung beans	8–10 hours	5 days	1 cup	4 cups
Comments: Mung beans sprout best if weighted down with a heavy dish and rinsed in very cold water. Sprout in darkness, and allow to grow two leaves before harvesting. Use the jar method.				
Mustard seeds	6 hours	4 days	3 tablespoons	3 cups
Comments: The paper-towel method works best. Try mixing these strong-flavored sprouts with other sprouts.				
Oats	8–10 hours	3 days	1 cup	2 cups
Comments: It can be difficult to find viable oats that will sprout. Also, excessive watering will spoil the oats. Use the jar method.				
Onion, chive, or garlic seeds	4–6 hours	4–5 days	1 tablespoon	$1\frac{1}{2}$–2 cups
Comments: These tasty sprouts are wonderful in salads. Use the paper-towel method.				
Pumpkin seeds	8 hours	1–2 days	1 cup	$1\frac{1}{2}$–2 cups
Comments: These seeds can be eaten after simply soaking. Use hulled seeds for sprouting.				
Quinoa	6 hours	2–3 days	1 cup	3 cups
Comments: Rinse several times before soaking. These seeds can be eaten after simply soaking. For sprouting, the jar or paper-towel method works best.				
Radish seeds	6 hours	3–5 days	3 tablespoons	3–4 cups
Comments: These sprouts have a warming, spicy flavor. They help break up phlegm. Use the jar method.				

Item	Soaking Time	Growing Time	Quantity	Yield
Rye	8–10 hours	3–4 days	1 cup	3 cups
Comments: Allow to grow two leaves before harvesting. These sprouts spoil easily in hot weather. Use the jar or tray method.				
Sesame seeds	6 hours	1 day	1 cup	1$\frac{1}{2}$ cups
Comments: Use unhulled seeds for sprouting. These sprouts will become bitter if left to grow too long. Use at $\frac{1}{16}$ inch. They are a good source of calcium. Use the paper-towel or jar method.				
Spelt	6 hours	1–2 days	1 cup	3 cups
Comments: Use the jar method, or grow like wheatgrass in a tray.				
Sunflower seeds	8 hours	2 days	1 cup	2 cups
Comments: Use hulled seeds for jar sprouting. Unhulled seeds can be grown in soil. These sprouts will become bitter if left to grow too long. (Use $\frac{1}{8}$ inch for the jar method.)				
Teff	3–4 hours	1–2 days	1 cup	2$\frac{1}{2}$–3 cups
Comments: Use the jar or paper-towel method.				
Triticale	12 hours	3 days	$\frac{1}{2}$ cup	1$\frac{1}{2}$ cups
Comments: Use the jar method, or grow like wheatgrass.				
Walnuts	4 hours	n/a	1 cup	1$\frac{1}{2}$ cups
Comments: Walnuts will not sprout. Soaking and rinsing, however, improves their digestability.				
Watercress seed	6 hours	3–5 days	1 tablespoon	1$\frac{1}{2}$ cups
Comments: The paper-towel method works best. These sprouts have a pungent flavor.				
Wheat	10–12 hours	2–3 days	1 cup	2–3 cups
Comments: These sprouts contain all eight of the essential amino acids and are a good source of antioxidants. People who are allergic to wheat usually do not have an allergic reaction to sprouted wheat. Wheatgrass can be grown using the tray method. Use the jar method to grow smaller wheat sprouts.				
Wild rice	9 hours	3–5 days	1 cup	2 cups
Comments: It can be difficult to find viable wild rice that will sprout. Most of it has been parched.				

JUICING

Raw fruits and vegetables contain an abundance of natural juices that can help dissolve impurities in the body. Fresh-pressed juice is better than commercial, pasteurized juice, because pasteurization involves heating to a high temperature, which destroys a juice's enzymes and breaks down many of its nutrients.

Because it is extracted from fruits and vegetables, juice contains many of their nutrients but not the fiber. It is easy for the body to assimilate and does not burden the digestive system. Juices can oxidize quickly and should be consumed within a few minutes of extraction. They should be sipped slowly, however, for optimal digestion. Gulping down juice bypasses the first agents of the digestive process: the digestive enyzmes in saliva. When you take the time to savor the taste of juice in your mouth, these enzymes have a chance to begin the digestive process.

The easiest way to make fresh juice from fruits and vegetables is to process them in a juicer. If you don't have a juicer, you can purée the produce with some water in a blender, and then strain the mixture through a sprouting bag. Avoid peeling fruits and vegetables with edible skins, such as apples and carrots, because in many cases the peels have unique nutritive components; also, some of the organisms that produce vitamin B_{12} are often found on the skins. Do peel those fruits and vegetables with tough or inedible skins, such as bananas, beets, avocados, and waxed produce.

Good Juices

The following fruits, vegetables, and greens make excellent juices. Try mixing up different combinations for truly delicious savory and sweet drinks.

- Apples
- Asparagus
- Beets*
- Cabbages
- Carrots
- Citrus fruits**
- Cucumbers
- Endive
- Fennel
- Garlic[†]
- Horseradish
- Leeks

- Mustard greens
- Onions[‡]
- Parsley[††]
- Parsnips
- Radishes[‡‡]
- Red bell peppers
- Romaine lettuce
- Spinach
- String beans
- Sweet potatoes
- Turnips
- Watercress

---

[*] drinking more than a full wineglass, undiluted, can cause dizziness and nausea

[**] best juiced with a citrus juicer

[†] use only in small amounts mixed with other juices

[‡] use only in small amounts mixed with other juices

[††] don't use more than 2 ounces undiluted

[‡‡] dilute with other juices

The Raw Facts

Carrots and beets are both high in sugars, and some raw foodists feel that their juices are too sweet to consume. However, if well diluted with water or mixed with other, less sweet juices, carrot and beet juices can be used on occasion.

Wild Juices

The juices of these wild greens are excellent. Instead of mowing and spraying your lawn, keep it organic and harvest these wild, wonderful weeds to heal and feed your needs!

- Alfalfa leaves
- Chickweed
- Dandelion leaves
- Lamb's-quarter
- Nettles
- Violet leaves

Juicing Supplements

These foods would not yield much liquid if run through a juicer, but they are ideal for puréeing and mixing in with other juices. Just combine the juice and your chosen supplemental food in a blender and process them. Generally, fruits taste best mixed with fruit juices and vegetables with vegetable juices.

- Apricots
- Avocados
- Bananas
- Cacti
- Cherries
- Kiwi
- Mangoes
- Nectarines
- Okra
- Papayas
- Peaches
- Plantains
- Seaweeds

Good Juicing Combinations

Here are a few to try—let your imagination fly!

- Carrot and celery
- Carrot, celery, and cucumber
- Celery, beet, and cucumber
- Celery and spinach
- Cucumber, beet, and spinach
- Nettle, celery, cucumber, and a bit of apple

Electrolyte Beverage

½ cup apple juice
½ cup celery juice
8 ounces water

Blood-Building Tonic

1 shot wheatgrass juice
1 cup beet juice

Disposing of the Pulp

Pulp left over from juicing can be stored in the refrigerator in a sealed container for three to five days. To save pulp for longer, dehydrate it: spread it on dehydrator sheets in a layer ¼–⅓ inch thick and dehydrate until it is totally dry (it will remain somewhat "tacky" to the touch). Once the pulp is dry, store it in glass containers in a cool, dark location, where it will keep for several months. If a recipe calls for 2 cups of fresh pulp, use only 1 cup of dehydrated pulp.

Use leftover juicing pulp to thicken soups, make vegetable patties, and add fiber to raw breads and crackers, or try it as a condiment. Many types of fresh pulp (especially carrot, celery, or cucumber) can be used on the skin as nourishing facials. Of course, pulp makes wonderful compost for the garden—if you can't eat it, at least return it to the earth!

DEHYDRATING

Dehydrating can provide the flavor of cooked food while protecting the enzymes and nutrients of raw food and reducing bacterial activity.

Preserving Food

Preservation techniques can allow you to keep foods beyond their season, but foods that are so preserved that they have a shelf life of decades are lacking life force. Canned spinach, for example, exhibits a loss of 80 percent of its magnesium, 70 percent of its cobalt, 40 percent of its zinc, and up to 91 percent of its vitamin B_6 content. Certainly, commercially preserved foods are free from bacterial contamination, as manufacturers boast. But if bacteria are not interested in a food, why would your body be?

Eating food fresh is best, of course. But if you wish to preserve food in its raw state, dehydrating, fermenting, and freezing are the preservation methods of choice.

Although it does cause some loss of nutrients, dehydrating is preferable to cooking or any other method of food storage. These foods require only one-sixth the storage space of fresh foods and so are great for travel and camping. Dried foods stored in glass containers in a dark area can last for several years (though it's best to consume them within six months). Remember, however, that fresh food is superior.

To prepare fruits and vegetables for dehydration, slice them thinly into pieces no more than $\frac{1}{2}$ inch thick. Small fruits such as grapes or berries can simply be cut in half. If you would normally peel the fruit or vegetable or remove its seeds, do so before dehydrating it.

When drying fruit that tends to discolor, soak it first in pineapple juice or diluted lemon juice to protect the color, if desired. Dried fruit can be soaked in water for a few hours to be reconstituted.

The Raw Facts

When purchasing dried fruit, be sure it has not been treated with preservatives, such sulfur dioxide and potassium sorbate. Preservative-treated fruits retain much of their bright color, whereas untreated fruits are browner or darker.

Air Drying

You can dry foods outdoors during warm, sunny weather or indoors in a warm, dry location. Just set the food on trays or racks that allow for air circulation underneath. Place cheesecloth or nylon mesh over the food to keep bugs away. Depending on the food and its thickness, dehydration could be completed in one to four days. Turn the items regularly so that they dry equally on all sides. If you're drying outdoors, bring the trays in during rainfall and at dusk, before dew settles. Return the trays to the sun the next day.

Using a Food Dehydrator

As mentioned earlier, your food dehydrator should have a temperature-control mechanism. Why? Because enzymes are destroyed at around 118°F, and most dehydrators without temperature-control mechanisms operate at temperatures higher than that. I recommend keeping a dehydrator set to under 100°F.

Food dehydrators are equipped with mesh trays or racks for holding the foods to be dried. The dehydrator circulates warm air around the foods, gradually evaporating the water content. For this reason, it's important not to overload the trays, as this might impede air flow and proper drying. If you're dehydrating a purée or some type of gooey food, you'll need to place it on solid trays that can then be slid right on top of the mesh trays or racks. Solid dehydrator trays, usually made of Teflex, are sometimes sold with dehydrators but may also be purchased separately. Because these solid trays won't allow air flow through them, you'll need to flip the items on them midway through the drying process to ensure that they dehydrate properly. In many cases, once the item is dry on one side and you're ready to flip it, you won't need the solid tray anymore, and you can place the item directly on the dehydrator rack.

Keep food that is nearest completion on the bottom dehydrator trays; moisture tends to rise and can be transferred to higher trays. You can also turn trays a quarter turn each time you check your food's progress to help ensure even drying.

Dehydrator-Dried Fruits and Vegetables

Air drying depends so much on temperature and humidity that it is impossible to give exact drying times for the process. Dehydrators offer a bit of standardization, although they too are affected by climate. The times given on page 132 are approximations. You'll know the foods are fully dried when they feel that way.

FERMENTING

Fermentation is one of the most ancient methods of food preservation. It requires no electrical equipment or high-tech materials. Fermenting can be done in a glass, ceramic, or hard plastic container with a press or heavy lid. I bought a simple pickle press from Gold Mine (see the Resources section) and I love using it to make sauerkraut from cabbage and wild greens.

The process of fermentation involves breaking down foods by using living microorganisms, such as enzymes. Fermented foods are rich in friendly bacteria, including *Lactobacillus brevis* and *L. planarum.* These bacteria convert starches and sugars into lactic acid and acetic acid. Fermented foods tend to be somewhat acidic and thus are beneficial for people who are overly alkaline.

Fermented foods also aid in the colonization of other beneficial bacteria that inhibit the overgrowth of unfriendly microorganisms, such as candida (yeast). They are easy to digest and bring a rich supply of enzymes into the body. They are a superb food for the elderly.

Miso, tamari, sauerkraut, apple cider vinegar, kim chee, yogurt, Rejuvelac, kombucha, and kefir are all fermented products. Chapter 5 includes recipes for sauerkraut (page 159) and Rejuvelac (page 151), which are both fermented foods.

DRYING TIMES FOR DEHYDRATOR-DRIED FRUITS

Recommended Fruit	Dehydrator Drying Time (in hours)	Recommended Fruit	Dehydrator Drying Time (in hours)
Apples	6–8	Grapes (sliced in half)	24–36
Apricots	8–12	Peaches	10–12
Bananas	6–8	Pears	12–18
Berries	12–24	Pineapples	24–36
Cherries (pits removed)	12–24	Plums	36–48
Cranberries (sliced in half)	12–24	Watermelon	24–36
Currants	12–24		

DRYING TIMES FOR DEHYDRATOR-DRIED VEGETABLES

Recommended Vegetables	Dehydrator Drying Time (in hours)	Recommended Vegetables	Dehydrator Drying Time (in hours)
Beets	4–8	Onions	12–14
Cabbages	12–15	Parsley	4–8
Carrots	12–18	Parsnips	8–12
Corn	8–12	Peas	12–18
Cucumbers	8–10	Peppers	8–12
Garlic	10–12	Summer squash	6–8
Leafy green vegetables	8–12	String beans	12–18
Horseradish	12–14	Tomatoes	6–8
Kohlrabi	18–24	Turnips	12–18
Leeks	4–8	Winter squash	12–18
Mushrooms	8–12		

FREEZING

Freezing is a viable means of food preservation when retaining enzymes is the goal. Enzymes cease working at very cold temperatures, but are not destroyed; they're ready to go back to work when temperatures normalize.

I don't eat frozen foods except for occasional homemade nut or banana icecream or a dessert that is firmed in the freezer. When food is frozen, its cell walls tend to burst due to the expansion that takes place when liquids freeze solid. Foods with lower water content are less adversely affected but nevertheless do experience some cellular breakdown. Frozen foods also lose much of their vitamin C content when they are thawed.

If you are going to eat frozen raw foods, I recommend eating only those you prepare yourself. Commercially frozen foods are often blanched (dipped in boiling water) to preserve their color beforehand, but blanching destroys up to 66 percent of the enzymes. When preparing produce for freezing, do not blanch it. Also, package foods to be frozen in typical serving sizes and in the form in which you would eat it (that is, cut corn kernels from the cob, peel bananas, and so on). Consume frozen foods within six months.

5

Raw Recipes

*B*efore you get started on a recipe, here are a few basic points to keep in mind:

- All ingredients should be raw, of course (raw carob powder, raw tahini, raw almond butter, unpasteurized miso, and so on). A few recipes in this chapter call for items that are not raw. These can be used for flavor, if desired, or omitted.

- Use organic produce whenever possible.

- Wash all produce.

- Peel what needs to be peeled (for example, bananas, avocados, jicama, papayas, and any waxed produce); otherwise, leave the peel on (for example, carrots, apples, and unwaxed cucumbers).

- Remove large, hard seeds, such as those of dates and prunes, and also some smaller ones, such as those of citrus fruits and papayas.

- Remove woody stems, such as those of figs and apples.

- Use pure water in any recipe that calls for water (or for soaking).

- When a recipe calls for soaking nuts or seeds, you'll typically soak them in twice as much water as their dry volume. Large nuts are generally soaked from eight to twelve hours. Small nuts and seeds are generally soaked from four to six hours. Rinse nuts and seeds in a colander after soaking, and drain them well and quickly before using them. Discard the nut soak water in the garden or use it to water plants. It is not for consumption. Dried fruit should be soaked in a small amount of water (just enough to cover) until it is tender. The soak water can usually be included to add moisture to a recipe. (Certain recipes may deviate from these guidelines.)

- Soaked dates are called for as a sweetener in many recipes; if you're using soft dates, however, you do not need to soak them.

- It's fine to substitute! Try using almonds for walnuts, raisins for dates, lemon juice for lime juice, and so forth.

- If what you are processing in the food processor or blender looks like it needs more water, add a little at a time.

- Feel free to omit any seasonings, including salt, from any of the recipes.

- The times given for food dehydration are not exact, as so much depends on the moisture of the food and of the surrounding climate. You are the best judge of when something in your dehydrator is ready.

- When dehydrating, keep the dehydrator's temperature set to just under 100°F.

- Many raw soups can also be used as salad dressings and as sauces for entrées or side dishes.

- Be joyous in your food preparation. Pray, sing, chant, and smile!

- It takes only a moment to decorate. Love, good cheer, and humor conveyed through beautiful food will inspire others to try it and like it!

- Use your imagination!

Eating Seasonally

Eating seasonally is the act of eating locally grown foods at the time in which they naturally ripen. This practice equates to saving money (food costs less when it's plentiful), supporting your own health (foods are most nutritious when and where they ripen), supporting local farmers, and reducing waste (locally grown foods do not have to be shipped great distances or overly packaged). Although it may be difficult to eat seasonally all the time, and although "local" may at times mean no more than "North American continent," making an effort to guide your diet at least partially by the seasons will vastly benefit you and your community.

The following are lists of the produce that is in season each month in the United States. These are only general guidelines; local market and weather conditions will also influence the seasonal selection available to you.

January
Avocados
Bananas
Cabbages
Cauliflower
Pears
Turnips
Winter squash

February
Avocados
Bananas
Broccoli
Cabbages
Cauliflower
Kumquats
Mangoes
Pears
Tangerines
Winter squash

March
Artichokes
Asparagus
Avocados
Bananas
Broccoli
Grapefruit
Kumquats
Lettuce
Mushrooms
Spinach

April
Asparagus
Bananas
Cabbages
Escarole
Onions
Pineapple
Radishes
Rhubarb
Spinach
Strawberries

May
Asparagus
Bananas
Celery
Papayas
Peas
Pineapple
Strawberries
Tomatoes
Watercress

June
Apricots
Avocados
Bananas
Cantaloupe
Cherries
Corn
Cucumbers
Figs
Limes
Mangoes
Nectarines
Onions
Peaches
Peas
Peppers
Pineapple
Plums
String beans
Summer squash

July
Apricots
Bananas
Blueberries
Cabbages
Cantaloupe
Cherries
Corn
Cucumbers
Eggplant
Figs
Nectarines
Okra
Peaches
Peppers
Prunes
String beans
Watermelon

August
Apples
Bananas
Beets
Berries
Cabbages
Carrots
Corn
Cucumbers
Eggplant
Figs
Melon
Nectarines
Peaches
Pears
Peppers
Plums
Summer squash
Tomatoes

September
Apples
Bananas
Broccoli
Carrots
Cauliflower
Corn
Cucumbers
Figs
Grapes
Greens
Melons
Okra
Onions
Pears
Summer squash
Tomatoes
Yams

October
Apples
Bananas
Broccoli
Coconut
Grapes
Peppers
Persimmons
Pumpkins
Yams

November
Apples
Bananas
Broccoli
Cabbages
Coconut
Cranberries
Dates
Eggplant
Pumpkins
Sweet potatoes

December
Apples
Avocados
Bananas
Coconut
Grapefruit
Lemons
Limes
Oranges
Pears
Pineapple
Tangerines

Breakfast

The saying that "breakfast is the most important meal of the day" is really just cereal-and-sausage propaganda. A light breakfast of fruit and/or freshly pressed juice will sustain you until noon. And before eating breakfast, it's best first to drink one of the following:

• Two 8-ounce glasses of water

• 8 ounces of water with the juice of half a lemon

• 8 to 16 ounces of Rejuvelac (see page 151)

• 8 to 16 ounces of freshly pressed juice (which can be diluted with the same amount of water)

In my home, we usually have fruit salad with avocado for breakfast. A breakfast of plain fruit salad might leave us hungry, but the addition of avocado gives us sustaining "go-power." However, sometimes a more substantial breakfast is appropriate, especially for active days, when guests visit, for people who are new to raw foods, or on special occasions. Here are some fantastic breakfast recipes for you to try.

Breakfast for Champions

This breakfast is a great day-starter when you're on the road or when fresh produce is unavailable.

Yield: 2 servings

$\frac{1}{4}$ cup mixed dried apricots, prunes, and dried figs,
soaked in $\frac{1}{2}$ cup water overnight

$\frac{1}{4}$ cup mixed shelled almonds, sunflower seeds,
and pumpkin seeds, soaked in $\frac{1}{2}$ cup water overnight,
then rinsed and drained

Combine nuts, seeds, and rehydrated fruit in a medium-sized bowl, and mix well. Store leftovers in a container in the refrigerator for up to three days.

Breakfast Patties

These patties can also be eaten for lunch or dinner.

Yield: about 15 patties

1 cup almonds, soaked overnight, then rinsed

1 cup Brazil nuts, soaked overnight, then rinsed

$\frac{1}{2}$ cup chopped onion

1 tablespoon Nama Shoyu

2 tablespoons Classic Herb Mix (page 115),
or a commercial poultry seasoning of your choice

$\frac{3}{4}$ cup water

1 tablespoon liquid smoke (optional; not a raw product)

Combine all ingredients in a food processor and purée. Shape the mixture into 2-inch round patties on solid dehydrator sheets and dehydrate for 3 hours. Remove the dehydrator sheets, flip the patties over onto the dehydrator tray, and continue dehydrating for another 3 hours. Store uneaten patties in the refrigerator, where they will keep for one to two days.

Brazil Nut-Banana Pancakes

*These might not be fluffy like traditional pancakes,
but they are light, crisp, and satisfying.*

Yield: about 15 pancakes

2 cups Brazil nuts, soaked overnight, rinsed,
then dehydrated 12 hours

2 peeled bananas

$1\frac{1}{2}$ cups water

Combine all ingredients in a food processor and pulse until the solids are chopped finely. Drop the mixture in 4-inch rounds onto solid dehydrator sheets and dehydrate for 12 hours. Remove the dehydrator sheets, turn the rounds over onto the dehydrator tray, and continue dehydrating for another 12 hours. Serve the pancakes with maple syrup (not a raw product), honey, sliced strawberries, blueberries, tahini, or Date Sauce (page 185). Store uneaten pancakes in the refrigerator, where they will keep for a week.

Groovin' Granola

This cereal is great as a snack, meal, or road food!
Serve with nut milk (see Almond Milk on page 144).

Yield: about 8 cups

1 cup almonds, soaked overnight, then rinsed

1 cup walnuts, soaked overnight, then rinsed

1 cup pumpkin seeds

1 cup sunflower seeds

2 cups dates, soaked for 20 minutes

1 cup raisins, soaked for 20 minutes

2 cored pears or peaches, sliced

2 tablespoons cinnamon

$\frac{1}{2}$ teaspoon Celtic salt

$\frac{1}{4}$ cup water

Combine all ingredients in a food processor and chop finely. Spread the mixture onto solid dehydrator sheets and dehydrate until crunchy (about 12 hours), occasionally breaking up large pieces into bite-sized morsels.

(You can also break up the granola by pulsing it a few times in a food processor.) Store uneaten granola in a glass jar in a cupboard, where it will keep for several weeks.

Winter Cereal

This cereal even stays crispy in milk!

Yield: 4 servings

2 cups buckwheat, sprouted 2–3 days using the jar method, then dehydrated until crisp (about 12 hours)

1 cup raisins

Combine the crisped buckwheat and raisins in a bowl and stir to mix. Serve the cereal with Almond Milk (page 144) and a sliced banana. Remaining cereal can be stored in a glass jar in the cupboard for a few months.

Breakfast Pudding

*This hearty breakfast is great
on a cold winter's morning.*

Yield: 2 servings

12 dried apricots, soaked overnight

2 cored apples, coarsely chopped

1 tablespoon tahini

$\frac{1}{2}$ teaspoon cinnamon

$\frac{1}{2}$ inch fresh gingerroot

$\frac{1}{4}$ cup raisins

Combine the apricots, apples, tahini, cinnamon, and gingerroot in a food processor and process until finely chopped and mixed. Pour the mixture over the raisins and stir. Chill the pudding for 1 hour before serving. Store uneaten pudding in the refrigerator, where it will keep for two to three days.

Cinnamon Buns

*These delicious buns have convinced
some of my friends to go raw!*

Yield: 24 buns

2 cups buckwheat, sprouted 2–3 days using the jar method

1 cup raisins

1 cup chopped dates, soaked for 20 minutes

2 teaspoons cinnamon

$\frac{1}{2}$ teaspoon cardamom

$\frac{1}{4}$ teaspoon Celtic salt

Combine all ingredients in a food processor and mince. Shape the mixture into 2-inch rounds on solid dehydrator sheets and dehydrate for 6 hours. Remove the dehydrator sheets, turn the rounds over onto the dehydrator tray, and continue dehydrating for another 6 hours. Frost the buns with Deluxe Frosting (page 245). Store uneaten buns in a container in the refrigerator, where they will keep for a week.

The "I Don't Do Dairy Department"

Dairy products tend to cause congestion, even in people who are not lactose intolerant or allergic to cow's milk. Soy milk is often touted as an alternative to cow's milk, but many people find soy milk difficult to digest. Rice milk and other packaged milk alternatives are heated to high temperatures during processing, which destroys many of their naturally occurring nutrients. Raw nut milks, on the other hand, are easy to digest, packed with nutrients, and adaptable to making many raw "dairy" products such as cheese, sour cream, and yogurt.

Almond Ricotta Cheese

This cheese is wonderful in raw Lasagna (page 196)
or as a spread on crackers.

Yield: 3 cups

3 cups almonds, soaked overnight,
then rinsed

2 tablespoons tahini

1 tablespoon chopped onion

1 tablespoon lemon juice

1 tablespoon miso

1 tablespoon nutritional yeast
(optional; not a raw product)

1 clove garlic

Combine all ingredients in a food processor and pulse until minced. Spread the mixture onto a solid dehydrator sheet and dehydrate. When the upper side appears dry, turn the cheese over onto the dehydrator tray, and continue to dehydrate until the cheese is mostly dry (4–5 total hours). Store uneaten cheese in the refrigerator, where it will keep for four to five days.

Almond Cheese

Cheese without congestion!

Yield: 3 cups

2 cups almonds, soaked for 12 hours
or overnight, then rinsed

1 cup Rejuvelac (page 151)

Combine the nuts and Rejuvelac in a blender and pulse until the nuts are minced. Pour the mixture into a sprout bag, set the bag in a bowl in a warm area, and let it drain for 2 hours. Place the drained bag in a warm location and let it ferment for 9 hours. (Placing a weight on the cheese in the sprout bag will create a firmer cheese.) Store uneaten cheese in an airtight container in the refrigerator, where it will keep for about two weeks.

I Can't Believe It's Not Feta

Add this cheese mix to salads and Mexican or Italian dishes.

Yield: I cup

1 cup firm Almond Cheese (see above)

1 tablespoon light miso

1 tablespoon nutritional yeast
(optional; not a raw product)

1 clove garlic

1 teaspoon lemon juice

$\frac{1}{2}$ teaspoon Celtic salt

Combine all ingredients in a food processor and purée. Scoop the mixture into a sprout bag, set the bag in a bowl, place a weight on top of the bag, and let it drain in the refrigerator for 3 hours. Store uneaten cheese in the refrigerator, where it will keep for one week.

Easy Cheese Spread

*Use this creamy cheese as a dip for vegetables
or as a spread on raw crackers.*

Yield: 2 $\frac{1}{2}$ cups

2 cups almond pulp left over from
making Almond Milk (see below)

$\frac{1}{2}$ cup extra-virgin olive oil

2 tablespoons lemon juice

$\frac{1}{2}$ teaspoon Celtic salt

2 tablespoons nutritional yeast
(optional; not a raw product)

1 tomato

Combine all ingredients in a food processor and purée. Store uneaten spread in the refrigerator, where it will keep for four to five days.

Almond Milk

*Why settle for a product in an aseptic package that has
a shelf life of three years? Choose vitality instead!*

Yield: I quart

1 cup almonds, soaked overnight,
then rinsed

1 quart water

1 tablespoon honey or 2 dates,
soaked for 20 minutes

Combine all ingredients in a blender and liquefy. Strain the liquid through a nut milk or sprout bag into another container. (Save the nut pulp for Easy Cheese Spread and other recipes.) Store unused milk in the refrigerator, where it will keep for four to five days.

Note: These directions can be followed to make cashew, hazelnut/filbert, sesame seed, sunflower seed, walnut, or pecan milk.

Raw Carob Milk

This flavored nut milk is a favorite with kids of all ages.

Yield: 2 servings

1 cup almonds, soaked overnight, then rinsed

1 quart water

3 tablespoons carob powder

2 tablespoons honey or 4 dates,
soaked for 20 minutes

Combine the almonds and water in a blender and purée. Strain the liquid through a nut milk or sprout bag into another container, squeezing the bag well. Rinse the blender and pour the strained milk back into it, along with the carob powder and honey or dates. Blend until thoroughly mixed. Store unused milk in the refrigerator, where it will keep for four to five days.

Almond Yogurt

This creamy blend is rich in both calcium and protein.

Yield: 5 cups

2 cups almonds, soaked for 24 hours, then rinsed

2 cups water

$\frac{1}{4}$ cup dates, soaked for 20 minutes

1 teaspoon vanilla extract
(optional; not a raw product)

Place the almonds and water in a blender and blend until smooth. Pour the mixture into a nut milk or sprout bag, set the bag in a bowl in a warm (not hot) area, and let it drain for 8–12 hours. Purée the dates and mix the purée with the almond pulp from the bag. Stir the vanilla extract into the mixture. Store uneaten yogurt in a glass jar in the refrigerator, where it will keep for four to five days.

Note: Yogurt can be made in the same manner using cashews, hazelnuts/filberts, pecans, sesame seeds, sunflower seeds, or walnuts.

Coconut Yogurt

Delicious and creamy.

Yield: 4 servings

$2/3$ cup pine nuts

Water of 2 young coconuts

Meat of 4 young coconuts

6 dates, soaked for 20 minutes

1 teaspoon vanilla extract (optional; not a raw product)

2 tablespoons coconut oil

Juice of 2 lemons

Combine all ingredients in a blender or food processor and blend into a smooth, creamy mixture. Store uneaten yogurt in a glass jar in the refrigerator, where it will keep for four to five days.

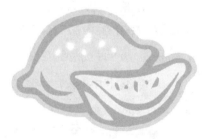

Sour Dream Cream

Simple and rich.

Yield: 3 cups

$1\frac{1}{2}$ cups macadamia nuts (or Brazil nuts),
soaked overnight, then rinsed

$3/4$ cup water

$1/4$ cup lemon juice

1 teaspoon Celtic salt

Combine all ingredients in food processor and pulse until the mixture is smooth.

Beverages

Raw beverages are both refreshing and healthful. They contain an abundance of nutrients and feature fruits, vegetables, herbs, and spices with wide-ranging potentials for healing. Rejuvelac is a fermented food that promotes healthy intestinal flora.

The following beverage recipes are also a great way to introduce children to raw foods, because the fruity drinks and sweet nut milk blends are just as delicious as the sugary juice blends promoted on television.

Enjoy these beverages as a snack or as a midday recharger—and don't forget to raise your glass in a toast to living foods!

Pink Lemonade

This no-sugar version is better than any lemonade you had as a kid.

Yield: 2 servings

2 cups water

1 cup orange juice

½ cup lemon juice

¼ cup strawberries, stems removed

Combine all ingredients in a blender, blend thoroughly, and enjoy.

Limeade

A cool and refreshing drink.

Yield: 2 servings

4 cups water

2 tablespoons honey

Juice of 6 limes

Mint sprigs

Combine the water, honey, and lime juice in a blender and blend until thoroughly mixed. Garnish with the mint sprigs.

Purple Haze

Get invigorated with this power punch.

Yield: 2 servings

3 dates, soaked for 20 minutes

1½ cups coconut water

1 cup blackberries

1 peeled banana

Combine all ingredients in a blender, blend thoroughly, and enjoy.

Orange Sunshine

Happy days are here again.

Yield: 2 servings

2 cups orange juice

1 peeled banana

1 medium papaya, peeled and seeded

Combine all ingredients in a blender and blend thoroughly. Sip, and merge with the universe.

Mango Lassi

This classic Indian drink is fit for the Hindu goddess Lakshmi herself.

Yield: 2 servings

2 cups Almond Milk (page 144)

2 mangoes, peeled and seeded

1 peeled banana

¼ cup dates, soaked for 20 minutes

¼ teaspoon cinnamon

¼ teaspoon cardamom seeds

1 teaspoon rosewater (optional; not a raw product)

Combine all ingredients in a blender and liquefy until the mixture reaches the consistency of a thin shake.

Coconut Milk

This drink is rich and nourishing.

Yield: 2 servings

3 dates, soaked for 20 minutes

3 cups coconut water

1 cup young coconut meat

Combine all ingredients in a blender, blend thoroughly, and enjoy.

If You Like Piña Colada

You're not missing out on anything with the raw version
of this popular beverage.

Yield: 2 large servings

$1/2$ cup macadamia nuts, soaked for 4 hours, then rinsed

$1/4$ cup chopped pineapple

1 orange, peeled and seeded

$1/4$ cup young coconut meat

$1 1/2$ cups water or coconut water

Combine all ingredients in a blender, blend thoroughly, and raise a toast to love!

Strawberry Shake

This shake creates true bliss.

Yield: 2 servings

2 cups Almond Milk (page 144)

6 dates, soaked for 20 minutes

1 cup strawberries, stems removed

1 peeled banana

$1/2$ teaspoon vanilla extract (optional; not a raw product)

Combine all ingredients in a blender and liquefy. Enjoy!

Banana Shake

This shake is an excellent children's drink.

Yield: I serving

1 cup Almond Milk (page 144)

2 dates, soaked for 20 minutes

1 peeled banana

1 teaspoon vanilla extract (optional; not a raw product)

Combine all ingredients in a blender, blend thoroughly, and enjoy.

Banana-Sesame Smoothie

Great for young children and the young at heart.

Yield: I serving

$\frac{1}{2}$ cup water

1 peeled banana

1 tablespoon tahini

Combine all ingredients in a blender, blend thoroughly, and enjoy.

Banana-Strawberry Rush

How could anyone drink a soda after this experience?

Yield: 4 servings

3 cups orange juice

2 cups strawberries, stems removed

1 peeled banana

Combine all ingredients in a blender, blend thoroughly, and enjoy.

Nut Nog

Welcome holiday guests with rawsome good cheer.

Yield: 4 servings

1 quart Almond Milk (page 144)

$1/4$ cup dates, soaked for 20 minutes

3 peeled bananas

$1/2$ teaspoon nutmeg

1 teaspoon cinnamon

1 teaspoon vanilla extract (optional; not a raw product)

$1/4$ teaspoon turmeric

Combine all ingredients in a blender and blend well. Serve the nog in festive glasses or mugs and sprinkly with a dash of cinnamon or nutmeg.

Apple-Ginger Juice

As Crosby, Stills, and Nash said, "Rejoice. Rejoice.
You have no choice."—Carry On

Yield: 2 servings

6 large apples, cored

2 inches fresh gingerroot

Juice of 2 lemons or limes

1 cup water

Run the apples and gingerroot through a juicer. Stir the citrus juice and water into the mixture. Rejoice!

Rejuvelac

Note: Rejuvelac can cause digestive discomfort in some people.
If that's the case for you, drink pure water instead.

Yield: 6 cups

2 cups soft wheat berries (rye, buckwheat, or millet can also be used)

Water

Soak the wheat berries overnight in a large jar of pure water. In the morning, drain the water from the wheat, but do not rinse. Allow the wheat to sprout for 2 days, still without rinsing. When white sprout tails begin to show, add 6 cups of pure water, cover the jar with cheesecloth, and set it in a warm location

(73°F is ideal) to ferment for 24 hours. Strain the Rejuvelac liquid into another container and store it in the refrigerator, where it will keep for several days.

The same batch of sprouts can be soaked three more times, in 4 cups of water rather than 6, to yield more Rejuvelac, and then they can be composted or thrown out to birds.

Rejuvelac Recharger

This recipe offers a more delicious way to enjoy the benefits of Rejuvelac.

Yield: 2 servings

2 cups Rejuvelac (page 151)

$\frac{1}{2}$ cup dried apricots, soaked for 1 hour

$\frac{1}{2}$ teaspoon vanilla extract (optional; not a raw product)

Combine all ingredients in a blender, blend thoroughly, and enjoy.

All About Rejuvelac

Rejuvelac is rich in enzymes, protein, carbohydrates, saccharides (sugars), lactobacilli (friendly bacteria that live in our digestive tract), B-complex vitamins, vitamins E and K, and antioxidants. It is a predigested beverage that is easily metabolized. It cleanses the intestines and helps provide the correct internal environment for the synthesis of nutrients.

Drink or use Rejuvelac in place of water, or add it to blended drinks or juices. I recommend starting a Rejuvelac routine by drinking 8 ounces a day, gradually working up to 1 quart daily. Start a new batch every three days to be well supplied.

When Rejuvelac is prepared correctly, it is cloudy with a faint yellow color. It should have a lemonlike tartness with a yeasty flavor. As the liquid is fermenting, tiny bubbles occasionally rise through it and can produce a slight carbonated quality. The formation of a white foamy layer on top of Rejuvelac is normal; this portion is not harmful to drink, but it can be strained off if desired.

If Rejuvelac ferments too long, it can develop a slight sourness. If the sprouting period is too long, the liquid can be either excessively sour or sweet. Sometimes the liquid becomes contaminated with the wrong bacteria, the grain is too old, or the weather is too humid. If your Rejuvelac doesn't taste right, just compost it and try again.

Salads

Eat one or two salads daily. If a salad is to be the main course for dinner, make enough that you can conveniently have some for lunch the next day. When you're preparing salads, tear greens into bite-sized pieces, rather than cutting them, as cutting greens with a metal knife tends to discolor them. Don't add cucumbers or tomatoes until you are ready to eat, because they will turn everything soggy; likewise, don't put them in any leftover salad that you're going to refrigerate overnight. To maintain the highest possible nutrient content, it is best to make salads no more than 1 hour before serving. Chill salads until serving time.

In addition to the standard varieties of lettuce and vegetables, include wild greens as well as edible flowers (see page 98) in your salads. Add garden herbs such as anise hyssop, arugula, basil, lemon balm, mizuna, parsley, peppermint, rosemary, and spearmint. Mix two or three different greens together. Many chefs make grand salads using tremendous numbers of different greens and vegetables; my own preference, however, is to use just a small number of ingredients in a salad. If you use only three ingredients at once, you can make an infinite variety of very different salads, whereas if you use ten ingredients at a time, every salad may seem similar to the last one you ate.

Asian Cucumber Salad

Enjoy this recipe with an Asian-themed raw entrée.

Yield: 2 servings

2 cucumbers, sliced

$1/2$ cup chopped fresh cilantro

3 tablespoons extra-virgin olive oil

2 tablespoons lime juice

1 teaspoon Curry Powder (page 116), or a curry powder of your choice

$1/2$ teaspoon Celtic salt

Combine all ingredients in a bowl and toss well.

Asian Salad

This mix is simple yet deluxe. Using 1 cup of red cabbage and 1 cup of white cabbage makes a nice presentation. Serve with Asian Dressing (page 164).

Yield: 2 servings

2 cups chopped cabbage

1 cup peeled, grated jicama

1 cup snow peas, each cut in half widthwise

$\frac{1}{2}$ inch fresh gingerroot, chopped

Combine all ingredients in a bowl and toss well.

Carrot Salad

Colorful simplicity—this is a favorite with children.

Yield: 2 servings

4 grated carrots

Juice of 1 orange

1 tablespoon extra-virgin olive oil

$\frac{1}{2}$ teaspoon Celtic salt

$\frac{1}{2}$ teaspoon freshly ground cumin

Combine all ingredients in a bowl and toss well.

Hey Beetnik!

Raw, red, and radical, with built-in dressing.

Yield: 2 servings

2 cups grated beets

2 tablespoons Nama Shoyu

2 teaspoons grated fresh gingerroot

1 teaspoon lemon juice

Combine all ingredients in a bowl and toss well.

Cole Slaw

This hearty salad makes a meal by itself,
especially when topped with a chopped avocado.

Yield: 4 servings

$1/2$ head red cabbage, shredded

$1/2$ head white cabbage, shredded

2 carrots, grated

1 cup chopped fresh parsley

$1/2$ cup extra-virgin olive oil

$1/4$ cup lemon juice

1 inch fresh gingerroot

$1/2$ teaspoon Celtic salt

1 teaspoon mustard powder

Toss the cabbage and carrots in a pretty bowl. Combine the remaining ingredients in a blender and blend until thoroughly mixed. Pour the mixture on top of the salad and stir.

Cool Cucumber-Mint Salad

This makes a light, refreshing salad for a summer's eve
or to cool the heat of spicy raw Indian fare.

Yield: 2–4 servings

2 cucumbers, chopped

$1/2$ cup finely chopped fresh spearmint

$1/4$ cup pine nuts

3 tablespoons water

1 tablespoon extra-virgin olive oil

1 tablespoon lemon juice

$1/4$ teaspoon Celtic salt

Place the cucumbers in a bowl. Blend the remaining ingredients in a blender. Pour the mixture over the cucumbers.

Caesar Salad

This rich salad with a built-in dressing can be a meal unto itself,
but it also makes a good accompaniment to Italian-style
dishes such as Pasta Primarawva (page 203).

Yield: 4 servings

1 head romaine lettuce, washed and dried

$\frac{1}{4}$ cup lemon juice

1 cup water

$\frac{1}{8}$ cup extra-virgin olive oil

2 teaspoons shredded kelp

$\frac{1}{2}$ teaspoon ground black pepper

$\frac{1}{2}$ teaspoon Celtic salt

$\frac{1}{2}$ teaspoon mustard powder

$\frac{1}{4}$ teaspoon turmeric

1 clove garlic

$\frac{1}{2}$ cup macadamia nuts or pine nuts, soaked for 4 hours, then rinsed

$\frac{1}{2}$ cup walnuts, soaked for 4 hours,
then dehydrated until crunchy (about 12 hours)

Tear the lettuce into bite-sized pieces and place in a pretty bowl. Combine the remaining ingredients except for the walnuts in a blender, blend well, and pour the mixture over the lettuce. Top the salad with the walnuts.

Mermaid Salad

This recipe brings to mind a favorite quote:
"I want to be where the people are. I want to be where there's singing and dancing." —ARIEL, FROM DISNEY'S THE LITTLE MERMAID.

Yield: 2 servings

1 cup arame, soaked for 20 minutes, then rinsed

2 tablespoons sesame seeds

2 teaspoons extra-virgin olive oil

1 teaspoon Nama Shoyu

Combine all ingredients in a bowl and toss well.

Corn Salad

This salad makes a great accompaniment to raw Mexican fare.

Yield: 2 servings

Kernels of 4 ears of corn (about 2 cups)

1 tomato, chopped

$\frac{1}{4}$ cup chopped fresh cilantro

2 tablespoons extra-virgin olive oil

$\frac{1}{2}$ teaspoon Celtic salt

Combine all ingredients in a bowl and toss well.

Italian Salad

Serve with Italian Dressing (page 164).

Yield: 2–4 servings

1 head romaine lettuce, washed, dried, and torn into bite-sized pieces

1 cup chopped fresh basil

$\frac{1}{4}$ cup pine nuts

20 sun-cured black olives, pitted

10 cherry tomatoes, sliced in half

Combine all ingredients in a bowl and toss well.

Mexican Salad

This salad makes the perfect lunch.

Yield: 2–4 servings

Kernels of 2 ears of corn

1 cup peeled, grated jicama

1 red pepper, chopped

$\frac{1}{2}$ cup chopped fresh cilantro

1 avocado, pitted, peeled, and chopped

1 head lettuce, washed and shredded

Combine all ingredients in a bowl and toss well. Serve with dressing of your choice.

Winter Waldorf Salad

This salad is both sweet and crunchy.

Yield: 2-4 servings

$\frac{1}{2}$ cup walnuts, soaked overnight, rinsed,
then dehydrated until crunchy (about 12 hours)

$\frac{1}{2}$ cup Almond Mayonnaise (page 180)

1 apple, finely chopped

2 stalks celery, finely chopped

2 cups grated carrots

$\frac{1}{2}$ cup raisins

$1\frac{1}{2}$ teaspoons grated fresh gingerroot

Combine all ingredients in a bowl, toss well, and serve.

Winter Solstice Salad

*The red and green hues of this salad are reminiscent
of the holiday symbols of eternal life.*

Yield: 2-4 servings

$1\frac{1}{2}$ cups finely chopped kale

$1\frac{1}{2}$ cups shredded beets

Make a circle with the chopped kale on a platter or in a bowl. Fill the center of the circle with the beets. Top the salad with a dressing of your choice. You can also shape this salad into a pie-tree shape on a large platter. Use small mounds of shredded beets or cherry tomatoes as the "decorations."

Rainbow Salad

Serve this and hear your friends say, "Wow!"

Yield: as many servings as you have vegetables

Grated beets, tomato, and red pepper (red)

Grated carrots or sweet potatoes (orange)

Grated yellow squash or rutabagas (yellow)

Chopped kale, broccoli, or avocado (green)

Pansy, borage, and/or chicory flowers (blue)

Chopped red cabbage (purple)

On a platter, shape the grated vegetables into layers of a rainbow, using the beets to make the top arc, and then layering the remaining ingredients in arcs under the beets.

Sauerkraut

Sauerkraut supports beneficial intestinal flora and provides vitamin C. In ancient times, seafarers ate sauerkraut to prevent scurvy (see "Citrus versus Scurvy" on page 49).

Yield: 8 servings

1 head white cabbage

1 head purple cabbage

4 teaspoons Celtic salt

1 tablespoon caraway seeds or dill seeds

Grate the cabbage (a food processor makes this easy) and toss it with the remaining ingredients. Place the mixture in a pickle press (see Gold Mine in the Resources section) and apply pressure with the press. Leave the press undisturbed for two weeks. When you open the press, you may find mold on top of the sauerkraut; scrape it off and discard it. Rinse the sauerkraut well in a colander. Store uneaten sauerkraut in the refrigerator, where it will keep for three to four weeks.

"Grate" Additions to Sauerkraut

Other chopped or grated fare can be mixed into cabbage sauerkraut, including apples, beets, broccoli, carrots, cauliflower, celery, onions, and daikon radishes. Aside from the traditional caraway and dill seeds, sauerkraut can also be flavored with 1 tablespoon per batch of chopped basil, chili peppers, garlic, gingerroot, dulse, kelp, or juniper berries.

Mediterranean Salad

Already dressed and delightful,
this salad can be an appetizer or a complete meal.

Yield: 4 servings as an appetizer or 2 servings as an entrée

4 tomatoes, chopped

2 cucumbers, chopped

1 cup chopped fresh parsley

$\frac{1}{2}$ cup chopped fresh basil

$\frac{1}{4}$ cup extra-virgin olive oil

$\frac{1}{4}$ cup sun-cured olives, pitted

$\frac{1}{2}$ teaspoon Celtic salt

Juice of 2 lemons

Combine all ingredients in a bowl and toss well.

Tabouli

Regular tabouli is made with cooked bulgur wheat.
This tabouli is wheat-free and, of course, raw.

Yield: 4–6 servings

1$\frac{1}{2}$ cups buckwheat, sprouted 2–3 days using the jar method,
then rinsed and drained

1 cup chopped fresh parsley

$\frac{1}{4}$ cup chopped fresh spearmint

1 tomato, diced

$\frac{1}{2}$ cup diced cucumber

2 scallions, sliced

$\frac{1}{4}$ cup lemon juice

$\frac{1}{4}$ cup extra-virgin olive oil

$\frac{1}{2}$ teaspoon salt

$\frac{1}{2}$ cup sun-cured olives, pitted

Combine the buckwheat, parsley, spearmint, tomato, cucumber, and scallions in a bowl and toss. Mix the lemon juice, olive oil, and salt into the salad, and garnish with the olives. Chill the salad for 30 minutes before serving.

Kale (or Collard Green) Salad

*This salad, inspired by gourmet raw chef Chad Sarno,
can be ready in an instant. Add a chopped tomato
and some sliced avocado and you have lunch!*

Yield: 2–4 servings

1 bunch kale or collard greens, finely chopped

2 tablespoons extra-virgin olive oil

2 tablespoons lemon juice

1 teaspoon chili powder

½ teaspoon Celtic salt

Place the kale or collard greens in a bowl. Mix the remaining ingredients together in a separate bowl, and then use your hands to "massage" the seasonings into the greens.

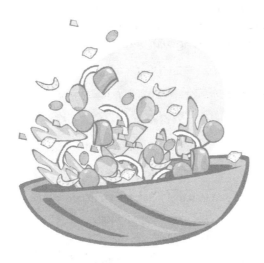

Dressings to Make Your Salads Sing

For optimal flavor and nutritional value, make salad dressings fresh, rather than making a week's supply at a time. However, if you make dressings ahead of time, store them in a glass container in the refrigerator for up to four to seven days. If you want to avoid using added oils, try blending together just a few raw ingredients, at least one of which is juicy or creamy. Three of my favorite, relatively oil-free dressings are made from equal parts of:

- Walnuts, cucumber, and orange
- Strawberry and avocado
- Tomato, red pepper, and sunflower seeds

Avoid Commercial Dressings

If you're making a salad at a salad bar, avoid the commercial dressings typically offered. Use plain lemon juice and olive oil instead. You can even bring your own raw dressing with you.

Russian Dressing

Raw and red.

Yield: 1½ cups

3 dates, soaked for 20 minutes
1 cup chopped tomato
½ cup extra-virgin olive oil
½ cup lemon juice
½ teaspoon Celtic salt
1 teaspoon paprika
1 clove garlic

Combine all ingredients in a blender and blend until smooth.

French Dressing

Un, deux, trois, voilà!

Yield: 2 cups

3 dates, soaked for 20 minutes

$1\frac{1}{2}$ cups extra-virgin olive oil

$\frac{2}{3}$ cup lemon juice

$\frac{1}{2}$ teaspoon celery seeds

$\frac{1}{2}$ teaspoon paprika

1 teaspoon chopped fresh basil

1 teaspoon Celtic salt

Combine all ingredients in a blender and blend until smooth.

Green Goddess Dressing

Cool, creamy, and dreamy.

Yield: 2 cups

2 avocados, pitted and peeled

1 cup water

$\frac{1}{4}$ cup lemon juice

1 teaspoon Celtic salt

Combine all ingredients in a blender and blend until smooth.

Honey-Lemon Dressing

This dressing is a favorite with kids.

Yield: 1 cup

$\frac{1}{2}$ cup lemon juice

$\frac{1}{2}$ cup honey

$\frac{1}{4}$ teaspoon Celtic salt

Combine all ingredients in a blender and blend until smooth.

Italian Dressing

A sure crowd-pleaser.

Yield: I cup

$3/4$ cup extra-virgin olive oil

$1/4$ cup lemon juice

$1/8$ teaspoon Celtic salt

1 teaspoon chopped fresh basil

Combine all ingredients in a blender and blend until smooth.

Asian Dressing

Flavor with flair!

Yield: I cup

$1/4$ cup Nama Shoyu

$1/4$ cup extra-virgin olive oil

$1/4$ cup water

1 tablespoon chopped fresh cilantro

1 inch fresh gingerroot

Combine all ingredients in a blender and blend until smooth.

Tahini Dressing

This dressing is rich in calcium.

Yield: about I $1/2$ cups

$1/2$ cup extra-virgin olive oil

Juice of 1 lemon

$1/4$ cup tahini

$1/3$ cup tamari

$1/4$ cup water

1 inch fresh gingerroot

Combine all ingredients in a blender and blend until smooth.

Ranch Dressing

A secret to eating raw is having some great salad dressings
in your life—and this recipe makes one of them.

Yield: about 1 1/2 cups

1 cup macadamia nuts, soaked overnight,
then rinsed

2 dates, soaked for 20 minutes

1 cup water

1/2 cup extra-virgin olive oil

1/4 cup chopped onion

1/2 teaspoon Celtic salt

1 teaspoon ground pepper

2 cloves garlic

Juice of 2 lemons

Combine all ingredients in a blender and blend until smooth.

Dressing for a Large Group

For those special occasions when
you have a big crowd to feed.

Yield: about 3 cups

8 dates, soaked for 20 minutes

1 cup water

1/2 cup lemon or lime juice

1/2 cup Nama Shoyu

1/2 cup tahini

1/4 cup extra-virgin olive oil

1 teaspoon Curry Powder (page 116),
or a curry powder of your choice

3 cloves garlic

Combine all ingredients in a blender and blend until smooth.

═══ *Soups* ═══

Raw soups are especially flavorful and, being puréed for the most part, are easier on the digestive system than solid foods are. Raw soups are particularly good for people with poor digestion, the elderly, or people recovering from illness. Serve a bowl of soup with a salad and some sprouted crackers for a sumptuous meal.

Most raw soups are best the day they are made. Refrigerator leftovers overnight but be sure to eat the soup the next day while it is still tasty and relatively fresh. Leftover soups can also be dehydrated and used for backpacking meals. Thick soups should be blended and dried as small wafers (3 inches wide, $\frac{1}{2}$ inch thick). Just add water and wild greens to rehydrate and rejuvenate your soup on the trail.

Coconut Soup

For a taste of the islands, try this flavorful soup.

Yield: 4 servings

$1\frac{1}{2}$ cups coconut water

$1\frac{1}{2}$ cups water

Meat of 2 young coconuts

1 avocado, pitted and peeled

1 clove garlic

1 inch fresh gingerroot

2 tablespoons white or yellow miso

2 tablespoons Nama Shoyu

Juice of 2 limes

1 tablespoon coconut oil

$\frac{1}{8}$ teaspoon cayenne powder

$\frac{1}{2}$ cup chopped fresh cilantro

$\frac{1}{2}$ cup chopped fresh basil

4 chopped tomatoes

Combine all ingredients except the tomatoes in a blender and purée. Pour the purée into soup bowls, top it with the chopped tomatoes, and serve.

Borscht (Beet Soup)

Allow the red rays to warm you on a winter's eve.

Yield: 4 servings

1 cup almonds, soaked overnight,
then rinsed

2 cups water

3 beets, peeled and chopped

$\frac{1}{4}$ cup chopped fresh dill

1 clove garlic

2 tablespoons extra-virgin olive oil

$\frac{1}{2}$ teaspoon Celtic salt

1 cup shredded cabbage

Place the almonds and two cups of fresh water in a blender and liquefy. Strain the liquid through a sprout bag to collect the almond milk into a large bowl. Add the remaining ingredients to the almond milk and stir. Pour half of the mixture from the bowl into the blender and blend until smooth. Pour the smooth mixture back into the bowl with the rest of the borscht and stir to mix. Enjoy!

Creamed Asparagus Soup

This soup is an excellent springtime entrée.

Yield: 4 servings

$\frac{1}{2}$ cup walnuts, soaked for at least 2 hours,
then rinsed

3 cups chopped asparagus
(remove tough bottom portion first)

2 cups water

3 stalks celery, each cut into thirds

$\frac{1}{2}$ teaspoon Celtic salt

Place the chopped asparagus in a large bowl. Combine the remaining ingredients in a blender and blend thoroughly. Pour the purée over the asparagus and serve. *Voilà!*

Cherry Soup

A seasonal delight.

Yield: 4 servings

$1/4$ cup dates, soaked for 20 minutes

2 cups cherries, pitted

$2^1/2$ cups water

2 tablespoons lemon juice or lime juice

Combine all ingredients in a food processor or blender and liquefy.

Cucumber Soup

Beat the heat with a cool bowl of this refreshing soup.

Yield: 2 servings

$1/4$ cup tahini

$1/2$ teaspoon Celtic salt

Juice of 1 lemon

3 tablespoons finely chopped fresh spearmint

1 large cucumber, chopped

Combine the tahini, salt, and lemon juice in a food processor and purée. Pour the purée into a bowl, add the chopped spearmint and cucumber, and stir to mix.

Carrot-Ginger Soup

This soup is superb food and great for building lung strength.

Yield: 3 servings

$1^1/2$ cups chopped carrots, divided

1 tablespoon white miso

1 teaspoon grated gingerroot

1 clove garlic

2 cups water

Place ³⁄₄ cup of the carrots in a bowl. Combine the remaining carrots and the rest of the ingredients in a blender and blend until smooth. Pour the blended mixture over the carrots in the bowl and serve.

Celery Soup

So simple, so satisfying.

Yield: 2 servings

4 stalks celery, chopped

1 cup water

1 avocado, pitted and peeled

1 tomato

Juice of 1 lemon or lime

1 teaspoon kelp

A handful of chopped fresh cilantro

Place the celery in a bowl. Combine the remaining ingredients in a blender and blend until smooth. Pour the purée over the chopped celery and stir to mix.

Corn Soup

This summer favorite will keep them coming back for more.

Yield: 4 servings

Kernels of 2 ears of corn

1¹⁄₂ cups Almond Milk (page 144) or sesame milk

¹⁄₂ avocado, pitted and peeled

¹⁄₄ teaspoon coriander seeds

¹⁄₄ teaspoon nutmeg

¹⁄₂ teaspoon Celtic salt

Place the corn kernels in a pretty bowl. Combine the remaining ingredients in a blender or food processor and purée. Pour the purée over the corn and stir to mix.

Curried Cauliflower Soup

It might be winter and it might be raw,
but this soup will warm you.

Yield: 4 servings

1 medium head cauliflower, finely chopped or grated

1 avocado, pitted and peeled

1$\frac{1}{2}$ cups water

1 clove garlic

$\frac{1}{4}$ cup lemon juice

4 tablespoons tahini

2 tablespoons Curry Powder (page 116),
or a curry powder of your choice

$\frac{1}{2}$ teaspoon turmeric

2 tablespoons Nama Shoyu

2 tablespoons white or yellow miso

Place the cauliflower in a pretty bowl. Combine the remaining ingredients in a food processor and purée. Pour the purée over the cauliflower and serve.

Tomato Cream Soup

This recipe is dedicated to my daughter Sunflower.
I craved cream of tomato soup when I was pregnant with her.
Now it is one of her favorite foods.

Yield: 2–4 servings

8 tomatoes, chopped

$\frac{1}{2}$ cup tahini or pine nuts

$\frac{1}{4}$ cup chopped fresh basil

1 teaspoon Celtic salt

$\frac{1}{2}$ onion, chopped

2 cups water

Combine all ingredients in a blender and pulse until the mixture reaches the desired consistency (creamy or still slightly chunky, whichever you prefer).

Gazpacho

This savory soup nourishes and refreshes.

Yield: 2 servings

5 medium tomatoes, finely chopped

1 red pepper, finely chopped

1 cucumber, finely chopped

$\frac{1}{4}$ onion, finely chopped

1 avocado, pitted, peeled, and chopped

1 cup water

$\frac{3}{4}$ teaspoon Celtic salt

$\frac{1}{2}$ cup chopped fresh cilantro

$\frac{1}{2}$ cup chopped fresh basil

$\frac{1}{2}$ cup lemon juice or lime juice

Combine all ingredients in a large bowl and toss. Pour half of the mixture into a food processor and pulse. Return the mixture to the bowl with the rest of the soup and mix well.

Miso Soup

*Garnish with some chopped scallions
for a tasty Asian treat.*

Yield: 2–4 servings

3 cups coconut water

2 tablespoons miso

1 inch fresh gingerroot

1 clove garlic

1 cup young coconut meat,
sliced into long noodles

$\frac{1}{2}$ red pepper, chopped

Combine the coconut water, miso, and gingerroot in a blender and purée. Pour the mixture into a pretty bowl, add the remaining ingredients, and mix.

Papaya Soup

Try papaya in a new way!

Yield: 2–4 servings

4 dates, soaked for 20 minutes

4 cups peeled, seeded, chopped papaya

3 cups water

1 cup pitted cherries

Juice of 2 limes

Combine all ingredients in a blender and blend thoroughly.

Energy Soup

Bless Ann Wigmore for this ultimate healing soup.

Yield: I serving

1 apple or a piece of watermelon with rind

1 cup Rejuvelac (page 151)

$\frac{1}{2}$ avocado, pitted and peeled

A large handful of sprouts and greens

1 teaspoon shredded dulse or kelp

Combine all ingredients in a blender or food processor and pulse until the soup is thoroughly chopped and mixed but still chunky in texture.

Sweet Potato Soup

This soup is rich in antioxidants and vibrant color.

Yield: 2 servings

2 cups peeled, chopped sweet potatoes

1 avocado, pitted and peeled

1 cup water

$\frac{1}{2}$ teaspoon Celtic salt

1 apple, peeled, cored, and chopped

Combine all ingredients in a blender and blend thoroughly.

Spinach Soup

Easy, gracious, and green.

Yield: 2 servings

4 cups chopped spinach

2 cups water

1 avocado, pitted and peeled

$\frac{1}{2}$ teaspoon Celtic salt

1 teaspoon lemon juice

2 tablespoons chopped fresh basil

$\frac{1}{4}$ teaspoon nutmeg

Combine all ingredients in a blender and purée.

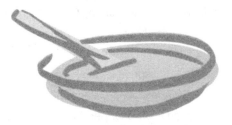

Winter Squash Soup

Raw winter squash may sound like a tough chew,
but when puréed, it becomes quite tender and flavorful.

Yield: 4 servings

1 acorn squash or butternut squash, peeled, seeded, and chopped

$\frac{1}{2}$ cup almond butter

1 tablespoon Curry Powder (page 116), or a curry powder of your choice

$\frac{1}{2}$ teaspoon nutmeg

4 cups water

$\frac{1}{2}$ inch fresh gingerroot

$\frac{1}{2}$ teaspoon Celtic salt

Combine all ingredients in a blender and blend thoroughly.

A Garden's Variety of Vegetable Dishes

Vegetables that turn you off when they are overcooked or canned and soggy take on a whole new life when prepared in tasty, raw dishes. Perhaps these recipes will even inspire you to grow your own vegetable garden—the best possible source of fresh, nutritious, delicious vegetables.

Green Bean Scene

Easy and elegant.

Yield: 2–4 servings

$1/2$ cup almonds, soaked overnight, rinsed,
then dehydrated until crunchy (about 12 hours)

3 cups chopped string beans

2 tablespoons extra-virgin olive oil

1 teaspoon lemon juice

$1/4$ teaspoon Celtic salt

1 teaspoon finely chopped fresh rosemary

Place the almonds in a blender or food processor and grind until broken into small pieces. Combine the almonds with the remaining ingredients in a bowl and stir to mix.

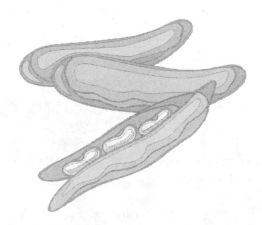

Sweet Potato Casserole

*You'll want to make this casserole
more often than just on holidays.*

Yield: 6 servings

$1\frac{1}{2}$ cups pecans, soaked overnight,
rinsed, then dehydrated

4 cups peeled, chopped sweet potatoes

$\frac{1}{2}$ cup water

$\frac{1}{2}$ cup dates, soaked for 20 minutes

1 teaspoon cinnamon

1 teaspoon vanilla extract
(optional; not a raw product)

$\frac{1}{2}$ teaspoon Celtic salt

$\frac{1}{4}$ cup honey

Place $\frac{1}{2}$ cup of the pecans and all of the sweet potatoes, water, dates, cinnamon, and vanilla in a food processor and purée. Pour the mixture into a casserole dish. In a separate bowl, combine the remaining pecans with the salt and honey and toss. Scatter the pecan topping over the casserole.

Pecan Parsnips

*Many people have never tried parsnips cooked, much less raw—but
this overlooked relative of the carrot deserves more recognition.*

Yield: 2–4 servings

1 cup pecans, soaked for 4 hours, then rinsed

1 cup water

1 cup chopped celery

$\frac{1}{2}$ teaspoon Celtic salt

6 parsnips, peeled and grated

Combine the pecans and water in a blender and purée. Toss the celery in a bowl with the salt. Add the parsnips to the celery, pour the pecan sauce over all, and stir to mix.

Oriental Broccoli

Until this dish came into my life, I had never tried raw broccoli.
What was I thinking all those years?

Yield: 4–6 servings

2 dates, soaked for 20 minutes

$\frac{1}{2}$ cup orange juice

1 teaspoon grated fresh gingerroot

$\frac{1}{4}$ cup Nama Shoyu

1 teaspoon toasted sesame oil
(optional; not a raw product)

$\frac{1}{4}$ cup extra-virgin olive oil

4 cups chopped broccoli

$\frac{1}{4}$ cup sesame seeds

Combine all ingredients except the broccoli and sesame seeds in a blender and purée. Combine the broccoli and sesame seeds together in a bowl and stir. Pour the purée over the broccoli and toss.

Stuffed Mushrooms

These mushrooms are an elegant finger-food for parties.

Yield: 4 servings

2 cups walnuts, soaked overnight, then rinsed

2 cups almonds, soaked overnight, then rinsed

2 tablespoons Classic Herb Mix (page 115),
or a commercial poultry seasoning of your choice

1 tablespoon miso

3 stalks celery, finely chopped

24 fresh shiitake mushrooms

Combine the walnuts, almonds, herb mix, and miso in a food processor and blend. Add the celery to the blended seasoning mixture and stir. Shape the mixture into 24 little balls and place one in each mushroom. Place the stuffed mushrooms on solid dehydrator sheets and dehydrate for 8 hours.

Summer Squash Supreme

Here's one idea for putting an abundant zucchini patch to good use.

Yield: 4–6 servings

2 cups macadamia nuts, soaked overnight,
then rinsed

4 sliced yellow squash or zucchini

$1/2$ cup light miso

1 teaspoon turmeric

1 cup water

2 tablespoons lemon juice

1 teaspoon Celtic salt

1 onion, finely chopped

1 teaspoon paprika

Place the summer squash or zucchini in a food processor fitted with a large grating blade and process until it is well chopped. Transfer the squash to a pretty dish. Combine the remaining ingredients in the food processor or blender and purée. Pour the purée over the squash. Serve the dish as is, or dehydrate for 3 hours to give it a crispy top.

Jicama Crunch Sticks

*Share a platter of these with a friend, and
you'll never miss French fries!*

Yield: 2 servings

1 jicama, peeled and cut into thin strips

2 tablespoons extra-virgin olive oil

1 tablespoon nutritional yeast
(optional; not a raw product)

1 teaspoon Chili Powder (page 115),
or a chili powder of your choice

$1/2$ teaspoon Celtic salt

Combine all ingredients, toss well, and serve.

Turnip Greens

*The seasoning in this recipe makes the
crunchy turnip greens simply delectable.*

Yield: 2–4 servings

1 bunch turnip greens, finely chopped

3 tablespoons extra-virgin olive oil

3 tablespoons lemon juice

$\frac{1}{2}$ teaspoon Celtic salt

Place the turnip greens in a bowl, top them with the olive oil, lemon juice, and salt, and mix, using your hands to "massage" the seasonings into the greens.

Herbed Turnips

*Turnips are a great fall and winter vegetable.
They keep well in cold storage and have a mellow flavor
that is complemented by green herbs.*

Yield: 4 servings

4 turnips or rutabagas, peeled and grated (about 4 cups)

Juice of 1 lemon

1 teaspoon Celtic salt

$\frac{1}{4}$ cup chopped fresh dill, parsley, or basil

3 tablespoons extra-virgin olive oil

Combine all ingredients, toss well, and serve.

Rice Replacements

The following vegetables can be grated (a food processor with a shredder works wonders) and used in place of rice:

- Jicama
- Turnips
- Zucchini
- Rutabagas
- Sweet potatoes

Season your "riced" vegetables with a bit of olive oil and Celtic salt.

Mashed Parsnips

*When you're serving a holiday meal, offer this delicious dish
in place of starchy mashed potatoes.*

Yield: 4–6 servings

1 cup macadamia nuts, soaked overnight, then rinsed

8 parsnips, peeled and chopped (about 6 cups)*

1 cup water

1 teaspoon Celtic salt

1/4 teaspoon fresh ground black pepper

Combine all ingredients in a food processor and pulse until the mixture is thick and smooth. Serve this dish with Nama Shoyu Gravy (page 184).

*Substitute rutabaga for the parsnips, if desired.

Corn on the Cob

This is the way to do corn!

Yield: 4 servings

1/2 cup extra-virgin olive oil

1 teaspoon Celtic salt

1/2 teaspoon turmeric

8 ears husked corn

Combine the oil, salt, and turmeric and mix. Brush the mixture on the corn. Place the corn on solid dehydrator sheets and dehydrate for 3 hours, turning the corn once every hour.

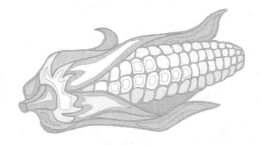

Sauces and Condiments

With the right sauce, a simple dish becomes unforgettable. The sauces and other condiments described here are good, traditional examples, but I encourage you to experiment with your own recipes for truly memorable culinary treats. Store leftover sauces in the refrigerator where they will keep for three to four days.

Almond Mayonnaise

Ooh la la. Why settle for anything less than the best?

Yield: about 1 cup

1 cup almonds*, soaked overnight, then rinsed

$\frac{1}{4}$ cup water

$\frac{1}{2}$ teaspoon Celtic salt

4 dates, soaked for 20 minutes

Juice of 1 lemon

$\frac{1}{4}$ cup extra-virgin olive oil

Combine all ingredients except the olive oil in a blender and blend until the ingredients are ground and thoroughly mixed. While blending, slowly drizzle in the olive oil as the mixture thickens.

*Substitute 1 cup almond pulp leftover from milk-making for the almonds, if desired.

Applesauce

Kids of all ages love this stuff.

Yield: 4 servings

6 large apples, cored and sliced

Juice of 1 lemon

8 dates, soaked for 20 minutes

$\frac{1}{2}$ teaspoon cinnamon

Combine all ingredients in a blender and purée.

Barbecue Sauce

Sweet, spicy, and smoky, this sauce is great with nut loaves and burgers. Try pouring it on a nut burger before dehydration, so that the burger and sauce fuse together in the dehydrator.

Yield: about 2 cups

1 $\frac{1}{2}$ cups sun-dried tomatoes,
soaked for 2 hours

1 cup chopped tomatoes

1 clove garlic

6 dates, soaked for 20 minutes

1 teaspoon Celtic salt

3 tablespoons lemon juice

1 $\frac{1}{2}$ teaspoons dry mustard powder

1 teaspoon Chili Powder (page 115),
or a chili powder of your choice

1 tablespoon liquid smoke
(optional; not a raw product)

Combine all ingredients in a blender and blend until smooth.

Raw Ketchup

Serve on nut burgers.

Yield: about 1 $\frac{1}{2}$ cups

1 cup chopped tomatoes

$\frac{1}{4}$ cup extra-virgin olive oil

3 dates, soaked for 20 minutes

1 tablespoon lemon juice

$\frac{1}{2}$ teaspoon Celtic salt

$\frac{1}{8}$ cup chopped onion

$\frac{1}{8}$ teaspoon celery seeds

$\frac{1}{8}$ teaspoon chopped fresh oregano

Combine all ingredients in a blender and blend until smooth.

Cranberry Sauce

A colorful accompaniment for a holiday feast,
this sauce can also be eaten as a snack anytime.

Yield: 8 servings

2 cups cranberries

2 medium oranges, peeled and seeded

$3/4$ cup dates, soaked for 20 minutes

2 teaspoons lemon juice

1 cup halved, seeded grapes

Combine all ingredients in a food processor and pulse until uniformly chopped and mixed. The sauce should be a bit chunky.

Curry Sauce

Serve as a condiment with Indian food.

Yield: $1/2$ cup

$1/4$ cup coconut oil

2 tablespoons tamarind (available at Asian markets),
soaked for 1 hour, or 2 tablespoons lemon juice

$1 1/2$ tablespoons Curry Powder (page 116),
or a curry powder of your choice

$1/2$ teaspoon Celtic salt

2 red peppers, chopped

Combine all ingredients in a blender or a food processor and purée.

Date Chutney

Like Curry Sauce, this chutney can be served
as an accompaniment to Indian fare.

Yield: 3 cups

3 cups dates, soaked for 20 minutes

1 teaspoon Curry Powder (page 116), or a curry powder of your choice

1 teaspoon Celtic salt

1 inch fresh gingerroot

1 clove garlic

1 teaspoon coconut oil

3 tablespoons water

Combine all ingredients in a food processor and purée.

Mango Chutney

This condiment is a treat with Indian or Mexican dishes!

Yield: 4 cups

2 cups peeled, seeded, chopped mangoes

2 cups chopped tomatoes

$\frac{1}{4}$ cup finely chopped onions

$\frac{1}{2}$ cup chopped fresh cilantro

Juice of 2 lemons

$\frac{1}{4}$ teaspoon Celtic salt

1 teaspoon finely chopped fresh jalapeño

Combine all ingredients in a food processor and pulse until the chutney is thoroughly mixed, with a chunky consistency.

Mint Chutney

Serve with Indian food, as a dip,
or as a spread for raw crackers.

Yield: 1$\frac{1}{2}$ cups

1 cup chopped fresh spearmint without stems

1 medium onion, chopped

4 tablespoons lime juice

2 dates, soaked for 20 minutes

Combine all ingredients in a food processor and pulse until the chutney is thoroughly mixed, with a chunky consistency.

Nama Shoyu Gravy

Serve on Mashed Parsnips (page 179).

Yield: I cup

¼ cup olive oil

¼ cup Nama Shoyu

¼ cup nutritional yeast (optional; not a raw product)

¼ cup water

Combine all ingredients in a blender and blend until smooth.

Garlic Butter

Try this spread on sprouted bread!

Yield: about ⅓ cup

¼ cup coconut oil

10 cloves garlic

¼ teaspoon Celtic salt

2 tablespoons chopped fresh parsley

Combine all ingredients in a blender or a food processor and blend until the mixture is smooth and creamy.

Herbal Butter

*Use as a spread on raw breads or crackers,
or as a sauce on raw "pasta" or "rice."*

Yield: ¼ cup

4 tablespoons coconut oil

1 teaspoon chopped fresh basil

¼ teaspoon Celtic salt

¼ teaspoon paprika

Combine all ingredients in a bowl and mix thoroughly.

Date Sauce

Use as a dip for fruit pieces on a skewer, like fondue.

Yield: 1 $\frac{1}{2}$ cups

$\frac{3}{4}$ cup dates, soaked for 20 minutes

1 cup water

1 teaspoon vanilla extract (optional; not a raw product)

Combine all ingredients in a blender or food processor and purée.

Sweet Mint Sauce

Drizzle on avocados, bananas, or strawberries.

Yield: 1 cup

$\frac{1}{2}$ cup chopped fresh spearmint

$\frac{1}{2}$ cup honey or $\frac{1}{2}$ cup dates, soaked for 20 minutes

Juice of $\frac{1}{2}$ lemon

Combine all ingredients in a blender or a food processor and purée until smooth.

Miso-Tahini Sauce

Great as a dip for Spring Green Rolls (page 213)
or as a condiment for other Asian fare.

Yield: 1 $\frac{1}{2}$ cups

$\frac{3}{4}$ cup water

2 tablespoons miso

$\frac{1}{2}$ cup tahini

$\frac{1}{2}$ teaspoon powdered miso

Juice of $\frac{1}{2}$ lemon

Combine all ingredients in a blender or a food processor and purée until smooth.

Holy Molé

A welcome addition to Mexican fare.

Yield: about 1/3 cup

4 tablespoons carob powder

2 teaspoons Chili Powder (page 115),
or a chili powder of your choice

1/2 teaspoon Celtic salt

1 small jalapeño

2 tablespoons flaxseeds

1/4 cup water

Combine all ingredients in a blender or a food processor and purée.

Carob Sauce

A delicious topping for fruit or other desserts.

Yield: 1 1/2 cups

1 cup coconut water

3 tablespoons almond butter

1/4 cup dates, soaked for 20 minutes

1/2 cup carob powder

1 teaspoon vanilla extract
(optional; not a raw product)

Combine all ingredients in a blender or a food processor and purée.

Red Pepper Sauce

*Try this sauce on Better-than-Crab Cakes (page 216).
It's also good as a vegetable dip.*

Yield: about 1 cup

1 medium red bell pepper, chopped

1/4 cup extra-virgin olive oil

3 tablespoons lemon juice

1 tablespoon Curry Powder (page 116),
or a curry powder of your choice

$\frac{1}{2}$ teaspoon Celtic salt

Combine all ingredients in a food processor and purée.

Sweet and Sour Sauce

A perfect complement to Asian dishes or nori rolls.

Yield: about 2 cups

$\frac{1}{2}$ cup dates, soaked for 20 minutes

$\frac{1}{2}$ cup dried apricots, soaked for 1–4 hours

1 teaspoon mustard powder

2 inches fresh gingerroot

$\frac{1}{3}$ cup orange juice

$\frac{1}{8}$ cup Nama Shoyu

$\frac{1}{8}$ cup flaxseeds

Combine all ingredients in a blender or a food processor and purée.

Tahini Sauce

Serve on Falafel Balls (page 210).

Yield: 1 $\frac{1}{2}$ cups

1 cup tahini

$\frac{1}{2}$ cup lemon juice

1 clove garlic

$\frac{1}{2}$ teaspoon Celtic salt

1 cup water

1 teaspoon cumin seeds

$\frac{1}{2}$ cup chopped fresh parsley

Combine all ingredients in a blender and blend until smooth.

Mustard Sauce

A wonderful condiment with Asian food.

Yield: ³/₄ cup

½ cup macadamia nuts, soaked overnight, then rinsed

1 tablespoon mustard powder

4 dates, soaked for 20 minutes

½ teaspoon turmeric

½ teaspoon Celtic salt

Juice of ½ lemon

Combine all ingredients in a blender or a food processor and purée.

Violet Honey

This recipe was inspired by one of my herbal teachers, Susun Weed. Use this special honey as a spread on sprouted crackers. It is an uplifting folk remedy for sorrow.

Yield: about 3 cups

2 cups violet flowers, collected in spring

1 cup honey

Juice of 1 lemon

Combine all ingredients in a blender and pulse until thoroughly mixed. Store the violet honey in a glass jar in the freezer.

Butterscotch Sauce

Serve over ice cream or fruit.

Yield: about 1 cup

½ cup dates, soaked for 20 minutes

¼ cup dried figs, soaked for 1 hour

Purée the fruit in a blender, adding just enough of the soak water to make a smooth mixture.

Dried-Fruit Jam

Jam on sprouted crackers with almond butter, anyone?
We're jammin'.

Yield: about 3 cups

$\frac{1}{2}$ cup raisins, soaked overnight

$\frac{1}{2}$ cup dried figs, soaked overnight

$\frac{1}{2}$ cup dried apricots, soaked overnight

Blend the fruit in a blender, adding just enough of the soak water to reach a jamlike consistency. Store the jam in the refrigerator, where it will keep for about two weeks.

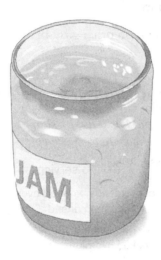

Dips and Pâtés

Dips and pâtés are puréed mixtures of healthy ingredients. They can encourage family members to try unfamiliar vegetables just by dipping in. There are so many things to do with pâté:

- Use as a filling for rolled nori sheets, collard leaves (with the middle vein cut out), or other greens.

- Use on top of a salad.

- Use as a dip.

- Use to stuff tomatoes, peppers, cucumbers, celery, and other vegetables.

- Dehydrate to make burgers.

- Serve on flax crackers or on other raw breads as a sandwich.

Southwestern Pâté

*Enjoy this pâté as a dip or shape it into patties
and dehydrate to make spicy burgers.*

Yield: 6 servings

1 cup almonds, soaked overnight,
then rinsed

1 cup sunflower seeds,
soaked overnight, then rinsed

1 tomato, chopped

1 clove garlic

½ cup chopped onion

½ teaspoon Celtic salt

1 tablespoon Chili Powder (page 115),
or a chili powder of your choice

1 teaspoon freshly ground cumin seed

⅛ teaspoon cayenne powder

1 tablespoon extra-virgin olive oil

Combine all ingredients in a blender or a food processor and purée.

Mexican Pâté

*This pâté can be spooned on top of a salad
or stuffed into a cabbage-leaf burrito.*

Yield: about 2 cups

1 cup sunflower seeds,
soaked overnight, then rinsed

1 carrot, chopped

1 tablespoon extra-virgin olive oil

1 tablespoon lemon juice or lime juice

1 teaspoon Celtic salt

1 teaspoon cumin seeds

2 teaspoons chopped fresh oregano
(or 1 teaspoon dried)

2 teaspoons chopped fresh basil
(or 1 teaspoon dried)

$1/4$ teaspoon cayenne powder

$1/2$ cup chopped onion

Combine all ingredients in a food processor and purée.

Sunflower Pâté

*Sunflower seeds are a nourishing adrenal tonic.
This pâté makes an excellent tuna-salad substitute
when mixed with chopped celery.*

Yield: $2 1/2$ cups

$1 1/2$ cups sunflower seeds,
soaked overnight, then rinsed

$1/2$ cup lemon juice

$1/4$ cup tahini

1 teaspoon Celtic salt

3 tablespoons chopped fresh parsley

1 inch fresh gingerroot

Combine all ingredients in a food processor and purée.

Pecan Cauliflower Pâté

This dish is always a favorite at potlucks.

Yield: about 4 cups

2 cups pecans, soaked for 4 hours, then rinsed

2 cups chopped cauliflower

$\frac{1}{2}$ inch fresh gingerroot

$\frac{1}{2}$ teaspoon Celtic salt

Combine all ingredients in a food processor and purée.

Olive Spread

Serve over zucchini pasta or as a dip.

Yield: 2 cups

$\frac{3}{4}$ cup walnuts, soaked overnight, then rinsed

1 cup pitted, chopped sun-cured olives

$\frac{1}{4}$ cup chopped celery

Combine the walnuts and olives in a food processor and purée. Stir the chopped celery into the mixture and serve.

Guacamole

This classic raw recipe can be served with slices of carrot, celery, jicama, or red pepper, or with your favorite raw crackers.

Yield: 1$\frac{1}{2}$ cups

2 avocados, pitted and peeled

1 tablespoon lemon juice

$\frac{1}{4}$ teaspoon Celtic salt

1 tomato, finely chopped

$\frac{1}{2}$ teaspoon Chili Powder (page 115)
or a chili powder of your choice

Mash the avocados with a fork. Add the remaining ingredients and mix well.

Salsa

Not only is this spicy blend a traditional accompaniment to Mexican food, but it is also bursting with antioxidants.

Yield: about 2 cups

5 tomatoes, chopped

1 clove garlic

$\frac{1}{2}$ cup chopped fresh cilantro

Juice of 1 lemon

2 scallions, chopped

$\frac{1}{2}$ teaspoon Celtic salt

1 teaspoon Chili Powder (page 115),
or a chili powder of your choice

Combine all ingredients in a bowl and mix well; or, if you prefer, combine all ingredients in a food processor, but pulse instead of puréeing to make sure the salsa's consistency stays chunky.

Hummus

Serve with raw vegetable chips.

Yield: about 2 $\frac{1}{2}$ cups

2 cups almonds,
soaked overnight, then rinsed

$\frac{2}{3}$ cup tahini

$\frac{1}{2}$ cup water

2 cloves garlic

Juice of 2 lemons

$\frac{1}{2}$ teaspoon Celtic salt

$\frac{1}{4}$ cup chopped fresh parsley

$\frac{1}{4}$ cup chopped fresh spearmint

Combine all ingredients in a food processor and purée.

Spinach Dip

Serve with sprouted crackers or vegetable chips. Invite a few friends over and watch this dip disappear.

Yield: about 2 cups

4 cups chopped spinach

$1/2$ cup tahini

1 tomato, chopped

$1/2$ cup chopped onion

3 tablespoons lemon juice

1 teaspoon Celtic salt

$1/2$ teaspoon nutmeg

Combine all ingredients in a blender or a food processor and purée.

Party-on Onion Dip

Serve with raw vegetable chips or flax crackers.

Yield: about 3 cups

2 cups Almond Cheese (page 143)

1 tablespoon miso

1 teaspoon garlic powder

3 teaspoons onion powder

$1/2$ –1 cup water (enough to make a diplike consistency)

$1/2$ teaspoon Celtic salt

Combine all ingredients and mix by hand or purée in a food processor, depending on the texture you prefer. Allow the dip to thicken for 1 hour before serving.

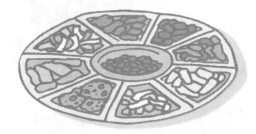

━━━ *Entrées* ━━━

These dishes can be enjoyed as the main event at lunches or dinners. Served with a salad or a vegetable side-dish, these entrées are filling, nutritious, and delicious. Meal preparation has never been so easy!

Nut "Meat" Balls

Serve with zucchini pasta and Tomato Sauce (page 205).

Yield: about 24 balls

$2/3$ cup walnuts, soaked overnight,
then rinsed

$2/3$ cup sunflower seeds,
soaked overnight, then rinsed

$2/3$ cup almonds, soaked overnight, then rinsed

1 teaspoon chopped fresh garlic

$1/2$ teaspoon Celtic salt

$1/4$ cup chopped fresh parsley

$1/4$ cup chopped celery

1 cup shiitake mushrooms (if dried,
soak for 2 hours first, then measure 1 cup)

$1/2$ cup water

1 inch fresh gingerroot

1 teaspoon chopped onion

2 teaspoons fresh rosemary
(or 1 teaspoon dried)

2 teaspoons fresh sage
(or 1 teaspoon dried)

$1/2$ teaspoon cumin seeds

$1/4$ cup extra-virgin olive oil

Combine all ingredients in a food processor and purée. Shape the mixture into about 24 small balls on solid dehydrator sheets and dehydrate for 8 hours, turning the balls regularly so they become crispy all around.

Lasagna

Serve this to company and they just might go raw themselves!

Yield: 6–8 servings

THE CHEESE

3 cups pine nuts

2 tablespoons tahini

1 tablespoon lemon juice

2 cloves garlic

1 tablespoon nutritional yeast
(optional; not a raw product)

THE VEGETABLES

4 cups spinach

4 zucchini

$\frac{1}{4}$ cup extra-virgin olive oil

1 tablespoon lemon juice

2 teaspoons fresh basil (or 1 teaspoon dried)

2 teaspoons fresh oregano (or 1 teaspoon dried)

$\frac{1}{4}$ teaspoon Celtic salt

$\frac{1}{4}$ teaspoon mustard powder

THE SAUCE

4 dates, soaked for 2 hours
(soak with the sun-dried tomatoes, below)

$1\frac{1}{2}$ cups sun-dried tomatoes, soaked for 2 hours

$1\frac{1}{2}$ cups chopped tomatoes

$\frac{1}{2}$ cup chopped fresh basil

2 tablespoons lemon juice

2 tablespoons extra-virgin olive oil

$\frac{1}{2}$ teaspoon Celtic salt

To make the cheese: Combine all ingredients in a food processor and purée. Spread the mixture about a half inch thick onto solid dehydrator sheets and dehydrate until firm (about 4 hours).

To prepare the vegetables: Wash and dry the spinach; set aside. Use a cheese slicer or mandoline to slice the zucchini horizontally into very thin, wide strips.

Combine the remaining ingredients from the "vegetables" list in a dish. Place the zucchini strips in the liquid mixture and let them marinate for 1 hour.

To make the sauce: Combine all sauce ingredients in a food processor and pulse until well blended but still chunky.

To finish: When all three components are ready, chop the spinach. Place a layer of the marinated zucchini on the bottom of a glass pan. Add patches of the cheese over it, followed by a layer of the chopped spinach and then a layer of the tomato sauce. Repeat the layering process until you have used up all the ingredients. Serve the lasagna fresh.

Rawvioli

So amazingly good! You can also use this recipe to make cannelloni;
just place a little filling on one end of a zucchini strip
and roll the zucchini up around it.

Yield: 6 servings

3 zucchini, sliced lengthwise into thin strips

1 cup pine nuts

1 cup young coconut meat
or an additional 1 cup pine nuts

2 tablespoons extra-virgin olive oil

2 tablespoons lemon juice

1 teaspoon Celtic salt

1 clove garlic

2 teaspoons fresh rosemary (or 1 teaspoon dried)

3 tablespoons chopped fresh basil

$\frac{1}{4}$ cup chopped fresh parsley

$\frac{1}{4}$ teaspoon ground black pepper

3 tablespoons water

Combine all ingredients except the zucchini in a food processor and blend. Place a spoonful of the mixture on half of a strip of zucchini and fold the zucchini over the filling, making a rectangle. Repeat with all the zucchini strips and all the filling. Place the stuffed zucchini rectangles on solid dehydrator sheets and dehydrate for 12 hours. Serve the rawvioli with a pesto or marinara sauce.

Vegetable Pot Pie

I often prepare this recipe in small, individual bowls as "pot tarts," adding the nut sauce as I serve each tart so everything stays crisp.

Yield: 6 servings

THE CRUST

1 cup pulp left over from making Almond Milk
(page 144)

1 tablespoon extra-virgin olive oil

½ teaspoon Celtic salt

THE FILLING

¼ cup each of chopped carrots, celery,
zucchini, spinach, and snow peas

THE SAUCE

½ cup pine nuts

1 cup water

To make the crust: Combine all crust ingredients and press the mixture into a glass pie plate. Place the pie plate in a dehydrator and dehydrate until the crust is dry (about 12 hours).

To make the filling: Place the chopped vegetables into the dehydrated crust.

To make the sauce: Combine all sauce ingredients in a blender or a food processor and purée.

To finish: When ready to serve, pour the sauce over the vegetables in the crust.

Nut Stuffing

For culinary accolades, serve this dish at your next holiday gathering.

Yield: about 15 servings

1 cup walnuts, soaked for 12 hours, then rinsed

1 cup pecans, soaked for 12 hours, then rinsed

1 cup almonds, soaked for 12 hours, then rinsed

1 cup hazelnuts/filberts, soaked for 12 hours, then rinsed

1 cup finely chopped onion

1 cup water

2 tablespoons fresh sage (or 1 tablespoon dried)

2 tablespoons fresh rosemary (or 1 tablespoon dried)

1 cup fresh parsley (or 2 tablespoons dried)

1 tablespoon Celtic salt

3 tablespoons flaxseeds, soaked in
6 tablespoons water for 15 minutes

Combine the walnuts, pecans, almonds, and hazelnuts/filberts in a food processor and grind them thoroughly. Pour the ground nuts into a bowl and mix in the remaining ingredients. Shape the mixture into two small, round loaves about $1/2$ inch thick on solid dehydrator sheets and dehydrate until crispy on one side (about 6 hours). Remove the dehydrator sheets, turn the loaves over onto the dehydrator tray, and continue dehydrating until both sides are crispy (about 4 more hours).

Nut Burgers

Aside from making a delicious burger meal, this mix can also be served as an appetizer in smaller pieces on sprouted bread, with Raw Ketchup (page 181) as a condiment.

Yield: about 12 burgers

1 cup pecans, soaked overnight, then rinsed

1 cup walnuts, soaked overnight, then rinsed

$1/2$ cup sunflower seeds, soaked overnight, then rinsed

1 onion, chopped

1 tablespoon miso or $1/2$ teaspoon Celtic salt

1 teaspoon Classic Herb Mix (page 115),
or a commercial poultry seasoning of your choice

$1/2$ cup sun-dried tomatoes, soaked for 2 hours

Combine all ingredients in a food processor and pulse until minced and thoroughly mixed. Shape the mixture into burger-sized patties on solid dehydrator sheets and dehydrate for 4 hours. Remove the dehydrator sheets, flip the patties over onto the dehydrator tray, and continue dehydrating for another 4 hours.

Savory Veggie Burgers

This mixture can be stuffed into peppers and tomatoes or used to top salads.

Yield: about 15 burgers

2 cups almonds, soaked overnight, then rinsed

4 dates, soaked for 20 minutes

2 cups chopped carrots

1 onion, sliced

1 tablespoon extra-virgin olive oil

2 tablespoons fresh sage
(or 1 tablespoon dried)

2 tablespoons fresh rosemary
(or 1 tablespoon dried)

1 teaspoon Celtic salt

3 tablespoons nutritional yeast (optional; not a raw product)

Combine all ingredients in a food processor and pulse until minced and thoroughly mixed. Shape the mixture into burger-sized patties and serve fresh. Alternatively, you can dehydrate the patties on solid dehydrator sheets for 4 hours, remove the dehydrator sheets, flip the patties over onto the dehydrator tray, and continue dehydrating for another 4 hours.

Sunburgers

Garnish with slices of tomato and parsley.

Yield: 4 servings

$\frac{1}{2}$ cup sunflower seeds, soaked overnight, then rinsed

1 cup pecans, soaked overnight, then rinsed

2 cups chopped cabbage

2 avocados, pitted and peeled

Combine all ingredients in a food processor and pulse until the mixture is minced and thoroughly mixed. Shape the mixture into patties and serve fresh.

Coconut Bacon

Coconut bacon is an excellent accompaniment to raw burgers. This recipe uses three condiments that are not raw; however, these condiments are used only in small amounts, and the result is so tasty it just might persuade meat-eaters to give up real bacon.

Yield: about 4 cups

Meat of 6 coconuts (best if the coconuts are mature and just past the "jelly" stage)

1 tablespoon liquid smoke (optional; not a raw product)

3 tablespoons nutritional yeast (optional; not a raw product)

1 tablespoon maple syrup (optional; not a raw product)

$\frac{1}{2}$ teaspoon Celtic salt

Cut the coconut meat into strips somewhat larger than traditional bacon strips. Place the strips in a bowl and add the remaining ingredients, stirring well. Dehydrate the strips on solid dehydrator sheets, turning the strips at least once, for about 24 hours or until crispy.

Roots Rock Reggae

For this recipe, thinly slice a variety of root vegetables such as carrots, sweet potatoes, onions, turnips, rutabagas, and parsnips.

Yield: 4 servings

6 cups chopped root vegetables

6 dates, soaked for 20 minutes

3 tablespoons Nama Shoyu

2 tablespoons extra-virgin olive oil

1 tablespoon chopped fresh rosemary

1 inch fresh gingerroot

Juice of $\frac{1}{2}$ lemon

Place the chopped root vegetables in a large bowl. Combine the remaining ingredients in a blender and purée. Pour the purée over the chopped roots and mix well. Place the mixture in a thin layer on solid dehydrator sheets and dehydrate for about 16 hours.

Pecan-Spinach Quiche

Raw quiche? You bet—and it won't clog your arteries.

Yield: 6 servings

2 cups pecans, soaked overnight, rinsed,
then dehydrated until crunchy (about 12 hours)

2 cups chopped spinach or wild greens

$\frac{1}{2}$ cup pine nuts

$\frac{1}{4}$ cup water

$\frac{1}{4}$ teaspoon nutmeg

$\frac{1}{2}$ teaspoon Celtic salt

2 tablespoons flaxseeds

Grind the pecans in a food processor. Press the ground pecans into a glass pie plate to form a crust. Combine the remaining ingredients in a food processor and purée. Pour the purée over the crust. Allow the quiche to set for 30 minutes before serving.

Holiday Mushroom Loaf

This loaf is just what you'll want for the holidays,
and is a sure reminder of childhood.

Yield: 8 servings

$1\frac{1}{2}$ cups almonds, soaked overnight, then rinsed

$1\frac{1}{2}$ cups pecans, soaked overnight, rinsed,
then dehydrated until crunchy (about 12 hours)

1 cup chopped fresh shiitake mushrooms (if dried, soak for 2 hours first)

1 tablespoon extra-virgin olive oil

1 teaspoon Celtic salt

1 tablespoon Classic Herb Mix (page 115),
or a commercial poultry seasoning of your choice

$\frac{1}{2} - \frac{3}{4}$ cup water

4 stalks celery, chopped

$\frac{1}{2}$ cup chopped onion

3 tablespoons flaxseeds, soaked in 6 tablespoons water for 15 minutes

Purée all of the ingredients, except the celery, onion, and soaked flaxseeds in a food processor until they are well ground. In a large bowl, combine the celery, onion, and flaxseeds with the rest of the ingredients and mix well. Shape the mixture into a shallow loaf on a solid dehydrator sheet and dehydrate for 12 hours.

Pasta Primarawva

Even hardcore fans of Italian food
will find this dish delicious and satisfying.

Yield: 2–4 servings

2 yellow squash

$\frac{1}{2}$ cup sun-dried tomatoes, soaked for 2 hours

3 tablespoons extra-virgin olive oil

1 tomato, chopped

$\frac{1}{2}$ cup sun-cured olives, pitted

$\frac{1}{4}$ cup chopped fresh basil

$\frac{1}{4}$ cup chopped fresh parsley

$\frac{1}{4}$ cup pine nuts

$\frac{1}{2}$ teaspoon Celtic salt

Slice the squash into long, thin noodles, or use a Spiralizer to "spiralize" it; set it aside. Combine the remaining ingredients in a food processor and pulse until well blended but still chunky. Toss the sauce with the squash noodles and serve.

Vegetable Pasta

A kitchen tool called a Spiralizer makes it easy to cut long, thin, angelhair pasta or flat, wide noodles from just about any kind of sturdy vegetable. Try making vegetable pasta from zucchini, yellow squash, rutabagas, daikon radishes, beets, carrots, or turnips. My friend Coco likes to "spiralize" sweet potato and then dehydrate it to make crunchy noodles as a topping for Asian dishes.

NoodleRoni and Cheese

When Rainbeau was pregnant, she craved macaroni and cheese.
Wanting to help her stay raw, we came up with this comfort food.

Yield: 2 servings

2 cups pine nuts or macadamia nuts

1 cup water

$\frac{1}{2}$ cup light (yellow or white) miso

$\frac{1}{2}$ cup sundried tomatoes,
soaked for 2 hours

2 teaspoons cumin

2 teaspoons tumeric

$\frac{1}{2}$ teaspoon Celtic salt

6 cups sunflower "grass"
cut into bite-sized pieces

Place nuts, water, miso, tomatoes, and spices in the blender and blend till smooth. Pour over bite-sized sunflower grass. Stir.

Buttered Noodles

Simple summer squash garnished with fine olive oil
and spices makes a satisfying repast.

Yield: 2–4 servings

4 cups zucchini pasta
(see "Vegetable Pasta" on page 203)

$\frac{1}{4}$ cup extra-virgin olive oil

$\frac{1}{2}$ teaspoon Celtic salt

$\frac{1}{4}$ cup pine nuts

$\frac{1}{4}$ cup chopped fresh parsley

Combine all ingredients in a large bowl and toss well.

Tomato Sauce

You can use this sauce on pasta or pizza.

Yield: 3 cups

$1/2$ cup sun-dried tomatoes,
soaked for 2 hours

3 dates, soaked for 20 minutes

4 large tomatoes

3 tablespoons extra-virgin olive oil

$1/4$ cup chopped fresh basil

2 cloves garlic

1 teaspoon aniseeds or fennel seeds

1 teaspoon Celtic salt

Combine all ingredients in a food processor and pulse until well mixed but still chunky.

Alfrawdo Sauce

Serve on vegetable pasta or pizza.

Yield: 4 servings

2 cups macadamia nuts,
soaked for 4 hours, then rinsed

$1/2$ cup pine nuts

2 cloves garlic

2 tablespoons lemon juice

$1 1/2$ cups water

$1/2$ teaspoon ground black pepper

2 teaspoons Celtic salt

1 teaspoon chopped fresh basil

Combine all ingredients in a blender or food processor and purée until smooth.

Pizza

*You can feel great about eating this pizza! I like to top it with
Almond Cheese (page 143), chopped basil, sun-dried tomatoes,
sun-cured olives, tomato slices, avocado slices, oregano, pine nuts,
edible flowers, and marinated eggplant or mushrooms.*

Yield: 6–8 servings

1½ cups buckwheat, sprouted 2–3 days using the jar method

¼ cup extra-virgin olive oil

⅔ cup chopped zucchini

2 tablespoons fresh basil (or 1 tablespoon dried)

2 tablespoons fresh oregano (or 1 tablespoon dried)

2 tablespoons fresh rosemary (or 1 tablespoon dried)

1 teaspoon Celtic salt

2 cloves garlic

⅔ cup flaxseeds, soaked in 1⅓ cups water for 15 minutes

Tomato Sauce (page 205), Herb Pesto (see below),
or Alfrawdo Sauce (page 205)

Toppings of your choice

Combine all ingredients except the flaxseeds in a food processor and purée.
Pour the purée into a bowl, add the flaxseeds, and mix well. Shape the mixture
into 2 large, round pizza crusts on solid dehydrator sheets and dehydrate for
7–8 hours or until crispy on one side. Remove the dehydrator sheets, turn the
pizza crusts over onto the dehydrator tray, and continue dehydrating for
another 7–8 hours or until dry. Spread a sauce of your choice over the crusts
and add any desired toppings.

The pizza crusts keep well, simply wrapped in an airtight bag for several weeks.
Once garnished, however, they are best eaten immediately.

Herb Pesto

Serve over vegetable pasta or a raw pizza crust.

Yield: 4–6 servings

1 cup pine nuts or walnuts, soaked overnight, then rinsed

3 cups chopped fresh basil (or arugula, young catnip, cilantro,
lemon balm, marjoram, parsley, rosemary, or sage)

5 cloves garlic

$3/4$ cup extra-virgin olive oil

1 teaspoon Celtic salt

Combine all ingredients in a blender or a food processor and purée until smooth.

Olive Pesto

Serve over vegetable pasta or on dehydrated crackers.

Yield: 2 servings

$1/2$ cup sun-cured black olives, pitted

$1/4$ cup chopped fresh basil

1 tablespoon lemon juice

1 tablespoon extra-virgin olive oil

$1/2$ teaspoon Chili Powder (page 115) or a chili powder of your choice

Combine all ingredients in a blender or a food processor and pulse until well blended but chunky.

Wild Thing Pesto

*I had been an herbalist a long time before I realized
how easy—and delicious—it is to eat raw nettles. This won't sting.*

Yield: $2 1/2$ cups

1 cup pine nuts or walnuts, soaked overnight, then rinsed

1 cup extra-virgin olive oil

7 cloves garlic

4 cups chopped nettles

$1/2$ teaspoon Celtic salt

Combine all ingredients in a blender or a food processor and pulse until the mixture has a pastelike consistency. Serve the pesto over fresh zucchini pasta or with dehydrated crackers.

Enchiladas

This raw version of a traditional Mexican dish is outstanding.
Serve it to dinner guests who are not accustomed
to raw food—they'll be amazed!

Yield: 8 servings

THE WRAPPING

8 cabbage leaves

THE FILLING

Kernels of 2 ears of corn

2 cups shredded zucchini or yellow squash

1 cup chopped fresh cilantro

2 tomatoes, chopped

2 avocados, pitted, peeled, and chopped

1 teaspoon Chili Powder (page 115),
or a chili powder of your choice

$\frac{1}{2}$ teaspoon Celtic salt

2 chopped red peppers

THE SAUCE

$\frac{1}{4}$ cup sun-dried tomatoes,
soaked in $\frac{1}{2}$ cup water for 2 hours

$\frac{1}{4}$ cup chopped tomato

1 tablespoon extra-virgin olive oil

$\frac{1}{2}$ teaspoon Celtic salt

To make the wrapping: Wash and pat dry the cabbage leaves.

To make the filling: In a large bowl, combine all filling ingredients and mix well.

To make the sauce: Place the sun-dried tomatoes in a food processor and purée. Pour the purée into a small bowl and stir in the remaining sauce ingredients.

To finish: Place a generous handful of the filling in the center of each cabbage leaf, and roll the cabbage leaf securely around it. Pour the sauce over the enchiladas and serve.

Flaxseed Burrito

*This surprisingly simple and delicious recipe
was inspired by Elaina Love Joy.*

Yield: 4 servings

4 large cabbage or lettuce leaves

1 cup whole flaxseeds, soaked in enough water to cover
in a glass baking dish for 48 hours (in warm conditions,
place the dish in the refrigerator after the first 12 hours)

2 cloves garlic

$\frac{1}{4}$ cup sun-dried tomatoes, soaked 2 hours

$\frac{1}{4}$ teaspoon Celtic salt

1 teaspoon Chili Powder (page 115), or a chili powder of your choice

Guacamole (page 192)

Salsa (page 193)

Wash and pat dry the cabbage or lettuce leaves; set them aside. Combine the garlic, tomatoes, salt, and Chili Powder in a food processor and purée. Stir the flaxseeds into the purée. Place one-quarter of the mixture on each cabbage or lettuce leaf and top with Guacamole and Salsa. Fold each leaf over the toppings and serve.

Spanish Rice

*This is a wonderful side dish to a Mexican-themed meal,
or enjoy it on its own.*

Yield: 2–4 servings

2 cups grated jicama

Kernels of 3 ears of corn

2 tomatoes, chopped

$\frac{1}{2}$ cup chopped fresh cilantro

1 clove minced garlic

$\frac{1}{4}$ cup extra-virgin olive oil or 1 avocado, pitted, peeled, and chopped

1 teaspoon Celtic salt

Combine the grated Jicama with the remaining ingredients and mix well.

Falafel Balls

This recipe is an example of the best of ethnic cuisine converted to raw form. Serve with Tahini Dressing (page 166).

Yield: 6 servings

$3/4$ cup almonds, soaked overnight, then rinsed

$3/4$ cup pecans, soaked overnight, then rinsed

$1/2$ cup sesame seeds

$1/4$ cup chopped fresh parsley

$1/4$ cup chopped fresh cilantro

$1/4$ teaspoon ground black pepper

2 tablespoons lemon juice

1 teaspoon cumin seeds

1 teaspoon Celtic salt

$1/4$ cup water

Combine all ingredients in a food processor and purée. Shape the purée into 1-inch-wide, $1/2$-inch-high patties on solid dehydrator sheets and dehydrate until crispy on both sides, turning the patties over when the top is crispy (8–12 hours total).

Vegetable Kabobs

So delicious—the mushrooms will satisfy even a meat-eater's cravings.

Yield: 20 kabobs

1 eggplant, peeled and cubed

2 small zucchini, cubed

1 box cherry tomatoes (about 36 tomatoes)

24 shiitake mushrooms (if dried, soak for 2 hours first)

$1/2$ cup extra-virgin olive oil

$1/2$ cup Nama Shoyu

3 dates, soaked for 20 minutes

1 tablespoon chopped fresh rosemary

Place the vegetables in a shallow glass pan. Combine the oil, tamari, and dates in a blender and blend until mixed. Stir the rosemary into the mixture. Pour the sauce over the vegetables and let the dish marinate in the refrigerator for 1 hour. Place the vegetables on skewers and set them on solid dehydrator sheets. Pour the leftover marinade over the skewered vegetables and dehydrate for 12 hours.

Chile Rellenos

These rich, nut-filled bell peppers are great Mexican-style fare. Try topping them with a dollop of Almond Cheese (page 143) before serving.

Yield: 2–4 servings

2 red peppers

1 cup walnuts, soaked overnight, then rinsed

1 cup almonds, soaked overnight, then rinsed

1 cup sun-dried tomatoes, soaked for 2 hours

1 clove garlic

$\frac{1}{2}$ teaspoon Celtic salt

1 teaspoon cumin seeds

2 teaspoons Chili Powder (page 115), or a chili powder of your choice

$\frac{1}{2}$ cup chopped onion

Cut each pepper in half, scoop out the inside, and cut each half into three equal pieces. Combine the remaining ingredients in a food processor and purée. Stuff each pepper slice with the purée, place on solid dehydrator sheets, and dehydrate for 5–6 hours or until the nut filling becomes dry on top.

Kitcheree

This nicely spiced recipe takes the place of Indian rice and vegetables.

Yield: 4 servings

1 cup shredded cabbage

1 small rutabaga, grated

$\frac{1}{2}$ cup chopped fresh basil

$\frac{1}{2}$ cup chopped fresh cilantro

2 teaspoons freshly ground cumin seeds

$\frac{1}{2}$ teaspoon turmeric

$\frac{1}{2}$ teaspoon coriander

$\frac{1}{4}$ teaspoon mustard seeds

$\frac{1}{8}$ teaspoon cayenne powder

$\frac{1}{2}$ teaspoon Celtic salt

$\frac{1}{8}$ cup coconut oil

In a large bowl, combine all ingredients and mix well. Serve the kitcheree with Palak (see below).

Palak (Creamed Spinach Curry)

If I couldn't have Indian food, the raw life would be a real challenge.

Yield: 4 servings

$\frac{1}{2}$ cup macadamia nuts, soaked 4 hours, then rinsed

2 tablespoons lemon juice

2 tablespoons coconut oil

1 inch fresh gingerroot

2 cloves garlic

4 cups chopped spinach

$\frac{1}{2}$ teaspoon Celtic salt

$\frac{1}{2}$ teaspoon nutmeg

1 teaspoon Curry Powder (page 116), or a curry powder of your choice

$\frac{1}{4}$ cup chopped onion

Combine all ingredients in a food processor and purée.

Tandoori Nut Balls

*Here's a recipe that brings crispiness to the table
without all the fat of deep frying.*

Yield: 4 servings

1 cup walnuts, soaked overnight, then rinsed

1 cup almonds, soaked overnight, then rinsed

1/2 cup sun-dried tomatoes, soaked for 2 hours

1/2 teaspoon Celtic salt

1 tablespoon Curry Powder (page 116), or a curry powder of your choice

1/2 cup chopped onion

1 red pepper, chopped

Combine all ingredients except the onion and red pepper in a food processor
and purée. Stir the onion and pepper into the purée. Shape the mixture into
1-inch balls on solid dehydrator sheets and dehydrate, turning the balls every
3 hours, until they are crisp on the outside (about 12–15 hours).

Spring Green Rolls

*Serve with a bit of Mustard Sauce (page 188)
and Sweet and Sour Sauce (page 187).*

Yield: 8 servings

8 collard green leaves, washed and cut in half
(strip away the middle stem)

2 avocados, pitted, peeled, and finely chopped

1 cup shredded carrots

1 cup chopped red pepper

1 cup almond butter

1/2 cup chopped fresh cilantro

1/2 cup chopped fresh basil

Lay the collard leaf halves on a plate. In a medium-sized bowl, combine the
remaining ingredients and mix well. Place a large spoonful of the mixture on the
end of each leaf, taking care to divide the mixture evenly among the leaves. Roll
up each leaf around its filling and serve.

Not Fried Rice

With this recipe, you'll never crave cooked fried rice again.

Yield: 6 servings

$\frac{1}{4}$ cup almonds, soaked overnight, then rinsed

1 peeled, riced jicama ("riced" means run through the
fine blade of a food processor so the result looks like rice;
see "Vegetable Pasta" on page 203)

2 tablespoons extra-virgin olive oil

$\frac{1}{2}$ cup chopped snow peas

2 tablespoons chopped fresh basil

2 tablespoons chopped fresh cilantro

$\frac{1}{4}$ cup chopped shiitake mushrooms
(if dried, soak for 2 hours first then measure $\frac{1}{4}$ cup)

$\frac{1}{2}$ teaspoon grated fresh gingerroot

1 tablespoon Nama Shoyu

Combine all ingredients in a bowl, mix well, and enjoy.

Oriental Noodles

*These vegetables taste like noodles with peanut sauce,
but without the aflatoxins!*

Yield: 4 servings

1 cup tahini

$\frac{1}{2}$ cup dates, soaked for 20 minutes

1 cup orange juice

$\frac{1}{2}$ cup Nama Shoyu

$\frac{1}{2}$ inch chopped or grated fresh gingerroot

4 daikon radishes, spiralized into wide noodles

1 cup snow peas, ends removed

$\frac{1}{4}$ cup sesame seeds

Combine the tahini, dates, orange juice, tamari, and gingerroot in a food
processor and purée. Pour the purée over the daikon strips. Stir the snow
peas into the mixture. Garnish the dish with the sesame seeds.

Asian Noodle Bowl

This dish is a cross between a soup and an entrée.
Serve it topped with a few chopped scallions.

Yield: 2–4 servings

4 cups water

2 teaspoons miso

1 tablespoon Nama Shoyu

$\frac{1}{2}$ teaspoon finely grated fresh gingerroot

1 cup finely shredded cabbage

2 small, slivered or "spiralized" yellow squash
("spiralized" means cut into strips with a Spiralizer)

$\frac{1}{4}$ cup chopped fresh cilantro

Combine the water and miso in a blender and purée. Combine this broth with the remaining ingredients in a large bowl and mix well.

Coconut Crisps

These crunchy noodles make a delicious topping for any
Thai, Indian, or other Asian dish.

Yield: about 5 cups

8 cups young coconut meat,
sliced into $\frac{1}{2}$-inch-thick noodles

$\frac{1}{4}$ cup Nama Shoyu

1 tablespoon Curry Powder (page 116),
or a curry powder of your choice

$\frac{1}{2}$ teaspoon cayenne powder

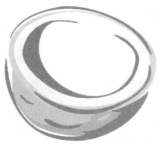

Combine all ingredients and stir to mix. Place the mixture in a thin layer on solid dehydrator sheets and dehydrate, turning the noodles over at least once, until crispy (about 24 hours).

Better-Than-Crab Cakes

This recipe has become one of our family favorites.
Try the cakes with Red Pepper Sauce (page 186).

Yield: about 15 patties

1 red pepper, chopped

1 zucchini or yellow squash, chopped

1 cup chopped carrots

1 cup chopped snow peas

1 1/2 cups pine nuts

3/4 cup almonds, soaked overnight

1 tablespoon fresh gingerroot

1/2 teaspoon Celtic salt

1/2 cup chopped fresh cilantro

1/2 cup water

Combine the red pepper, zucchini or squash, carrots, and snow peas in a food processor fitted with a shredding blade, and pulse until grated and mixed. Remove the mixture to a separate bowl. Combine the pine nuts, almonds, gingerroot, salt, cilantro, and water in the food processor, now fitted with an S-blade, and purée. Stir the purée into the grated vegetables. Shape the mixture into 1/2-inch-thick patties on solid dehydrator sheets and dehydrate until dry, turning the patties over when they are dry on top (about 12 hours total).

Samosas

This raw version of the deep-fried pastries offered
in Indian restaurants has a zesty spicy flavor.

Yield: 8 servings

2 cups walnuts, soaked overnight, rinsed,
then dehydrated until crunchy (about 12 hours)

2 cups chopped cauliflower

1 sweet potato, peeled and chopped

1/2 onion, chopped

1 zucchini, chopped

Juice of 1 lemon

2 teaspoons Curry Powder (page 116),
or a curry powder of your choice

1 teaspoon Celtic salt

2 cloves garlic

$\frac{1}{8}$ teaspoon cayenne powder

$\frac{1}{2}$ cup water

1 cup snow peas, each cut in thirds horizontally,
or 1 cup organic, frozen peas

Place the walnuts in a food processor and pulse until powdered; set aside. Place the remaining ingredients except the peas in the food processor and purée. Add the peas to the purée and stir. Shape the mixture into 8 round or 8 triangle shapes. Coat the shapes in the powdered walnuts, place them on solid dehydrator sheets, and dehydrate for about 12 hours, turning when dry on one side.

Thai Vegetables

It takes less time to make this dish than to fetch Thai take-out.

Yield: 6 servings

2 cups chopped purple cabbage

2 cups chopped white cabbage

2 cups chopped cauliflower

$\frac{1}{2}$ cup cilantro

1 avocado, pitted, peeled, and chopped

1 inch grated fresh gingerroot

1 clove garlic

1 tablespoon grated organic orange peel

4 tablespoons maple syrup (not a raw product),
or 2 tablespoons honey diluted in 1 tablespoon water

4 tablespoons Nama Shoyu

$\frac{1}{4}$ cup extra-virgin olive oil

A dash of cayenne powder

Combine all ingredients in a large bowl and toss. Top the dish with grated coconut (fresh or dried) or raw macadamia nuts, if desired.

Pad Thai

Don't feel guilty that this is so delicious to eat yet so easy to make.

Yield: 4 servings

THE NOODLES

2 cups white cabbage

2 cups purple cabbage

2 cups noodlelike slivers of young coconut meat

$\frac{1}{2}$ cup chopped fresh cilantro

$\frac{1}{2}$ cup chopped fresh basil

THE SAUCE

1 inch fresh gingerroot

6 dates, soaked for 20 minutes

2 tablespoons tamarind paste (soaked for 20 minutes in
3 tablespoons water; do not drain), or lemon juice or lime juice

2 tablespoons Nama Shoyu

$\frac{1}{2}$ cup orange juice

$\frac{1}{4}$ teaspoon cayenne

$\frac{1}{4}$ cup tahini or almond butter

$\frac{1}{2}$ cup cashews or pine nuts, as garnish

Hand chop or use the large blade on the food processor to grate the cabbage.

To make the base: Combine coconut, cabbage, and herbs in a large bowl and toss.

To make the sauce: Combine all sauce ingredients in a blender or food processor and purée.

To finish: Pour the sauce over the coconut and cabbage noodles and garnish with nuts.

Nori Rolls

See pages 190–192 for some great pâté recipes to use in these nori rolls. Avoid wet fillings, as they make the rolls somewhat slimy.

Yield: 1 serving per filled nori sheet

Nori seaweed sheets

Pâté of choice

Fillings of choice

Fill one end of a nori sheet with a line of pâté, add a few other filling ingredients, and roll the sheet up. When it is rolled, wet the edge of the nori sheet on the side that goes underneath the roll and press it together to close.

Tasty Nori Roll Fillings

Nori rolls can serve as a raw sandwich—a meal in itself. They can also be sliced into bite-sized rounds as hor d'oeurves for parties. Here are some tasty fillings:

chopped avocado	pitted sun-cured olives	wild greens	fresh cilantro
chopped onions	grated fresh gingerroot	sprouts	grated beets
grated carrots	red pepper slices	fresh basil	

Raw-Style Ribs

My relatives from the South love this dish!

Yield: 6 servings

2 cups walnuts, soaked overnight, then rinsed

2 cups pecans, soaked overnight, then rinsed

1 cup sunflower seeds, soaked overnight, then rinsed

1 cup sun-dried tomatoes, soaked for 2 hours

1 onion, finely chopped

1 tablespoon miso

2 teaspoons cumin seeds

1 teaspoon Celtic salt

$\frac{1}{2}$ cup water

Barbecue Sauce (page 181)

Combine all ingredients except the Barbecue Sauce in a food processor and purée. Shape the purée into 6 burger-sized patties, place them on solid dehydrator sheets, brush them with Barbecue Sauce, and dehydrate for 4 hours. Turn the patties, brush them with Barbecue Sauce, and continue dehydrating for another 4 hours.

The Better-Than-Bread
Unbakery

Many people who try to initiate a diet of almost any kind, whether for weight loss or just plain health improvement, find that bread is a constant temptation and a sure obstacle to the desired goal. Baked bread, being very starchy, contributes to carbohydrate overload and blood sugar spikes. Breads made from unsprouted wheat, rye, oats, and barley also contain gluten, a common allergen.

The recipes that follow, however, offer tasty raw alternatives to baked bread. These unbaked goods can be served with meals, broken into pieces for dipping, or used to make raw sandwiches.

Nut Pyramids

These pyramids make a great party snack,
lunch, or travel food.

Yield: about 40 pyramids

2 cups almonds or hazelnuts/filberts,
soaked overnight, then rinsed

1 large tomato, cut into fourths

2 stalks celery, cut into thirds

1 carrot, cut into thirds

$1/4$ cup chopped onion

2 tablespoons fresh rosemary (or 1 tablespoon dried)

2 tablespoons fresh sage (or 1 tablespoon dried)

1 teaspoon Curry Powder (page 116),
or a curry powder of your choice

$1/2$ teaspoon Celtic salt

2 tablespoons lemon juice

6 sheets nori seaweed

Combine all ingredients except the nori in a food processor and purée; set aside. Cut the nori sheets into triangles (approximately 6 triangles from a sheet). Place a spoonful of the filling on half of the triangles. Cover each with another triangle and press down lightly on the cover triangles so they'll stick securely. Place the pyramids on solid dehydrator sheets and dehydrate overnight. Store the pyramids in an airtight container, where they will keep for several weeks (even unrefrigerated).

Flax Crackers

I once threw a soggy flax cracker out in the yard,
and it grew into hundreds of flax plants. Now that's live food!

Yield: 2–3 trays of crackers

2 cups flaxseeds

4 cups water

$\frac{1}{4}$ cup dried kelp

Soak the flaxseeds in the water for 15 minutes. Stir the dried kelp into the water and seeds. Spread the mixture onto 2–3 solid dehydrator sheets and dehydrate for 4 hours. Remove the dehydrator sheets, flip the crackers over onto the dehydrator tray, and continue dehydrating until they are crisp (about 4–6 more hours). Break crackers into pieces as needed. When dry, these crackers will keep indefinitely.

Variations on Flax Crackers

Any of the following ingredients can be substituted for kelp in the Flax Crackers recipe:

Basil (1 tablespoon)	Cilantro (1 tablespoon)
Celtic salt (1 teaspoon)	Cinnamon (1 teaspoon)
Chili powder (1 tablespoon)	Corn kernels ($\frac{1}{4}$ cup)
Chives (1 tablespoon)	Garlic (1 tablespoon)
Chopped onions ($\frac{1}{4}$ cup)	Raisins ($\frac{1}{4}$ cup)
Chopped red peppers ($\frac{1}{4}$ cup)	Sliced apples ($\frac{1}{4}$ cup)
Chopped tomatoes ($\frac{1}{4}$ cup)	Sliced bananas ($\frac{1}{4}$ cup)

Chapatis

Enjoy these crisps as an accompaniment to Indian dishes.

Yield: about 15 chapatis

2 cups almonds, soaked overnight, then rinsed

$1/2$ cup chopped fresh cilantro

1 teaspoon cumin seeds

3 dates, soaked for 20 minutes

1 teaspoon coriander seeds

1 teaspoon Celtic salt

Combine all ingredients in a food processor and purée. Shape the purée into flat, 3-inch rounds on solid dehydrator sheets and dehydrate for 6 hours. Remove the dehydrator sheets, turn the chapatis over onto the dehydrator tray, and continue dehydrating for another 6 hours.

Corn Chips

You'll want plenty of these chips on hand
for guacamole and other raw dips.

Yield: 2 dozen chips

1 cup sunflower seeds, soaked overnight, then rinsed

Kernels of 6 ears of corn

$1/2$ teaspoon Celtic salt

1 teaspoon Chili Powder (page 115),
or a chili powder of your choice

2 tablespoon flaxseeds,
soaked in 4 tablespoons water for 15 minutes

$1/2$ cup water

Combine all ingredients except the flaxseeds in a blender or food processor and purée. Stir in the flaxseeds. Drop the mixture by the spoonful onto solid dehydrator sheets in thin, flat, 4-inch rounds (flatten them with the back of the spoon, if necessary) and dehydrate until the chips are crisp on one side. Turn the chips over and continue dehydrating until they are dry on the other side (12–15 total hours).

Berry Good Scones

Bring a couple of these scones to school or work—
and bring an extra to share, because you'll need it.

Yield: 24 scones

2 cups buckwheat, sprouted 3 days using the jar method

2 peeled bananas

$3/4$ cup dates, soaked for 20 minutes

1 teaspoon cinnamon

$1/2$ teaspoon cardamom

1 teaspoon vanilla extract (optional; not a raw product)

1 cup blueberries

Combine all ingredients except the blueberries in a food processor and blend. Stir the blueberries into the mixture. Drop the mixture in scone shapes (rounded triangles) onto solid dehydrator sheets and dehydrate for 4 hours. Remove the dehydrator sheets, turn the scones over onto the dehydrator tray, and continue dehydrating for another 4 hours or until dry.

Apple-Raisin Scones

Better than doughnuts!

Yield: about 20 scones

4 cups buckwheat, sprouted 3 days using the jar method

1 cup dates, soaked for 20 minutes

1 teaspoon vanilla extract (optional; not a raw product)

2 apples, cored and sliced

1 cup raisins, soaked for 20 minutes

Place all ingredients except the raisins in a food processor and purée. Stir the raisins into the purée. Shape the mixture into rounds $1/2$-inch high and about 3 inches in diameter on solid dehydrator sheets and dehydrate for 4 hours. Remove the dehydrator sheets, turn the scones over onto the dehydrator tray, and continue dehydrating for another 6–8 hours or until the scones are dry on top.

Corn Bread

This bread is dense and filling.
Serve it sliced as an accompaniment to raw soups.

Yield: 2 loaves

2 cups spring wheat, soaked overnight, rinsed,
drained, sprouted 1 day using the jar method,
then dehydrated until crispy (about 12 hours)

2 cups buckwheat, sprouted 4 days
(using the jar method), dehydrated until crispy
(about 12 hours), then powdered into flour

1 cup pine nuts

$\frac{3}{4}$ cup water

1 teaspoon Celtic salt

$\frac{1}{4}$ cup extra-virgin olive oil

$\frac{1}{4}$ cup water

1 tablespoon Chili Powder (page 115),
or a chili powder of your choice

2 cups corn kernels

Combine all ingredients except the corn in a food processor and purée. Pour
the purée into a large bowl and stir the corn into it. Spread the mixture $\frac{1}{3}$-inch
thick on solid dehydrator sheets and dehydrate until the bread is dry on one
side. Remove the dehydrator sheets, turn the bread over onto the dehydrator
tray, and continue dehydrating until both sides are dry (about 15 total hours).

Tostadas

It's worth keeping these tostadas on hand—
it takes just a few minutes to cover them with
pâté and fresh vegetables for a quick lunch.

Yield: about 20 tostadas

1 cup flaxseeds

4 cups water

1 tomato

Kernels of 4 ears of corn

1 red pepper, chopped

1 teaspoon cumin seeds

$\frac{1}{4}$ cup chopped fresh cilantro

$\frac{1}{2}$ teaspoon Celtic salt

$\frac{1}{2}$ onion, chopped

Soak the flaxseeds in the water for 15 minutes; set aside. Combine the remaining ingredients in a food processor and purée. Stir the flaxseeds into the purée. Pour the mixture in 8-inch rounds onto solid dehydrator sheets and dehydrate until the rounds are dry on one side (about 6 hours). Remove the dehydrator sheets, turn the tostadas over onto the dehydrator tray, and continue dehydrating until they are dry on the other side (4–6 more hours).

Garlic Toast

Yes, it's true: garlic bread is still on the menu, even with a raw diet.

Yield: 24 rounds

3 cups almond pulp left over from
making Almond Milk (page 143)

1 cup flaxseeds, soaked in 2 cups water
for 15 minutes

$\frac{1}{4}$ cup extra-virgin olive oil

$\frac{1}{2}$ teaspoon Celtic salt

$\frac{1}{4}$ cup chopped garlic

$\frac{1}{4}$ cup chopped fresh basil

2 tablespoons fresh rosemary
(or 1 tablespoon dried)

$\frac{1}{2}$ cup water

Combine all ingredients in a bowl and mix well. Mold the mixture into rounds $\frac{1}{4}$-inch thick on solid dehydrator sheets and dehydrate until the rounds are dry on one side. Remove the dehydrator sheets, turn the rounds over onto the dehydrator tray, and continue dehydrating until the toast is crisp on both sides (12–15 total hours).

Almond Crackers

Simple, elegant, and golden.

Yield: 24 crackers

6 tablespoons flaxseeds

12 tablespoons water

2 cups almonds, soaked overnight,
or 2 cups almond pulp left over from
making Almond Milk (page 144)

1 cup chopped carrots

1 teaspoon Celtic salt

$\frac{1}{2}$ cup chopped onion

$\frac{1}{2}$ cup water

Soak the flaxseeds in the water for 15 minutes. The seeds will soak up this water and will not need to be drained. Combine the remaining ingredients in a blender or food processor and purée. Stir the flaxseeds and the soak water into the purée. Drop the mixture in 3-inch, flat rounds onto solid dehydrator sheets and dehydrate until the rounds are crisp on one side. Remove the dehydrator sheets, turn the crackers over onto the dehydrator tray, and continue dehydrating until they are crisp on both sides (12–15 total hours).

Almond Shortbread

Rich and raw.

Yield: 2 large sheets

4 cups almond pulp left over from
making Almond Milk (page 143)

$\frac{1}{2}$ cup coconut oil

1 cup flaxseeds, soaked in 2 cups water for 15 minutes

$\frac{1}{2}$ cup dates, soaked for 20 minutes

1 inch fresh gingerroot

1 teaspoon cinnamon

$\frac{1}{2}$ teaspoon cardamom

1 teaspoon Celtic salt

Combine all ingredients (except the flaxseeds) in a food processor and purée. Stir in the flaxseeds. Press the purée into 2 square or round loaves, $^1/_2$-inch thick, on solid dehydrator sheets and dehydrate for 4 hours. Flip the shortbread over on the dehydrator sheets and continue dehydrating for another 4 hours or until it is crisp on both sides.

Essene Bread

This bread can be made with a multitude of possible ingredients.

Yield: 2 loaves

2 cups grain (kamut, rye, spelt, wheat, or a combination thereof), sprouted using the jar method

1 cup grated vegetables (beets, cabbages, carrots, peeled jicama, or peeled sweet potatoes)

$^3/_4$ cup chopped onion (or apples, raisins, dates, sunflower seeds, sesame seeds, or tomatoes)

2 tablespoons seasoning (something that complements the other ingredients, such as cinnamon for apples, basil for tomatoes, rosemary for sesame seeds, or caraway for rye and sunflower seeds)

Combine all ingredients in a food processor and purée. Shape the purée into 2 round loaves, no higher than $^3/_4$ inch, on solid dehydrator sheets and dehydrate until the top crust is dry. Remove the dehydrator sheets, turn the loaves over onto the dehydrator tray, and continue dehydrating until both sides of the loaves are dry (15–20 total hours).

Sandwich Ideas

You can make raw sandwiches using dehydrated, sprouted-grain breads, green wraps (romaine lettuce, kale, and collard greens work well), or hollowed-out tomatoes or peppers that you can stuff. My favorite sandwich fillings include:

Sprouts	Avocados	Avocados and tomatoes
Tahini	Hazelnut/filbert butter	Almond butter
Cucumbers	Honey and bananas	Almond butter (and dates or jam)

Take-It-with-You Bar

An ideal food for the road or the lunchbox.

Yield: 10 bars

1 cup almonds, soaked overnight, then rinsed

$\frac{1}{2}$ cup raisins, soaked for 20 minutes

2 apples, cored and chopped

Combine all ingredients in a food processor and purée. Shape the purée into blocks (about the size of traditional granola bars) on solid dehydrator sheets and dehydrate for 6 hours. Remove the dehydrator sheets, flip the bars over onto the dehydrator tray, and continue dehydrating for another 6 hours or until the bars are dry on both sides.

On-the-Road-Again Bars

Like the bars from the previous recipe, these travel well.

Yield: 10 bars

1 cup hazelnuts/filberts,
soaked for 12 hours or overnight, then rinsed

$\frac{1}{2}$ cup dried apricots, soaked for 4 hours

10 dates, soaked for 20 minutes

2 cups chopped, cored apples

$\frac{1}{4}$ cup water, if needed for moisture

Combine all ingredients in a food processor and pulse until well blended but still chunky. Shape the mixture into blocks (about the size of traditional granola bars) on solid dehydrator sheets and dehydrate, flipping the bars over when they are dry on one side (about 10 total hours).

═══ ᗪesserts ═══

For some folks, desserts are reserved for occasional treats and celebrations. Others enjoy them often, especially when new to the raw life. Even so, no matter which you prefer, these raw desserts are more nutritious than what many Westerners eat for an entrée.

▰▰▰▰▰ _Nutty Fruitcake_ ▰▰▰▰▰

This is the kind of fruitcake you'll actually want to eat and share with others.

Yield: 12 servings

2 cups almonds, soaked overnight, rinsed,
then dehydrated until crunchy (about 12 hours)

2 cups hazelnuts/filberts, soaked overnight, rinsed,
then dehydrated until crunchy (about 12 hours)

2 cups pecans or walnuts, soaked overnight, rinsed,
then dehydrated until crunchy (about 12 hours)

$1/4$ teaspoon Celtic salt

1 cup dates, soaked for $1/2$ hour

$1/4$ cup honey

1 cup raisins

1 cup chopped prunes

1 cup chopped dried apricots

1 tablespoon grated organic orange peel

2 cups fresh coconut

$1/4$ cup flaxseeds

Combine all ingredients except the flaxseeds in a large bowl and stir to mix. Remove half of the mixture to a food processor and purée. Return the purée to the bowl with the other half of the mixture and stir well. Stir the flaxseeds into the mixture. Shape the dough into 2 round loaves about $1/2$ inch high on solid dehydrator sheets and dehydrate until the loaves are dry on one side. Remove the dehydrator sheets, turn the loaves over onto the dehydrator tray, and continue dehydrating until completely dry (15–18 total hours).

Berries and Nut Cream

Simple yet elegant, a classic dessert.

Yield: 4 servings

1 ½ cups macadamia nuts,
soaked for 4 hours, then rinsed

½ cup orange juice

6 dates, soaked for 20 minutes

½ teaspoon vanilla extract
(optional; not a raw product)

1 cup in-season berries, such as blueberries,
strawberries, raspberries, or blackberries

Combine the nuts, juice, dates, and vanilla in a food processor and purée. Stir the berries into the purée. Serve the berries and cream in bowls garnished with a sprig of fresh mint or edible flowers, if desired.

Carob Brownies

This dessert is a truly great treat.

Yield: 12 servings

2 cups pecans, soaked overnight, then rinsed

1 cup almonds, soaked overnight, then rinsed

1 cup pine nuts

1 cup dates, soaked for 20 minutes

½ cup carob powder

1 peeled banana

1 teaspoon vanilla extract (optional; not a raw product)

Combine all ingredients in a food processor and purée. Place the dough in a layer about ½-inch thick on solid dehydrator sheets and dehydrate for 6 hours. Remove the dehydrator sheets, turn the brownie layers over onto the dehydrator tray, and continue dehydrating for another 4 hours. When done, cut the brownies into squares or rectangles.

Carob Crunch Balls

*Keep a batch of these goodies in the freezer
and you'll always have a tasty treat to offer guests.*

Yield: about 24 balls

1 cup walnuts, soaked overnight, then rinsed

1 cup almond butter

1 cup dates, soaked for 20 minutes

$\frac{1}{2}$ cup carob powder

$\frac{1}{2}$ cup buckwheat, sprouted 3 days using the jar method,
then dehydrated until crispy (about 12 hours)

Combine all ingredients except the buckwheat in a food processor and purée.
Stir the buckwheat into the purée. Shape the mixture into 1-inch balls and store
them in the freezer. Serve frozen.

Cosmic Carob Fudge

Even chocolate lovers find this fudge delicious.

Yield: 24 pieces

2 cups Brazil nuts, soaked overnight, rinsed,
then dehydrated until crunchy (about 12 hours)

2 cups dates, soaked for 20 minutes

4 tablespoons carob powder

1 cup water

1 cup flaxseeds

1 cup walnuts, soaked overnight, rinsed,
then dehydrated until crunchy (about 12 hours)

Combine the Brazil nuts, dates, carob powder, and water in a food processor
and blend. Stir the remaining ingredients into the mixture. Press the mixture
into a glass baking dish and store it in the freezer. Cut the fudge into squares
when ready to serve.

Orange-Berry Un-Gelatin

This recipe makes a light, refreshing dessert.
It's a great treat for someone recovering from a cold or sore throat.

Yield: 6 servings

3 tablespoons agar flakes

1 cup cold water

1 cup hot water

1 cup orange juice

1/2 cup honey or 1/2 cup dates, soaked for 20 minutes,
then puréed in a blender

2 cups in-season berries, such as raspberries,
blackberries, blueberries, or strawberries

Stir the agar into the cold water, allow it to set 1 minute, and add the hot
water. Bring the agar mixture to a boil, let it simmer for 2 minutes, and let it
cool. In a separate bowl, stir together the juice, honey or dates, and berries.
Pour the cooled agar liquid over the fruit mixture and stir to mix. Refrigerate
the "gelatin" for at least 1 hour before serving.

Poppyseed Pastry

You can also enjoy this pastry for a special brunch.

Yield: 8 servings

2 cups walnuts, soaked overnight, rinsed,
then dehydrated until crunchy (about 12 hours)

6 dates, soaked for 20 minutes

1 teaspoon grated organic orange peel

1/2 teaspoon Celtic salt

1 cup poppy seeds

1 cup raisins, soaked for 1/2 hour

Combine the walnuts, dates, orange peel, and salt in a food processor and
purée. Press the mixture into a glass pie plate. Combine the poppy seeds
and raisins in the food processor and purée. Fill the crust with the purée.
Slice and serve.

Macadamia-Apricot Cookies

These cookies are a great comfort food.

Yield: about 24 cookies

1 cup dried apricots,
soaked for 2 hours, then chopped

1 cup macadamia nuts,
soaked overnight, then rinsed

1 cup pine nuts

$\frac{1}{2}$ cup dates, soaked for 20 minutes

1 teaspoon vanilla extract
(optional; not a raw product)

Combine all ingredients in a food processor and purée. Shape the mixture into flat, 3-inch rounds on solid dehydrator sheets and dehydrate until the top side is dry. Remove the dehydrator sheets, turn the cookies over onto the dehydrator tray, and continue dehydrating until the cookies are dry on both sides (8–12 total hours).

Sunflower Power Balls

A delicious way to use one of Nature's supreme seeds.

Yield: 24 balls

2 cups sunflower seeds, divided

$\frac{1}{2}$ cup carob powder

$\frac{1}{2}$ cup almond butter or tahini

$\frac{1}{2}$ cup dates, soaked for 20 minutes, then puréed

1 teaspoon vanilla extract
(optional; not a raw product)

$\frac{1}{2}$ teaspoon cinnamon

$\frac{1}{2}$ cup raisins

In a large bowl, combine 1 cup of the sunflower seeds with the remaining ingredients and mix well. Shape the mixture into $\frac{1}{2}$-inch balls, roll them in the remaining cup of sunflower seeds to cover, and store them in the freezer. Serve frozen.

Lemon Delight

Light and lively, this recipe makes a most refreshing dessert.

Yield: 12 slices

2 cups dates, soaked for 20 minutes
in 1 cup lemon juice (reserve the juice)

2 cups walnuts, soaked overnight, then rinsed

1 tablespoon chopped organic lemon peel

2 cups sesame seeds

Combine the dates, lemon juice, walnuts, and lemon peel in a food processor and purée. Press the mixture into a glass pie plate. Cover the mixture with the sesame seeds, pressing the seeds gently into the surface, and store it in the freezer. Serve the Lemon Delight frozen and sliced.

Fruit Aspic

This dessert is light and refreshing, and not too sweet.

Yield: 6–8 servings

$1\frac{1}{2}$ tablespoons agar flakes

$\frac{1}{2}$ cup water

2 peeled bananas

2 cups apple juice or orange juice

2 cups blueberries

Mix the agar into the water and allow it to soak for 1 minute. Bring the agar mixture to a boil and simmer for 1 minute; set aside (see "The Raw Facts" on page 235). Combine the banana and apple juice or orange juice in a blender and purée. Place the blueberries in a pretty bowl or a ring-shaped dish. Stir the agar broth into the puréed juice and banana, and then pour the mixture gently over the blueberries. Allow the aspic to gel in the refrigerator for 1 hour before serving. Decorate the aspic with fruit slices and edible flowers, if desired.

The Raw Facts

Agar (also known as agar agar) is a gelatin derived from several types of seaweeds. It can be used as a thickening agent in place of commercial gelatin (which is made from animal hooves and bones). Agar must be soaked and then heated before it will solidify.

Simple Fruit Leather

This snack can go in your kid's lunchbox—or yours.

Yield: 1 tray

6–8 apples, apricots, or peaches, or 2 cups smaller fruit such as blueberries, strawberries, or figs, or any combination thereof

Place the fruit in a food processor and purée. Spread the purée in a layer about $1/4$-inch thick on a solid dehydrator sheet and dehydrate for 6–12 hours, until the top of the leather is dry. Remove the dehydrator sheets, turn the leather over onto the dehydrator tray, and continue dehydrating for another 6–12 hours or until the leather is completely dry. Roll up the leather in waxed paper and store it in the refrigerator, where it will keep for about 1 month.

Variations on Simple Fruit Leather

Be creative! Try apples or bananas mixed with apricots, berries, dates, peaches, plums, or prunes. Adding a squeeze of lemon or a pinch of grated citrus peel is a nice touch. Try mixing in sesame or sunflower seeds, tahini or almond butter (1 cup to each 4 cups of fruit), carob powder, coriander, ginger, or vanilla. If the mixture needs to be thickened, add 1 tablespoon of flaxseeds for each cup of blended fruit. For a more substantive snack, spread raw tahini or almond butter into the bottom third of a sheet of fruit leather, roll it up tightly, and slice the roll into 8–10 rounds.

Live Holiday Nuts

*Make a batch of these tasty nuts to take to the movies
so you won't be tempted by popcorn.*

Yield: about 5 cups

1 cup almonds, soaked overnight, then rinsed

1 cup hazelnuts/filberts, soaked overnight, then rinsed

1 cup pecans, soaked overnight, then rinsed

1 cup sunflower seeds, soaked overnight, then rinsed

1 tablespoon extra-virgin olive oil

1 tablespoon Nama Shoyu

1 teaspoon Chili Powder (page 115), or a chili powder of your choice

2 tablespoons nutritional yeast (optional; not a raw product)

Place the nuts and sunflower seeds in a bowl. Stir the remaining ingredients
into the nuts and seeds and toss the mixture, using your hands if necessary to
make sure it is uniformly coated. Place the mixture on solid dehydrator sheets
and dehydrate for 8–10 hours or until the nuts and seeds are crisp, stirring
them occasionally.

Sesame-Spirulina Bars

Don't you love how a dessert can also be a super-powered tonic?

Yield: 12–16 servings

½ cup coconut oil

⅓ cup honey

½ teaspoon Celtic salt

1 teaspoon vanilla extract (optional; not a raw product)

¼ cup spirulina powder

¾ cup sesame seeds (I use black sesame seeds,
but regular, unhulled sesame seeds are fine)

¾ cup pine nuts

Combine all ingredients in a bowl and mix thoroughly. Press the mixture into an
8" x 10" glass pan. Refrigerate the mixture for 1 hour and cut it into squares
before serving.

Super Sesame Bars

These are a cross between a cookie and a cracker.

Yield: About 24 bars

1 cup dates, soaked 20 minutes

2 cups sesame seeds

1 teaspoon vanilla extract (optional; not a raw product)

$1/2$ cup flaxseed

$1/4$ teaspoon Celtic salt

Place the soaked dates in a blender and purée. In a bowl mix together the dates and pour onto dehydrator sheets, turning after about 8 hours. Finish drying on the dehydrator tray.

All-Raw Apple Pie

This classic American dessert gets even better when it's raw.

Yield: 8 servings

THE CRUST

2 cups almonds, soaked for 12 hours, rinsed,
then dehydrated until crunchy (about 12 hours)

$1/2$ cup dates, soaked for 20 minutes

THE FILLING

7 apples, peeled and chopped

1 banana, peeled and sliced

1 cup dates, soaked for 20 minutes

$1/2$ cup raisins, soaked for 30 minutes

1 teaspoon cinnamon

Juice of 1 lemon

To make the crust: Combine the almonds and dates in a food processor and pulse until evenly ground and mixed. Press the mixture into a glass pie plate.

To make the filling: Combine all filling ingredients in a food processor and purée.

To finish: Spoon the filling into the pie crust and serve.

Blueberry Pie

Besides being delicious, blueberries are the number-one antioxidant food; in particular, they are considered to be very beneficial for the eyes.

Yield: 8 servings

THE CRUST

2 cups almonds, soaked for 12 hours, rinsed, then dehydrated until crunchy (about 12 hours)

$\frac{1}{2}$ cup dates, soaked for 20 minutes

THE FILLING

$\frac{1}{2}$ cup dates, soaked for 20 minutes

2 peeled bananas

3 cups blueberries

To make the crust: Combine the almonds and dates in a food processor and pulse until evenly ground and mixed. Press the mixture into a glass pie plate.

To make the filling: Combine the dates and bananas in a food processor and purée.

To finish: Place the blueberries in the crust. Pour the purée over the berries and serve.

Sweet Potato Pie

Serving this pie is a great way to get kids of all ages to eat more beta-carotene-rich vegetables.

Yield: 8 servings

THE CRUST

2 cups pecans, soaked overnight, rinsed, then dehydrated until crunchy (about 12 hours)

$\frac{1}{2}$ cup dates, soaked for 20 minutes

THE FILLING

2 large sweet potatoes, chopped

1 cup macadamia nuts, soaked overnight, then rinsed

6 dates, soaked for 20 minutes

1 teaspoon cinnamon

$\frac{1}{2}$ teaspoon cardamom

$\frac{1}{4}$ teaspoon nutmeg

To make the crust: Combine the pecans and dates in a food processor and purée. Press the mixture into a glass pie plate.

To make the filling: Combine all filling ingredients in a food processor and purée.

To finish: Spoon the filling into the crust and serve.

Key Lime Pie

Everyone wants seconds of this dessert!

Yield: 8 servings

THE CRUST

2 cups pecans, soaked overnight, rinsed,
then dehydrated until crunchy (about 12 hours)

$\frac{1}{2}$ cup dates, soaked for 20 minutes

THE FILLING

1 avocado, pitted and peeled

$\frac{1}{2}$ cup coconut water

Pulp of 1 young coconut

$\frac{1}{3}$ cup lime juice

Grated peel of half an organic lime

1 teaspoon vanilla extract (optional; not a raw product)

$\frac{1}{4}$ teaspoon Celtic salt

$\frac{1}{2}$ cup dates, soaked for 20 minutes

2 tablespoons flaxseeds

To make the crust: Combine the pecans and dates in a food processor and pulse until evenly ground and mixed. Press the mixture into a glass pie plate.

To make the filling: Combine all filling ingredients in a food processor and purée.

To finish: Pour the filling into the crust. Chill the pie for 1 hour before serving.

Pecan Pie

Love that country pie!

Yield: 8 servings

THE CRUST

1½ cup pecans, soaked overnight, rinsed,
then dehydrated until crunchy (about 12 hours)

½ cup dates, soaked for 20 minutes

THE FILLING

1½ cup pecans, soaked overnight, rinsed,
then dehydrated until crunchy (about 12 hours)

1 cup dried figs, soaked for 1 hour

½ cup dates, soaked for 20 minutes

1 tablespoon flaxseeds,
soaked in 2 tablespoons water for 15 minutes

1 peeled banana

1 teaspoon cinnamon

½ teaspoon nutmeg

¼ teaspoon cardamom

1 teaspoon vanilla extract
(optional; not a raw product)

To make the crust: Combine the pecans and dates in a food processor and pulse until evenly ground and mixed. Press the mixture into a glass pie plate.

To make the filling: Combine all filling ingredients except the pecans and flaxseed in a food processor and purée. Stir in flaxseed.

To finish: Layer the pecans in the crust. Cover the pecans with the filling and serve.

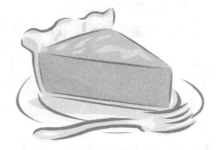

━━━━━ *Pumpkin Pie* ━━━━━

*I like to decorate this pie with a jack o' lantern face
made of raisins or almonds.*

Yield: 8 servings

THE CRUST

2 cups pecans, soaked overnight, rinsed,
then dehydrated until crunchy (about 12 hours)

$\frac{1}{2}$ cup dates, soaked for 20 minutes

THE FILLING

2 cups peeled, seeded, chopped pumpkin meat

1 cup dates, soaked for 20 minutes

$\frac{1}{2}$ cup almond butter

2 teaspoons cinnamon

1 teaspoon grated fresh gingerroot

$\frac{1}{2}$ teaspoon cloves

$\frac{1}{2}$ teaspoon nutmeg

$\frac{1}{4}$ teaspoon cardamom

$\frac{1}{4}$ cup water or apple juice

To make the crust: Combine the pecans and dates in a food processor and pulse until evenly ground and mixed. Press the mixture into a glass pie plate.

To make the filling: Combine all filling ingredients in a food processor and purée.

To finish: Spoon the filling into the crust and serve.

━━ *Red, White, and Blue Fruit Salad* ━━

This festive fruit dish is also great for breakfast.

Yield: 2 servings

1 cup sliced strawberries, stems removed

2 peeled bananas, sliced

1 cup blueberries

Combine all ingredients in a bowl and serve.

Creamy Carob-Coffee Pie

*This smooth, creamy pie will make you glad
to have been turned on to the raw foods diet.*

Yield: 8 servings

THE CRUST

2 cups walnuts, soaked overnight, rinsed,
then dehydrated until crunchy (about 12 hours)

$\frac{1}{2}$ cup dates, soaked for 20 minutes

$\frac{1}{4}$ teaspoon Celtic salt

THE FILLING

1 $\frac{1}{2}$ cups macadamia nuts,
soaked for 4 hours, then rinsed

1 peeled banana

$\frac{1}{2}$ cup dates, soaked for 20 minutes

$\frac{1}{2}$ cup dried figs, soaked for 1 hour

$\frac{1}{4}$ cup carob powder

2 teaspoons coffee extract (optional; not a raw product)

1 teaspoon caramel extract (optional; not a raw product)

To make the crust: Combine all crust ingredients in a food processor and purée. Press the mixture into a glass pie plate.

To make the filling: Combine all filling ingredients in a food processor and purée.

To finish: Spoon the filling into the crust. Chill the pie for 1 hour before serving.

Carob Layer Cake

*You can make this cake for birthdays
or to celebrate any day you choose.*

Yield: 12 servings

4 peeled bananas

2 cups dates, soaked for 20 minutes

1 cup walnuts, soaked overnight, then rinsed

2 cups carob powder

$1/2$ cup water

Combine all ingredients in a food processor and purée. Pour the batter in 2 rounds of equal size onto solid dehydrator sheets and dehydrate until dry on one side (about 6 hours). Remove the dehydrator sheets, turn the rounds over onto the dehydrator tray, and continue dehydrating for another 3 hours or until the rounds are dry. Decorate the cake layers with Carob Frosting (page 245), if desired.

Very Vanilla Cake

Decorate this cake with frosting and fresh berries.

Yield: 12 servings

1 cup pecans, soaked overnight, rinsed, then dehydrated until crunchy (about 12 hours)

1 cup walnuts, soaked overnight, rinsed, then dehydrated until crunchy (about 12 hours)

1 cup almonds, soaked overnight, rinsed, then dehydrated until crunchy (about 12 hours)

$1/2$ cup dates, soaked for 20 minutes

$1/4$ teaspoon Celtic salt

1 tablespoon vanilla extract (optional; not a raw product)

$1/2$ cup water

$1/2$ cup flaxseeds

Combine all ingredients except the flaxseeds in a food processor and purée. Stir the flaxseeds into the purée. Shape the mixture into 2 large, round loaves, each about $1/2$ inch high, on solid dehydrator sheets and dehydrate for 4 hours. Remove the dehydrator sheets, turn the loaves over onto the dehydrator tray, and continue dehydrating for another 4 hours.

Amazing Cake

This cake does include a few spoonfuls of real chocolate powder,
which is not a raw product, but I've noticed that some raw
restaurants often include chocolate in a few desserts.
For those of us who absolutely love it,
an occasional chocolate dessert is a supreme treat.
This recipe is for my husband, Tom.

Yield: 12 servings

THE BASE

5 cups walnuts, soaked overnight, rinsed,
then dehydrated until crunchy (about 12 hours)

3 cups dates, soaked for 20 minutes

3 tablespoons sugar-free chocolate powder

1 teaspoon vanilla extract
(optional; not a raw product)

$1/4$ teaspoon Celtic salt

THE FILLING

2 cups raspberries or chopped strawberries,
stems removed

THE TOPPING

1 cup tahini

$1/2$ cup dates, soaked for 20 minutes

3 tablespoons chocolate powder

1 teaspoon vanilla extract
(optional; not a raw product)

To make the base: Combine all base ingredients in a food processor and purée. Pat the purée evenly over the bottom of a glass cake pan.

To make the filling: Spread the berries over the base.

To make the topping: Combine all topping ingredients in a food processor and purée.

To finish: Spread the topping over the nut and berry base. Garnish the cake, if desired, with edible flowers or a fresh fruit mandala.

Carob Frosting

This raw life is so amazing.
We get to enjoy so much goodness—like this recipe!

Yield: 1 1/2 cups

1 avocado, pitted and peeled

1 cup dates, soaked for 20 minutes

1/2 cup carob powder

1 teaspoon vanilla extract (optional; not a raw product)

Combine all ingredients in a food processor and purée.

Holiday Frosting

Beets lend this mixture a bright red hue.

Yield: 1 1/2 cups

1 cup macadamia nuts, soaked 4 hours, then rinsed

1/4 cup beet powder

1 cup dates, soaked for 20 minutes

1/4 cup water

1 teaspoon vanilla extract (optional; not a raw product)

Combine all ingredients in a food processor and purée.

Deluxe Frosting

This frosting makes any cake taste sensuously rich.

Yield: 1 1/2 cups

1/2 cup coconut butter

1/2 cup dates, soaked for 20 minutes

1/2 cup pine nuts

1 teaspoon vanilla extract (optional; not a raw product)

Combine all ingredients in a food processor and purée.

Orange Frosting

Spread this frosting on the cake of your choice.

Yield: 1½ cups

1½ cups macadamia nuts, soaked 4 hours, then rinsed

1 cup dates, soaked for 20 minutes

Juice of 1 orange

1 tablespoon rosewater (optional; not a raw product)

1 teaspoon vanilla extract (optional; not a raw product)

Combine all ingredients in a food processor and purée.

Apricot Pudding

Nothing could be easier.
Try garnishing the pudding with pine nuts.

Yield: 2 servings

1 cup dried apricots, soaked in 1 cup water for 4 hours

Place the rehydrated apricots in a food processor and purée. Serve pudding in cups.

Natural Food Colorings

The following products can be used to dye coconut, frostings, and puddings:

Red: Beet powder

Green: Chlorofresh Capsules made by Nature's Way (prick 2–3 capsules with a pin and squeeze out the contents)

Yellow: Turmeric

Blue green: Spirulina

Orange: Beet powder and turmeric

Lemon Pudding

With recipes like this, it's quick, easy, and delicious
to make healthful snacks.

Yield: 2 servings

1 cup Brazil nuts, soaked overnight, then rinsed

8 dates, soaked for 20 minutes

Juice of 3 lemons

1 teaspoon grated organic lemon peel

Combine all ingredients in a food processor and purée. Serve pudding in cups.

Lime Pudding

If you love limes, this dessert is a wish come true.

Yield: 2 servings

2 cups avocado, pitted, peeled, and chopped

1 $\frac{1}{2}$ cups lime pulp (no seeds or skin)

Juice of 2 limes

2 cups dates, soaked for 20 minutes

Combine all ingredients in a food processor and purée. Serve pudding in cups.

Butterscotch Pudding

An extraordinary version of the ultimate comfort food.

Yield: 4 servings

1 cup dried apricots, soaked overnight in water

2 peeled bananas

8 dates, soaked for 20 minutes

1 teaspoon vanilla extract (optional; not a raw product)

$\frac{1}{4}$ cup almond butter

Combine all ingredients in a food processor and purée, using as much of the soak water as needed for a pudding-like consistency. Serve pudding in cups.

Vanilla Pudding

This pudding is a wonderful treat for children.

Yield: 3 servings

Meat of 2 young coconuts

1 cup dates, soaked for 20 minutes

1 teaspoon vanilla extract (optional; not a raw product)

$\frac{1}{4}$ cup coconut water

Combine all ingredients in a food processor and purée. Serve pudding in cups.

Carob Pudding

Garnish this pudding with a mint leaf or strawberry slice.
Add some pine nuts for crunch.

Yield: 2 servings

$\frac{1}{2}$ cup almonds, soaked overnight, then rinsed

2 peeled bananas

$\frac{1}{2}$ cup water

2 tablespoons carob powder

$\frac{1}{2}$ cup dates, soaked for 20 minutes

Combine all ingredients in a blender or food processor and purée.

Coconut Pudding

We love to drink coconut water and always want to make something
with the leftover young coconut meat. This pudding fits the bill.

Yield: 2 servings

1 cup fresh young coconut meat

Juice of 4 lemons

7 dates, soaked for 20 minutes

$\frac{1}{2}$ teaspoon vanilla extract (optional; not a raw product)
or 1 inch vanilla bean

Combine all ingredients in a food processor and purée. Serve pudding in cups.

Apricot Ice Cream

You can also make this recipe with fresh peaches.

Yield: about 5 cups

1 quart Almond Milk (page 144)

$\frac{1}{2}$ cup dates, soaked for 20 minutes

7 fresh apricots or 14 dried Turkish apricot halves,
soaked for 2 hours

1 peeled banana

Combine all ingredients in a blender and blend well. Chill the mixture for 1 hour. Place the mixture in an ice cream maker and process until frozen.

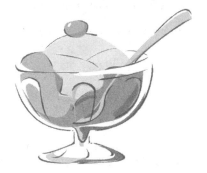

Lime-Avocado Ice Cream

Here's something special for the discriminating palate.

Yield: about 4 cups

$1\frac{1}{4}$ cups coconut water

$\frac{1}{4}$ cup lime juice

$\frac{1}{2}$ cup dates, soaked for 20 minutes

$\frac{1}{4}$ cup coconut oil

1 medium avocado, pitted and peeled

$\frac{1}{4}$ teaspoon Celtic salt

$\frac{1}{2}$ peel of an organic lime

Combine all ingredients in a blender and blend well. Chill the mixture for 1 hour. Place the mixture in an ice cream maker and process until frozen.

Mango-Papaya Ice Cream

*This recipe combines two of nature's most luscious fruits
in one great dessert.*

Yield: about 6 cups

1 quart Almond Milk (page 143)

1 mango, peeled and seeded

1 cup peeled, seeded, chopped papaya

$\frac{1}{2}$ cup dates, soaked for 20 minutes

1 teaspoon cinnamon powder

Combine all ingredients in a blender and blend well. Chill the mixture for
1 hour. Place the mixture in an ice cream maker and process until frozen.

Banana Split

A better split than any dairy concoction.

Yield: 2 servings

2 scoops raw ice cream of your choice

1 large peeled banana, split lengthwise

4 tablespoons Carob Frosting (page 245)

3 tablespoons walnuts, soaked overnight, rinsed,
then dehydrated until crunchy (about 12 hours)

Arrange the ice cream between the banana halves. Top the split with the carob
sauce and walnuts.

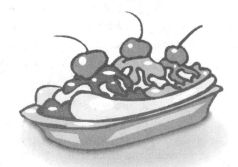

6

Eating Raw with Family and Friends

opefully in the near future, restaurants and catered affairs will offer a raw selection just as they usually offer vegetarian fare. In the meantime, this chapter provides a few ideas for being flexible in social settings.

RESTAURANTS AND PARTIES

Americans consume some 65 percent of their meals outside the home. People who are most concerned with the healthfulness of their diets may not live up to this statistic, tending instead to eat meals prepared by their own hand at home, but life does bring occasions when eating out is necessary, whether at a restaurant, at a dinner party, or on the road. Before you start worrying about the hassle this could be, be assured—eating raw away from home can be a simple proposition. The following tips should help.

Restaurants

Raw restaurants are a growing trend (see the list in the Resources section), and if there's one in your area, you're in luck—you can arrange to have most of your restaurant outings there. However, whether for the sake of companions who are not raw or because there isn't a raw restaurant in the area, at some point you'll find yourself venturing through the doors of a "cooking" restaurant.

Your best raw bet in a non-raw restaurant is a salad. If the restaurant doesn't have a salad bar, examine the salads on the menu, being sure to read the lists of ingredients carefully and asking the waitstaff to omit anything cooked when you order. For salad dressing, ask for olive oil and lemon juice, or you can easily bring your own raw dressing from home. I often order a salad as an appetizer and another type of salad as an entreé. Adding your own chopped avocado or nuts to a restaurant salad makes it feel more like a meal.

For breakfast, ask for a fresh fruit platter. Tell the waitperson you want more fruit instead of the usual cottage cheese. You might consider bringing along some dates to add to it. No fruit platter? Perhaps they have a ripe melon.

Do your best, but be prepared to compromise, and be gracious with the waitstaff, who will have to go out of their way to answer your questions and procure your special requests.

Dinner Parties

When you are invited to a dinner party that will not be raw, inform your host of your food program as soon as you receive the invitation, but tell him or her not to fret or go to any trouble to accommodate you; offer to bring to the party a raw dish that you can eat as a main course and that others can try, if they wish, as a side dish.

When you're talking to your host or to your friends, avoid preaching the benefits of the raw diet. Once you've told them that you're on a raw diet, they may ask about it, but if they do not, don't force the details on them. When you are the host of your own dinner party, you can introduce your guests to the delights of a raw diet without any lecturing at all, simply by offering a wide range of delicious raw foods. Good party fare includes:

- Raw vegetable chips (fresh, or dehydrated with a touch of olive oil and Celtic salt) of carrots, jicama, Jerusalem artichokes, sweet potatoes, and zucchini

- Flax crackers

- Raw dips for the chips and crackers

- Canapes

- Guacamole

- Pâtés spread on cucumbers, celery sticks, or sprouted breads or crackers

- Watermelon boat

- Shish kabobs on toothpicks

- Slices of cucumber or zucchini with nut butters

- Cherry tomatoes

- Guacamole

- Nuts and seeds

- Marinated vegetables

- Fruit slices

- Nori rolls

- Pizzas

- Dates stuffed with almond butter

- Fruit fondue (bite-sized portions of apples, bananas, pears, and mangoes with various sweet dipping sauces)

- Vegetable fondue (bite-sized portions of carrots, bell peppers, cucumbers, and zucchini with various sweet or savory dipping sauces)

See Chapter 5 for more recipes and ideas.

Presentation of food is highly important, and perhaps even more so with raw foods. It's always best to prepare dishes as close as possible to the time of consumption so that the fresh foods won't wilt or discolor. Serve foods on beds of colorful greens, grated carrots, or sliced cabbage. Use garnishes that complement the dishes in flavor and color, such as:

- Cucumber slices

- Radish roses

- Cherry tomatoes

- Cauliflower buds

- Carrot curls

- Sprouts

- Avocado balls (scooped out with a melon baller)

- Buckwheat lettuce

- Sunflower greens

- Lemon slices

- Watercress

- Chopped nuts

- Olives

- Chopped red pepper

- Berries

- Slices of citrus fruits

- Pomegranate seeds

- Star fruit slices

- Fresh herbs (basil, chives, cilantro, dill, fennel, oregano, mint, parsley, or rosemary)

- Edible flowers

Geometric designs offer another option for creative food presentation. You can place a lacey, paper doily or a large maple leaf on the food, sprinkle on paprika, cinnamon, or another powdered seasoning, and then carefully remove the doily or leaf, leaving behind an interesting design. Nuts, dried fruit, or edible flowers can be used to make a mandala design on your presentation. Cookie cutters are useful for making interestingly shaped sprouted crackers, and pretty rings or molds add an extra flair to raw cakes and pâtés. Finally, serve your food on beautiful plates, bowls, and platters to make it a feast for the eyes as well.

Traveling

Being raw will lower the cost of traveling, because raw foods are generally less expensive than cooked foods. In fact, you can even plan your vacation around your raw diet: travel to a fruit-filled, tropical paradise during mango or durian season; visit the wilds of Maine during blueberry season; and enjoy the hospitality of the South during peach or orange season.

When traveling by car, bring an ice chest to carry your raw salad dressings; during hot weather, keep your fruits and vegetables in the chest, too. A cutting board, knife, sprout bag, bowls, and utensils are also useful.

Prepare dried fruits and vegetables before a trip. Take flax crackers, raw granola, sunflower and pumpkin seeds, and sun-cured olives. Keep a small container of unpasteurized miso with you; it can be stirred into a bit of purified water to make a soup broth. Travel with superfoods such as powders or tablets of barley grass, wheatgrass, spirulina, or blue-green algae for the nutrients and energy they provide, especially if you can't count on being able to find fresh vegetables.

Make it part of the fun of your journey to find health foods stores and restaurants that serve salads. Stop at roadside markets. Take the opportunity to eat simply. Have an adventure!

INTRODUCING RAW TO YOUR FAMILY

You might be ready for the raw life, but perhaps not everyone in your family is. When you begin, ask your family members for—and thank them for—their support. Let them know that you are not expecting them to join you in your new diet, but that you look forward to having more raw foods available at meals, so that you can all still eat together. If being raw is a new thing in the household, slowly increase the amount of raw food on the table. Serve salad before anything cooked. Find out what kinds of foods other family members enjoy, and make raw versions of them.

Most importantly, let go of the need to change others. You will impress people more with your health and vitality than you ever will with preaching. Be a living example of your beliefs.

Living Raw with Children

Children can enjoy a raw foods diet from the moment of birth. Breast milk is, after all, the supreme raw food. It is fresh, nutritious, safe, free of contamination, and always the right temperature, and it comes in lovely containers! Breast milk is ideal for a baby's first six months to one year of age. The World Health Organization is currently encouraging women to nurse for at least two years, and many mothers nurse for even longer.

Diluted carrot juice can be introduced to babies between four and six months of age. After six months, diluted, noncitrus fruit juices can be given on occasion. For nursing babies, limit their juice intake to 3–4 ounces daily, so they focus on breast milk. Coconut water is excellent for young children and can be given after six months. Green vegetable drinks can be introduced between six to nine months of age; if they taste strongly, they can be sweetened with apple or carrot juice or diluted 50 percent with water. Nut and seed milks can be introduced around eight months, and smoothies can be given to babies from nine months and up. Citrus fruits and juices can be given when the child is at least one year of age.

Solid foods can be started around six months, when the baby is able to hold his or her head up independently or has doubled his or her birth weight. A blender or grinder can be used to mash raw foods into suitable baby fare. It is wisest to introduce only one new food a week; try mixing a bit of the new food with a food that is already familiar to the child. Bananas are an ideal first solid food. Other raw foods that make excellent, blended baby foods include:

- Apples
- Apricots
- Avocados
- Berries
- Cherimoyas
- Cherries
- Coconut meat (fresh and young)
- Mangoes
- Melon
- Papayas
- Peaches
- Pears
- Peas
- Plums
- Spinach
- String beans
- Sweet potatoes
- Winter squash
- Yellow squash
- Zucchini

If any of these foods need to be sweetened, blend in some soaked raisins or dates.

When the child reaches toddlerhood, he or she will appreciate solid finger-food. Peel those foods that can be peeled and introduce solid foods only under supervision, as babies choke easily, whether their food is raw or not. Good finger-foods include:

- Apples
- Bananas
- Berries
- Mangoes
- Melon
- Peaches
- Pears
- Plums
- Summer squash

Spirulina can be given in small amounts, about ¼ teaspoon daily, to a child over seven months old. Spirulina is a good source of protein and chlorophyll.

The Raw Facts

Do not give honey to babies less than two years of age, as there is a slight danger of botulism; children over the age of two will not be susceptible to it. Use soaked dates, apricots, or figs for sweetening, if needed. Better yet, offer unsweetened foods that are naturally delicious.

Once a child has adequate teeth to chew well and begins to show an interest in what adults are eating, he or she is ready to explore the full palate of adult food. At this point, one way to encourage your child to eat more vegetables is to serve a tasty dip along with them. Tahini, which is made from ground sesame seeds, is rich in protein and calcium, tastes pleasant, and makes a good vegetable dip. Ground sunflower and pumpkin seeds are rich in the mineral zinc and are excellent for kids who are slow to grow. Sea vegetables are a great source of minerals for developing bones; use kelp or dulse in dressings and as seasonings. Often it is the texture of a vegetable that children dislike, not the flavor of the vegetable, so try a variety of forms and textures to see what your kids like best.

If your child is a picky eater, ask him or her for suggestions. Rather than announcing that broccoli is on the dinner menu, try asking the child if he or she would rather have broccoli or zucchini, and honor his or her preference. If your children are quick to assert that they hate broccoli, remind them that they might have disliked it when they were four (for example), but now that they are six, and much bigger, they might find that they like it. Children appreciate the opportunity to show their maturity.

Take your child shopping with you and ask him or her to select one produce item for every color of the rainbow that he or she would like to eat.

Decoration, presentation, and humor are particularly effective tools in living raw with children. Delight your kids by making food in shapes such as their initials, hearts, animals, or flowers. Use raisins, nuts, or sliced fruit to design a happy face or mandala on a salad, a bowl of sprouted cereal, or an open-faced, sprouted-almond butter sandwich. Create theme menus: a jungle meal, for example, or a meal featuring foods from a particular country. Invite young ones into the kitchen to help; participating, even in simple tasks like stirring, pouring, or decorating, can give a child a sense of having contributed to the family's meal.

Almost all children like sweets and to deny them will only cause arguments, so be sure to provide homemade, raw sweets. Make fresh-frozen treats from mashed watermelon, orange juice, or apple juice. Freeze some Raw Carob Milk (see page 145) for "fudgey-sicles." Use fruit and dried fruit in place of candy.

Rather than forbidding kids to eat certain foods, explain to them why these are foods your family chooses to avoid. But don't expect your children to be totally raw their entire lives. They'll have friends, school lunches, and restaurants to tempt them with non-raw food, and they'll want to try it. It's not worth a big argument if your kids decide to eat unraw; in fact, you're likely to turn them off the raw foods diet if you are maniacal about it. Just make sure your kids have healthy, raw food available at all times, so that

Raw for Your Pets

Dogs and cats are often among the members of a family. They are not naturally vegetarian, of course, but in nature all animals do eat their food raw. Your household pets can, too. At the very least, they can benefit from some raw foods being introduced into their diet. Cats often like avocados, sprouts, tomatoes, cucumbers, nutritional yeast, spirulina, and garlic powder. Dogs tend to like avocados, bananas, apples, grated carrots, nutritional yeast, garlic powder, sea vegetables, and tahini.

For more information about a raw foods diet for pets, see _Natural Remedies for Dogs and Cats_ by C. J. Puotinen, or _Reigning Cats and Dogs_ by Pat McKay.

they have a choice. When dealing with children and nutrition, humor and sincerity are the best approach. If you lay the groundwork for a healthy lifestyle early, your kids will return to eating healthy foods when they are old enough to make their own decisions.

THEME DINNERS

Dinners with a theme are especially fun for parties, holidays, and special celebrations. You don't need to make all the dishes suggested for a theme, of course, but try at least a few for a varied, scrumptious meal. You can also throw a potluck dinner, and have each attendee make one of the dishes from the theme group. (Check the index for page numbers.)

All-American

Sunflower Pâté, with celery added

Mashed Parsnips with Nama Shoyu

Nut Burgers, Savory Savory Veggie Burgers, or Sunburgers, with Raw Ketchup

Vegetable Pot Pie

All-Raw Apple Pie

Orange-Berry Gelatin

Red, White, and Blue Fruit Salad

Caribbean

Coconut Soup or Papaya Soup

Mango Salsa

Roots Rock Reggae

Not-Fried Rice

Vegetable Kabobs

Key Lime Pie

Mango-Papaya Ice Cream

French

Mediterranean Salad with French Dressing

Creamed Asparagus Soup

Green Bean Scene

Stuffed Mushrooms

Summer Squash Supreme

Pecan-Spinach Quiche

Very Vanilla Cake with Super Frosting and fresh berries

German

Celery Soup

Kale Salad

Sauerkraut

Breakfast Patties

Brazil Nut-Banana Pancakes

Applesauce

Poppyseed Pastry

Noodle Roni and Cheese

Holiday

Nut Nog

Hey Beetnik!

Cranberry Sauce

Winter Waldorf Salad

Winter Solstice Salad

Borscht

Sweet Potato Casserole

Holiday Mushroom Loaf

Nut Stuffing

Mashed Parsnips

Nama Shoyu

Pumpkin Pie

Pecan Pie

Very Vanilla Cake with Holiday
　Frosting

Nutty Fruitcake

Indian

Mango Lassi

Cool Cucumber-Mint Salad

Coconut Soup

Kitcheree

Palak

Curry Sauce

Date Chutney

Mint Chutney

Samosas

Tandoori Nut Balls

Chapatis

Mango-Papaya Ice Cream

Coconut Pudding

Italian

Caesar Salad or Mediterranean
　Salad with Italian Dressing

Garlic Butter

Garlic Toast

Olive Spread

Tandoori

Lasagna

Rawvioli

Buttered Noodles

Primavera Pasta with Olive Pesto,
　Tomato Sauce, Alfredo Sauce,
　Herb Pesto, or Wild Thing
　Pesto

Mexican

Corn Salad or Mexican Salad

Gazpacho

Jicama Crunch Sticks

Mexican Pâté

Guacamole

Corn Chips

Holy Molé Sauce

Salsa

Enchiladas

Chili Rellenos

Spanish Rice

Tostadas

Lemon Delight

Key Lime Pie

Middle Eastern

Mediterranean Salad or Tabouli
   Salad

Hummus

Falafel Balls with Tahini Sauce

Vegetable Kabobs

Coconut Pudding

Lemon Delight

Oriental

Asian Salad or Mermaid Salad

Coconut Soup

Asian Broccoli

Spring Green Rolls with Mustard
   Sauce and Sweet and Sour
   Sauce

Not-Fried Rice

Thai Noodles

Thai Vegetables

Oriental Noodles

Nori Rolls

Miso-Tahini Sauce

Lemon Delight

Southern

Limeade

Kale (or Collard Green) Salad

Corn on the Cob

Raw-Style Ribs

Barbecue Sauce

Pecan Pie

Sweet Potato Pie

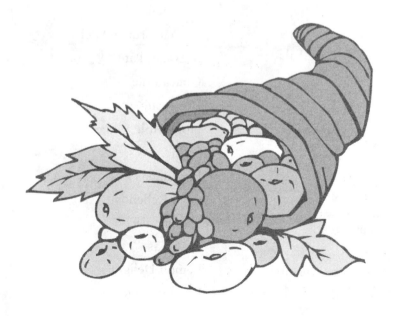

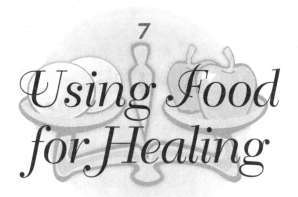

7
Using Food
for Healing

R aw foods have an important role in healing. This chapter discusses the balancing properties of various foods, the use of foods in color therapy, and the physiological effects of the "five flavors." It also discusses the role of fasting and how to do it safely. A discussion on the philosophy of food combining closes the chapter. Isn't it wonderful to be able to heal your body while enjoying nature's bounty?

ACIDITY AND ALKALINITY

Acidity and alkalinity can be measured by the pH scale, a numerical range from 0 to 14: 7 is neutral, lower numbers indicate increasing acidity, and higher numbers indicate increasing alkalinity. In layman's terms, pH is a measure of hydrogen-ion concentration or activity. Acidity is a state of excess hydrogen, and alkalinity is a state of insufficient hydrogen. "Excess" and "insufficient" are, of course, relative terms; pure water has a pH of 7, whereas the human body is, overall, slightly alkaline.

Acid is associated with *yin* qualities and alkali with *yang* qualities. An acidic condition, thus, could also be described as a yin *excess, and an alkaline condition could be described as a yang* excess. Taking this concept one step further, those foods that are acid-forming in the body stimulate *yin*, while those foods that are alkaline-forming stimulate *yang*.

Electrolytes can affect the body's pH balance. Electrolytes are minerals (including calcium, lithium, magnesium, phosphorus, and potassium) that, when in solution, conduct electricity. Alkaline elements attract a negative charge, and acid elements attract a positive charge.

Acidosis

When excess hydrogen atoms are present in the body, this is a state called acidosis, in which the excess hydrogen can combine with oxygen to create water. This process depletes the body of oxygen; as a result, lactic acid builds up, the system become even more acidic, and cellular function is diminished. Acidosis can cause the mind to work more slowly, as well as causing inflammation, puffiness, and tissue tightness. An overly acidic condition is a breeding ground for cancer, diabetes, parasites, and immune deficiencies. Acidosis is also a major factor contributing to drug addiction.

Signs of acidosis include:

- Craving coffee, alcohol, marijuana, cocaine, and other drugs
- Stress headaches
- Anger and short temper
- Muscle stiffness and spasms
- Sinus congestion
- Irritability
- Lethargy
- Negative thought patterns
- Itchy skin
- Acne
- White lines or flecks in the iris of the eyes

Chlorine, iodine, nitrogen, phosphorus, silicon, and sulfur are the most common acid-forming elements. Acidic compounds of these elements tend to be present in the roots and seeds of plants and the muscles of animals.

Alkalosis

When less hydrogen is present in the blood and tissues, this is a state of increased alkalinity, or alkalosis. Alkaline elements and compounds are prevalent in the body and are required in bodily fluids, including blood. In fact, healthy cells are slightly alkaline. Most people will find that their health and well-being benefit from becoming more alkaline through diet; being overly alkaline, however, is unhealthy.

Symptoms of alkalosis include:

- Anxiety
- Overexcitability
- Spaciness
- Laziness
- Chronic coldness
- Muscle spasms
- Slow recovery from injury
- Muscle tension and pain

- Lack of ambition
- Passivity

- Low tolerance for stimulation
- Heartburn

Calcium, iron, magnesium, manganese, potassium, silicon, and sodium are the most prevalent alkaline elements. These elements tend to be present in the leaves and stems of plants and in the bones of animals.

The Raw Facts

Although many fruits are known to have an acidic flavor, they may, in fact, promote alkalinity in the body. For example, many think of lemons and oranges as being acidic; however, they have an alkalinizing effect in the body.

Acid-Producing Foods

In general, consume acid-producing foods in greater moderation than alkali-forming foods.

FRUITS		
Blueberries	Pineapple (if picked unripe)	Strawberries
Cranberries (slightly acid-producing)	Plums and prunes	

VEGETABLES		
Rhubarb	Sauerkraut	

GRAINS		
Barley	Oats	Spelt
Buckwheat	Rice (slightly acid-producing)	Wheat
Kamut	Rye	

BEANS		
Azuki beans	Kidney beans	Navy beans
Black beans	Lentils	Pinto beans
Garbanzo beans	Mung beans	Red beans

NUTS AND SEEDS		
Brazil nuts	Macadamias	Pistachios
Cashews	Peanuts	Pumpkin seeds
Hazelnuts/filberts	Pecans	Sunflower seeds

FLAVORINGS

Artificial sweeteners	Pepper	Vegetable oils (except olive oil)
Curry	Salt	White vinegar
Molasses	Sugar	

Alkali-Producing Foods

To become more alkaline and less acidic, incorporate the following foods into your diet. Limit your intake of meats, fats, and sugars. Try drinking wheatgrass juice—it's very alkalinizing.

FRUITS

Apples	Grapes	Passionfruit
Apricots	Guava	Peaches
Avocados	Kiwi	Pears
Bananas (ripe)	Kumquats	Persimmons
Berries (except blueberries)	Litchi	Pineapple (ripe)
Cantaloupe	Mangoes	Plums
Citrus fruits	Melons	Pomegranates
Currants	Nectarines	Raisins
Dates	Olives	Tamarinds
Figs	Papayas	Watermelon

VEGETABLES

Algae	Endive/Escarole	Peas (fresh)
Artichokes	Garlic	Peppers
Asparagus	Herbs	Potatoes
Beets	Horseradish	Pumpkins
Broccoli	Jerusalem artichoke	Radishes
Brussels sprouts	Kale	Rutabagas
Burdock	Kelp	Spinach
Cabbages	Kohlrabi	Spirulina
Carrots	Leeks	Sprouts
Cauliflower	Lettuce	Squash (summer and winter)
Celery	Mushrooms	String beans
Collard greens	Mustard greens	Sweet potatoes
Corn (fresh)	Okra	Swiss chard
Cucumbers	Onions	Tomatoes
Dulse	Parsley	Turnips
Eggplant	Parsnips	Watercress

GRAINS		
Buckwheat	Millet	Sprouted grains

BEANS		
Lima beans	Mung bean sprouts	Soybeans

NUTS AND SEEDS		
Almonds	Coconut	Sesame seeds

FLAVORINGS		
Acidophilus	Goat's milk	Olive oil
Apple cider vinegar	Honey	Tamari
Bee pollen	Miso	Umeboshi plum paste
Carob	Nutritional yeast	

COLOR THERAPY

Color is the radiant reflection of luminous energy in various wavelengths, with the power to affect both the body and soul. Color therapy, or the conscious implementation of color to encourage well-being and healing, has been used in schools, hospitals, workplaces, and other institutions for decades. Science has shown that blood pressure, pulse, and respiratory rate are decreased by exposure to cool colors, such as green, blue, and black, and increased by warm colors, such as red, orange, and yellow.

We often select our clothing to invoke certain moods: light, bright colors to complement the hues of spring, or deep, dark colors for somber occasions. We decorate our homes with paints, pillows, tapestries, and lights of different colors in an effort to evoke certain atmospheres. Our choices of color in terms of our diet have a similar power. Colors in plant foods not only indicate the presence of certain nutritional compounds but, when ingested, yield a vibrational energy that can be used to nourish both our physical and emotional selves.

For optimum health, eat foods in a wide range of colors. Your meals should be a riotous rainbow of color, rather than a bland palette of whites or browns. Celebrate life by celebrating color!

Red

Red, the most physical and sensual of the colors, vibrates the most slowly and has the longest wavelength in the visible spectrum. Red is stimulating, hot (*yang*), and exciting; it is associated with vitality, strength, passion, and willpower.

Red stimulates the sympathetic nervous system. It can be used to treat anemia, colds, low blood pressure, erectile dysfunction, fatigue, weakness, and depression. It helps one feel present and grounded. Use red when feeling run down, to improve athletic performance, and when quick energy bursts are required. A study done on athletes at the University of Texas indicated that viewing red light increased strength by 13.5 percent and produced 5.8 percent more electrical muscle activity.

When red is present in food, it often denotes ripeness or sweetness, as well as the presence of lycopenes, quercetin, and vitamin C. Because red is so energizing, it should be avoided in decorating eating areas, as it makes diners feel hurried. In packaging, however, red is attention getting and highly visible, so you'll find it often on supermarket shelves.

Red Foods

- Beets
- Cayenne
- Cherries
- Cranberries
- Dulse
- Hibiscus flowers
- Kidney beans
- Pink grapefruit
- Radishes
- Raspberries
- Red apples
- Red cabbages
- Red currants
- Red peppers
- Red plums
- Rhubarb
- Rose hips
- Strawberries
- Tomatoes
- Watermelon
- Whole wheat

Orange

Orange is the blending of red (physical action) with yellow (wisdom). It symbolizes enthusiasm, outgoingness, optimism, confidence, joyfulness, and courage.

Orange can lift spirits, foster humor, and loosen repression. Orange is associated with the sexual center, skin, kidneys, pancreas, spleen, and bronchial tubes. Use orange to help relieve asthma, bronchitis, constipation, diarrhea, gas, hemorrhoids, and hypoglycemia.

In plant foods, orange is often an indicator of high carotene content. Being a social color, orange is useful for decorative highlights in places where people gather, such as family rooms. Fast-food restaurants use orange to attract lots of people without encouraging them to linger.

Orange Foods

- Almonds
- Apricots
- Cantaloupe
- Carrots
- Coriander
- Cumin
- Dates
- Ginger
- Mangoes
- Nectarines
- Oranges
- Papayas
- Paprika
- Peaches
- Persimmons
- Pumpkins
- Sweet potatoes
- Tangerines
- Walnuts
- Winter squash

Yellow

Yellow is warm (*yang*) and is associated with things sunny, cheerful, joyous, optimistic, practical, confident, and illuminating. It is also associated with wisdom, knowledge, logic, and the mind.

Yellow is used to benefit the adrenal glands, gallbladder, liver, muscles, nervous system, pancreas, and stomach. Illnesses that can be treated with yellow are allergies, arthritis, asthma, constipation, coughs, depression, diabetes, eczema, gallstones, gas, hiatal hernia, hypothyroidism, indigestion, lymphatic congestion, motion sickness, and obesity. Yellow is a nerve stimulant; it can be helpful with depression, fear, and tension, and can soothe mental exhaustion.

Yellow in food often indicates the presence of lutein, magnesium, and vitamin C and limonene. Because it is a sharpening color that enhances alertness, concentration, communication, and focus, you will often find yellow on food packaging.

Yellow Foods

- Anise seeds
- Bananas
- Chamomile
- Cinnamon
- Corn
- Dill
- Evening primrose flowers
- Golden apples
- Grapefruit
- Honey
- Lemons
- Lemongrass
- Marigold flowers
- Nuts
- Parsnips
- Pineapple
- Saffron
- Vegetable oils
- Whole grains
- Yams
- Yellow peppers
- Yellow squash

Green

Green is made by combining yellow (wisdom) with blue (spirituality). Being in the middle of the color spectrum, it is neither hot nor cold. Green is the color of the heart center, healing, balance, compassion, love, transformation, growth, generosity, and peace.

Green is rejuvenating and anti-inflammatory. Green can help calm anger and improve memory, paranoia, and nervous exhaustion. It affects the lungs, heart, thymus gland, and immune system. Use green for backaches, heart trouble, immune disorders, lupus, allergies, head colds, shock, and trauma, and to lower blood pressure.

Green in plants signifies the presence of chlorophyll. We see green as clean, crisp, and refreshing, and so it is often used to market cleaning products.

Green Foods

- Alfalfa
- Asparagus
- Avocados
- Broccoli
- Brussel sprouts
- Celery
- Chives
- Comfrey
- Cucumbers
- Green grapes
- Green peppers
- Kiwi
- Leafy green vegetables
- Lettuce
- Limes
- Mint
- Nettles
- Okra
- Oregano
- Parsley
- Peas
- Rosemary
- String beans
- Tarragon
- Wheatgrass
- Zucchini

Blue

Blue is cool (yin), crisp, clean, and refreshing. Blue is associated with spirituality, serenity, truth, communication, revelation, trust, and faith. Its effect is calming and instills gentleness and composure. Blue can be used to counteract violence, restlessness, agitation, hyperactivity, violence, and insomnia.

Being a counterirritant, blue is the color of choice to soothe pain and suffering. It causes the brain to secrete tranquilizing chemicals. Blue can be used to lower blood pressure, pulse rate, and brain wave activity, and to quiet menstrual cramps. Use blue for a fever, sore throat, ear infection, toothaches, bee stings, hyperthyroid, colic, burns, itches, and rashes. It is also used in hospital neonatal wards to facilitate the breakdown of bilirubin in jaundiced babies.

Blue foods are often rich in flavonoids. Blue is not always a good color for decorating a social area due to its quieting, cooling effect.

Blue Foods

- Blue corn
- Blue grapes
- Blue potatoes
- Blueberries
- Borage flowers
- Catnip
- Chicory flowers
- Hyssop
- Juniper berries
- Kelp
- Pansy flowers

Indigo

Indigo, a regal, dark blue-violet, is cool (*yin*) and calming. It is associated with our psychic awareness, intuition, and memory.

Indigo is soothing and antiseptic. It can help balance fear, frustration, and negative emotions; it helps one to be less aware of pain yet fully conscious. Use indigo for pain, poor motor skills, posture, menstrual irregularities, hair loss, and eye and ear disorders.

In foods, indigo appears as blue with a black overtone, as in black beans, blackberries, or plums. Indigo foods are often good sources of vitamin K and lycopene.

Indigo Foods

- Black beans
- Blackberries
- Black cherries
- Black currants
- Black olives
- Black soybeans
- Boysenberries
- Plums
- Prunes
- Raisins
- Tamari
- Vanilla beans
- Violet flowers

Violet

Violet is a mix of blue (spirituality) and red (passion), is considered regal, dignified, and exclusive. It is cooling (*yin*), cleansing, antiseptic, soothing, and narcotic. Violet symbolizes creative imagination and spiritual attainment, and corresponds to psychic protection, artistry, and mystery. It correlates to cosmic consciousness; with violet, we can be more open to divine power.

Violet helps normalize hormonal activity, curb appetite, and regulate metabolism. It is said to be more sexually stimulating to women. Use violet to treat migraines, epilepsy, parasites, dandruff, and baldness, to soothe serious mental conditions, and to relieve the side effects of chemotherapy.

Violet foods are often rich in vitamin D.

Violet Foods

- Amaranth
- Basil flowers
- Dulse
- Eggplant
- Elderberries
- Lavender
- Marjoram
- Mint flowers
- Mulberries
- Passionflower
- Passionfruit
- Purple cabbages
- Purple grapes
- Purple onions
- Purple plums
- Rosemary flowers
- Sage flowers
- Thyme flowers

Black

Black foods are associated with the kidneys and bladder in Asian medicine. Foods that are black in color are usually rich in minerals.

Black Foods

- Black beans
- Black quinoa
- Black sesame seeds
- Seaweeds
- Wild rice

White

White is associated with the top of the color spectrum (crown chakra) and, in Asian medicine, with strengthening to the lungs and large intestines. White foods are often rich in sulfur and quercetin.

White Foods

- Cauliflower
- Garlic
- Horseradish
- Jicama
- Radish
- White onion

THE FIVE FLAVORS

Our taste buds are capable of deciphering five different flavors: sour, bitter, sweet, pungent (spicy), and salty. (The Ayurvedic tradition, however, includes a sixth flavor, astringent; see the description of sour, below.) When we eat, our taste buds transmit signals about the type and potency of the flavors they are experiencing; when our brain receives those signals, it recognizes the flavors.

According to Oriental medicine, the experience of each flavor stimulates various physiological functions. Salty, sour, and bitter are considered *yin* or cooling, with a downward-moving energy. *Yin* flavors tend to arise and subside quickly. Sweet and pungent are considered *yang* or warming, with an upward-moving energy. *Yang* flavors are slower to be sensed and remain longer in the mouth.

These are vast generalizations, of course, and exceptions exist. Most foods contain a combination of flavors. Cinnamon, for example, is both pungent and sweet, whereas apples are both sweet and sour. Having a diet balanced in all five flavors helps keep the body in balance; omitting one flavor from the diet is like removing a color from the rainbow, leaving you with a less beautiful, less harmonized experience. Unfortunately, the typical Western diet tends to overemphasize the sweet and salty flavors while abandoning the bitter, pungent, and sour flavors.

It's also important to eat a diet that varies in potency of flavor. Some foods, like watercress, have strong flavors, and some, like lettuce, are mild. Eating a diet of only mild, bland foods can make the personality thus. Choosing only strongly flavored foods may support an overly intense personality. As is so often the case, moderation and variety are the keys to health and well-being. Savor the many flavors of life!

The Raw Facts

To improve your sense of taste, chew food thoroughly to allow more molecules to interact with your smell and taste receptors. The back of the tongue is most receptive to bitterness; the sides react most sensitively to salty and sour flavors; and the tip of the tongue reacts most to sweetness.

Sour

The sour flavor is cooling, drying, and astringent. It is usually due to the presence of acids such as ascorbic, citric, and malic acid.

Sourness stimulates the liver, gallbladder, appetite, and salivary function, and can aid in fat metabolism. It can restrict secretions such as seminal fluid, sweat, urine, blood, and diarrhea. It helps tonify tissue and may benefit conditions such as varicosities and hemorrhoids. Excessive sourness, however, can weaken the muscles, impair digestion, and make one's flesh tough.

Some examples of sour foods are lemons, lemongrass, orange peel, raspberries, rhubarb, rose hips, sorrel, tomatoes, Rejuvelac, seed-milk yogurt, and apple cider vinegar.

The astringent flavor is a powerful version of sour. It is very drying and cooling.

Examples of astringent foods include pomegranates, cranberries, beans, lentils, broccoli, cabbages, cauliflower, celery, spinach, and cinnamon.

Bitter

The bitter flavor is considered cooling, drying, strengthening, draining, and anti-inflammatory. This flavor usually indicates the presence of some type of alkaloid.

Bitterness stimulates the small intestines, pancreas, and digestive secretions. It helps strengthen the heart, lower cholesterol and fevers, deter parasites, improve the metabolism of fats, and strengthen people with food allergies. Bitterness helps eliminate heat and phlegm, especially from the lungs, and is often indicated in cases of inflammation and health conditions involving excess dampness. It is also beneficial for people who are lethargic as well as hot and aggressive. Too much bitterness, however, can be drying and contractive, causing skin withering and hair loss. People who are cold, dry, or suffering from ulcers should limit the bitter flavor in their diet.

Examples of bitter foods include celery, endive, escarole, hops, kale, parsley, spinach, and yarrow.

Sweet

The sweet flavor is an indicator of sugars in a food. Sweetness nourishes the *yin*, or fluids, of the body; they, in turn, help build up the person who is dry, has a weak immune system, or is frail.

The sweet flavor is regarded as a general tonic that is especially nourishing to the stomach and spleen. It mitigates acute symptoms, increases tolerance for stress and pain, and both energizes and calms. Excessive sweetness, however, can lead to lethargy and congestion, slow down digestion, and cause aching in the bones and joints.

Examples of sweet foods include bananas, dates, figs, prunes, mangoes, peaches, pears, raisins, apple juice, orange juice, honey, stevia (an herb that is used as a natural sweetener), winter squash, and sweet potatoes.

Pungent (Spicy)

The pungent or spicy flavor is warming and dispersing. Most pungent foods contain some sort of essential oil that moves internal energy to the surface, and they are said to be cooling to the interior of the body while warming to the exterior. Many pungent foods have antimicrobial activity.

The pungent flavor affects the lungs and large intestines in particular. It induces perspiration, stimulates the nerves, and promotes circulation. It also stimulates hydrochloric acid production and thus aids digestion. Pungent foods are especially beneficial for those with cold constitutions. Too much pungency can decrease flexibility, impair digestion, and lead to erectile dysfunction and exhaustion. Limit pungent flavors in the diet in cases of general debilitation, dizziness, burning sensations (such as sweating, heat in the mouth, or even hot flashes), and neuralgia.

Examples of pungent foods include basil, cayenne, cinnamon, garlic, ginger, horseradish (especially wasabi), mustard greens or seeds, onions, oregano, peppermint, radishes, and rosemary.

Salty

The salty taste is cold, softening, draining, and diuretic. It indicates the presence of mineral salts.

Salt especially affects the nerves, kidneys, and bladder. It aids fluid metabolism and helps strengthen the nerves. If used in moderation, salt can have a cleansing effect in the body; for example, it can help soften hardened masses, such as tumors. The overuse of salt, however, can contribute to fluid retention, erectile dysfunction, gray hair, loose teeth, eczema, and high blood pressure. Craving salt excessively may indicate adrenal exhaustion.

Celery, dill, and sea vegetables like kelp and dulse are good examples of salty foods.

THE DOCTRINE OF SIGNATURES

The Doctrine of Signatures is a philosophy that appears in almost every world culture. Its foundation is the concept that every living thing is marked with a "signature" (however subtle it may be) that tells its use, function, or role in the world. The signature is a function of the organism's features and environment. This philosophy holds, for example, that by observing a plant closely and taking note of the color of its flower, the shape of its leaf, and how and where it grows, we can determine its place in the universal plan.

According to the Doctrine of Signatures, plants that thrive in a particular environment are meant to be used—in the diet or as healing medicines—by the denizens of that environment. Plants that grow right outside your back door, for example, may be saying, "Use me. Use me a lot." Plants that are rare in a particular environment might be asking to be used with caution and respect. Plants available only in the spring or fall might be appropriate for just that time of year.

Would you believe that kidney beans, which are shaped like a human kidney, are good for the kidneys? That beets, with their blood-red color, help build the blood? That cauliflower, with its cerebrum-shaped head, nourishes the brain? Although this reasoning may sound superstitious, it often turns out to be true. We must simply discover the connection between plant and effect. Some might say that the attribution of signature comes after the fact, as a result of the discovery of a plant's use: "Ah, yes, we have seen that cauliflower nourishes the brain. And oh my—cauliflower looks like a brain, too! Obviously, it was trying to tell us what we have just discovered." But such skepticism begs the question of which came first: the discovery of cauliflower's brain-nourishing powers, or of its particular form and shape?

If you have trouble believing in the philosophy and its implications, you can at least consider it a system of memory cues. Once you've learned that beets build the blood, for example, you can commit that fact to memory by linking their blood-red color with their blood-building properties. And whether or not one is to give any credit to the Doctrine of Signatures, consider the terminology associated with cooking: fried, burned, baked, toasted, grilled, roasted, scrambled, scorched, seared, irradiated, parched, scalded, smoked, sizzled, and so on. These are all terms associated with pain, fire, and destruction. Wouldn't you rather avail yourself of the life energy of raw foods: fresh, crisp, alive, vital, natural, active, and colorful?

FASTING

If the medical professionals courageously popularized the fast among their patients, there would be infinitely less suffering than there is now. That many would be saved who now die through the drug and feeding treatment is a certainty.

—Gandhi (1945)

The ancient practice of fasting is the safest, quickest, and least expensive method of healing. It accelerates both physical and spiritual purification and rejuvenation. Although your immune system will function at optimal strength while you're on a raw foods diet, if you should happen to become ill, fasting offers a quick way to recover.

Fasting provides the following benefits:

- Conserves energy
- Causes colds and flus to vanish rapidly
- Gives overburdened organs a chance to rest
- Improves the intestines' ability to digest and assimilate
- Facilitates the breakdown, absorption, and elimination of abnormal growths and obstructions in the body
- Frees energy for creativity and mental focus
- Helps a body accomplish, in just a few days, healing that might otherwise take weeks or never happen
- Allows the organs of elimination to discharge accumulated material and inorganic chemicals
- Can help one quickly let go of addictions
- Allows for a restful time for the body to heal itself
- Can help the body eliminate deep illness
- Fine-tunes mental faculties
- Creates a state of heightened awareness

Some people have a tradition of fasting at the seasonal equinoxes. Many like to begin a fast at the new moon, long associated with new beginnings. A fast can be begun at any time, although there are certain logistical details to consider. Rest and relaxation are important during a fast, so it's important to schedule your fast for when you can take time away from the hustle of your ordinary life.

If you have never fasted before, you may want to begin by simply skipping a meal. Then, try fasting one day a week or for thirty-six hours. Once you have grown accustomed to these shorter fasts and are ready for a three-day fast, start fasting on the last day of your work week, and then take the weekend to complete the fast. Hunger usually disappears by the third day. When your mouth tastes fresh and sweet and perspiration becomes fragrant, you'll know that your body has cleansed itself.

Note: Unless you are experienced with fasting, you should not undertake a fast of longer than three days without proper guidance from an experienced healthcare practitioner.

While you are fasting, drink plenty of pure water. Sip, rather than gulp, to avoid swallowing air and causing gastrointestinal distress. If you become hungry, do five to ten minutes' worth of vigorous exercise, such as jumping jacks. In general, mild exercise, such as walking or working in the garden, is appropriate, but you should avoid exertion. When you bathe, the water temperature should be lukewarm; cold showers or baths can lower blood pressure and cause dizziness, and hot baths and showers can be weakening. Before bathing, encourage the elimination of toxins by dry-brushing your skin with a natural-fiber brush: start at the limbs and work inward from the feet and hands, making five to ten circular strokes in each area.

When Not to Fast

Fasting is not recommended in cases of hernia, paralysis, advanced cancer (especially of the liver), diabetes, hypoglycemia, tuberculosis, lead poisoning, advanced osteoporosis, inflammation, or wasting disease. Do not fast if you are emotionally distressed, overly cold or hot, more than 10 pounds underweight, pregnant, or nursing. Fasting is also not encouraged during very cold seasons because it diminishes body heat.

While you are fasting from food, fast also from junk television, junk literature, and using foul language. Clean your space, closets, and cupboards. By making these outer changes, you will be reminded of your inner cleansing. Allow fasting to be a tool for evolution, so that you return to your ordinary life a better person.

Juices and Cleansing Beverages

Although the water-only fast is considered the true and best method of fasting, you can also drink water flavored with freshly squeezed lemon juice. Fresh-pressed diluted juices, though not part of a true fast, can nourish, cleanse, and provide raw materials for healing. Consider diluted carrot, beet, celery, cucumber, watermelon, and wheatgrass juices. Coconut water is excellent for a fast, truly healing, and absolutely delicious. If you are fasting on juices, make sure they are freshly made and not pasteurized (as pasteurized juices lack enzymes).

The Master Cleanser

*Try drinking this beverage during a fast
to facilitate cleansing of your body systems.
(My gratitude goes to Stanley Burroughs, author
of* The Master Cleanser, *and creator of this recipe.)*

1 gallon water

1/2 cup lemon juice

1/4 teaspoon cayenne powder

Maple syrup (not a raw product),
raw honey, or soaked dates

Combine all ingredients, using the maple syrup,
honey, or soaked dates to sweeten. Drink as
much of this cleanser as desired.

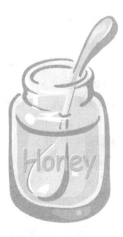

Citrus Juice Cleanser

*Like the Master Cleanser, this beverage promotes system
cleansing and can be consumed during a fast,
in addition to plain water.*

Juice of 12 oranges

Juice of 6 lemons

Juice of 6 grapefruit

Spring water

Combine the citrus juices in a glass gallon jar.
Fill the jar to the top with spring water.
Drink a glass of this cleanser every
hour or as desired.

Breaking the Fast

Break your fast with something easy to digest: a diluted juice or a light, refreshing organic fruit such as cantaloupe or pear. Continue eating only fruit for several meals. Then have a salad for a meal, and gradually progress back to eating a regular raw foods diet.

FOOD COMBINING

The philosophy of food combining, in which certain foods are said to complement or oppose each other in the digestive process, is based primarily on cooked food. When you are following a raw foods diet, which is bountiful in the enzymatic activity that aids digestion, proper food combining is not as critical. It does become critical, however, for people with poor assimilation, digestion problems, or low energy. If you are eating a completely raw diet and are still experiencing any of these health concerns, the food-combining guidelines below may be helpful.

Mixing foods that require different digestive times and enzymes can cause food digestion to be difficult or slow. Starch digestion, for example, begins in the mouth and requires alkaline digestive secretion; but protein digestion begins in the stomach, where acid secretions such as hydrochloric acid and pepsin are found. When mixed, the alkaline and acidic secretions neutralize each other, resulting in poor digestion of both starch and protein.

Avoid drinking beverages simultaneously with meals to avoid diluting your digestive juices. Ideally, drink one half-hour before a meal or one and a half hours after.

Fruits and vegetables are generally best not mixed. The exceptions to this rule are avocado (a fruit), which combines well with vegetables, and celery and lettuce, which combine well with fruit. Avoid combining acidic fruits such as grapefruit with sweet fruits such as raisins, because acidic and sweet fruits require different digestive times and secretions. People who find that fruit gives them gas can blame it on improper combining or the fact that the fruit is cleansing bacterial overgrowth from the digestive tract.

It is best not to eat fruit for at least one to two hours after a meal. Fruit is digested quickly and can ferment if it's held up in the digestive process by other, more complex foods that are difficult to digest. When eating several fruits, save the sweetest fruits for last, as their higher concentration of sugars will facilitate the digestion of the less-sweet fruits.

For optimal digestion, eat light foods before heavy foods, because the lighter foods (being more watery) will be digested more quickly. Eat fats and proteins at separate meals. Save raw desserts such as cakes, cookies, and puddings to be eaten at least an hour after a meal and only a couple of times a week.

Some raw foodists eat only one food at a time, which is probably ideal for digestion. However, I love the fact that simply eating raw, even when I don't follow all the food-combining rules, has brought me and my family better health and excellent digestion.

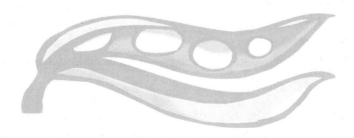

APPENDIX

Nutrients and Source Foods

In Chapters 1 through 7, we examined the characteristics of a wide range of fruits, vegetables, nuts, grains, and other components of a raw foods diet. Here you'll find explanations of the terminology that came up in those chapters, with discussions of the actions and benefits of particular nutritional compounds. The description of each compound is followed by a list of foods in which it can be found. If you wish to focus on a particular nutrient, be sure to eat adequate amounts of the foods that are listed with it. Of course, you must also be sure to eat a wide range of foods in order to meet your body's overall nutritional requirements. Choosing a varied diet of raw foods will enable you to build an optimal nutritional foundation without having to rely heavily on supplements.

Carotenoids

Carotenoids prevent vision problems, improve skin health, help repair the lining of the respiratory and digestive tracts, enhance immunity, and help protect against pollution. There are many different kinds of carotenoids, from alpha to zeta. Monoterpene carotenoids, for example, in addition to having the above characteristics, are antioxidant and protect against cancer and heart disease.

Alpha-Carotene

Berries (all)　　　　　　　　Oranges
Broccoli　　　　　　　　　　Peaches
Carrots　　　　　　　　　　 Pumpkins
Corn　　　　　　　　　　　　Seaweeds
Leafy green vegetables (all)　Sweet potatoes

■Beta-Carotene

Apricots (fresh and dried)
Broccoli
Cabbages
Cantaloupe
Grapefruit
Leafy green vegetables (all)
Lamb's-quarter
Mangoes
Nori
Oranges

Orange vegetables (especially pumpkins, sweet potatoes, and yams)
Papayas
Parsley
Peppers (especially green)
Persimmons
Tomatoes
Watermelon
Winter squash
Yellow squash

■Cryptoxanthin

Apples
Apricots (fresh and dried)
Corn
Green peppers
Lemons

Oranges
Papayas
Paprika
Persimmons
Starfruit

■Gamma-Carotene

Tomatoes

■Lutein

Apples
Apricot
Beets
Broccoli
Brussels sprouts
Calendula flowers
Carrots
Collard greens
Corn
Cranberry
Hibiscus
Kale
Kiwi
Lettuce
Marigold flowers

Mustard greens
Orange juice
Orange peel
Paprika
Peach
Peas
Potatoes
Pumpkins
Raisins
Red grapes
Red peppers
Spinach
Spirulina
Taro root
Tomatoes

Turnip greens
Winter squash

Zucchini

▪Lycopene

Apricots (fresh and dried)
Carrots
Green peppers
Guava

Pink grapefruit
Tomatoes
Watermelon

▪Monoterpenes

Basil
Broccoli
Carrots
Citrus fruits (all)
Eggplant

Parsley
Peppermint
Tomatoes
Yams

▪Phytoene

Tomatoes

▪Phytofluene

Tomatoes

▪Zeaxanthin

Bell peppers
Corn
Grapes
Leafy green vegetables (all)
Kiwi
Marigold flowers

Oranges
Paprika
Raisins
Spirulina
Squash (winter varieties)
Zucchini

▪Zeta-Carotene

Tomatoes

B-Complex Vitamins

This group of vitamins functions as coenzymes (a substance necessary for enzyme functioning) and is especially important in the metabolism of fats, carbohydrates, and proteins. B-complex vitamins are needed for cellular reproduction, including production of red and white blood cells. Individual B vitamins, described below, also offer particular benefits.

Each of the following foods contains the entire group of B-complex vitamins:

Alfalfa leaf

Beans (especially pea)

Brown rice

Brussels sprouts

Leafy green vegetables (all)

Nuts (all)

Nutritional yeast

Whole grains (all)

▓ *Vitamin B$_1$ (Thiamine)*

Vitamin B$_1$, or thiamine, is necessary for a sense of well-being. It promotes muscle tone in the digestive tract, improves nutrient assimilation, and stabilizes the appetite.

Apricots (fresh and dried)

Asparagus

Avocados

Broccoli

Leafy green vegetables (all)

Nutritional yeast

Nuts (especially almonds, Brazil
  nuts, pine nuts, and pistachios)

Peas

Pineapple

Seeds (especially chia, flax, pumpkin,
  sesame, and sunflower)

Soy

Watermelon

Whole grains (especially brown
  rice, millet, oats, and rye)

▓ *Vitamin B$_2$ (Riboflavin)*

Vitamin B$_2$, or riboflavin, supports growth and energy. It promotes healthy vision by preventing dry eyes and cataracts, and is also needed for the health of skin, hair, and nails. Cracks around the corners of the mouth can indicate a riboflavin deficiency.

Asparagus

Avocados

Beans (all)

Bee pollen and royal jelly

Black currants (fresh and dried)

Broccoli

Leafy green vegetables (especially
  collard greens and spinach)

Mushrooms

Nutritional yeast

Nuts (all)

Okra

Soy

Sunflower seeds

Whole grains (especially brown rice)

▓ *Vitamin B$_3$ (Niacin)*

Vitamin B$_3$, or niacin, is necessary for production of adrenal and sex hormones. In addition to aiding the metabolism of fats, carbohydrates, and proteins, this nutrient helps regulate blood sugar levels and lowers cholesterol.

Asparagus
Avocados
Broccoli
Cantaloupe
Dates
Figs (fresh and dried)
Leafy green vegetables (all)
Mushrooms
Plums and prunes
Raspberries
Sesame seeds

Beans (all)
Bee pollen
Soy
Squash
Strawberries
Sunflower seeds
Tempeh
Tomatoes
Watermelon
Whole grains (especially barley, millet, and brown rice)

Vitamin B$_6$ (Pyridoxine)

Vitamin B$_6$, or pyridoxine, is required for the production of stomach acids and the absorption of vitamin B$_{12}$. It is also important for hormonal balance and supports immune system function.

Apples
Asparagus
Avocados
Bananas
Barley
Beans (especially garbanzo, lentil, lima, navy, pea, and soy)
Bee pollen
Blueberries
Brown rice
Buckwheat
Cabbages
Cantaloupe
Carrots
Corn
Flaxseeds
Grapes and raisins
Leafy green vegetables (all)

Mangoes
Mushrooms
Nutritional yeast
Nuts (especially Brazil nuts, chestnuts, hazelnuts/filberts, and walnuts)
Onions
Oranges
Plums and prunes
Sesame seeds
Soy
Squash
Sunflower seeds
Sweet potatoes
Tomatoes
Walnuts
Watermelon
Whole wheat

Biotin

Biotin can be provided through the diet, but this B vitamin is also produced by healthy intestinal flora.

Almonds   Mushrooms
Bananas   Nutritional Yeast
Beans   Soy
Grapes and raisins   Walnuts
Leafy green vegetables (all)   Whole grains (all)

Folic Acid

Folic acid helps in RNA and DNA production, and is necessary for the development of the nervous system in embryos.

Almonds   Grapes and raisins
Artichokes   Leafy green vegetables
Asparagus   (especially spinach)
Avocados   Nutritional yeast
Barley   Oranges
Beans   Papayas
  (especially garbanzo and soy)   Pecans
Bee pollen   Plums and prunes
Beets   Rice
Blackberries   Rye
Brussels sprouts   Soy
Cabbages   Sunflower seeds
Cantaloupe   Sweet potatoes
Dates   Walnuts
Fenugreek seeds   Whole wheat

Para-Aminobenzoic Acid (PABA)

Para-aminobenzoic acid, or PABA, is a constituent of folic acid. PABA aids in the assimilation of pantothenic acid and supports healthy intestinal flora. It is also considered an antioxidant that protects the skin from cancer and sunburn.

Beans (all)   Spinach
Mushrooms   Whole grains (all)
Nutritional yeast

▇ Vitamin B₅ (Pantothenic Acid)

Pantothenic acid is found in most foods, plants, and animals. It is needed by the adrenal glands for hormone production and is also important in energy production.

Asparagus
Avocados
Beans (especially lentil, pea, and soy)
Bee pollen and royal jelly
Broccoli
Cabbages
Corn
Leafy green vegetables (all)
Nutritional yeast

Nuts (especially cashews, hazelnuts/ filberts, and pecans)
Papayas
Pineapple
Seeds (especially flax, sesame, and sunflower)
Shiitake mushrooms
Watermelon
Whole grains (especially buckwheat)
Yams
Yogurt

▇ Choline

Choline is necessary for the transmission of nerve impulses from the brain throughout the nervous system. Choline regulates gallbladder function, liver function, and hormone production. It also helps break down cholesterol, thereby normalizing cholesterol levels.

Avocados
Beans (especially garbanzo, lentil, pea, and soy)
Cabbages
Cauliflower
Corn
Green beans

Leafy green vegetables (all)
Nutritional yeast
Nuts (all)
Seeds (all)
Whole grains (especially brown rice and oats)

▇ Inositol

Inositol is needed for hair growth. It also helps reduce cholesterol, prevents hardening of the arteries, helps the liver metabolize fats, and has a calming effect.

Beans (all)
Cabbages
Fruit (all)
Leafy green vegetables (all)
Nutritional yeast

Nuts (all)
Seeds (all)
Sprouts (all)
Whole grains (all)

■ Vitamin B_{12} (Cyanocobalamin)

Vitamin B_{12}, or cobalamin, is probably considered the most controversial of vitamins. It is needed for digestion, nutrient assimilation, and protein synthesis. Vitamin B_{12} helps prevent anemia, aids folic acid in regulating the production of red blood cells, improves iron utilization, and promotes normal growth and fertility. It also prevents nerve damage by helping to manufacture the protective fatty insulation that surrounds the nerves. A deficiency in vitamin B_{12} can cause fatigue, nerve degeneration, clumsiness, depression, memory loss, and, in severe cases, death.

Vitamin B_{12} is produced by bacteria, so the B_{12} we're able to consume through our diet is derived from the bacteria on the plants and animals we eat. We also have B_{12}-producing bacteria living throughout our bodies, especially between the teeth and gums, on the tonsils and tongue, and in the nasal area and small intestines. To properly absorb B_{12}, we must have a healthy pancreas and strong gastric secretions. Once absorbed, the vitamin is not stored in the blood but in the liver and other organs.

There is conflicting information about the vitamin B_{12} content of different foods (especially fermented foods) and how much our bodies require, and more research is needed. Generally speaking, however, eating small amounts of unwashed, organic fruits and vegetables provides all the B_{12} we need. The most likely dietary sources of B_{12} are listed below. Some raw fooders choose to supplement B_{12} with a pill.

Alfalfa leaves	Nutritional yeast
Bananas	Plums and prunes
Barley grass	Sauerkraut (unpasteurized)
Bee pollen	Seaweeds (especially kelp and nori)
Comfrey leaves	Spirulina
Concord grapes and raisins	Sprouts (all)
Ginseng	Sunflower seeds
Hops	Yogurt
Miso (unpasteurized)	Wheatgrass
Mustard greens	

■ Vitamin B_{15} (Pangamic Acid)

Vitamin B_{15}, or pangamic acid, is needed to reduce histamine levels in the body, and also helps supply oxygen to the tissues.

Almonds	Brown rice
Apricot seeds	Nutritional yeast

Vitamin B$_{17}$ (Laetrile)

Vitamin B$_{17}$, or laetrile, is believed to inhibit the activity of cancer cells.

Almonds
Apple seeds
Apricot seeds
Barley
Blackberries
Brown rice
Buckwheat
Cherry seeds
Chia seeds
Cranberries (fresh and dried)
Elderberries
Flaxseeds
Garbanzo beans (sprouted)
Lentils (sprouted)
Macadamia nuts

Millet
Mung beans (sprouted)
Nectarine seeds
Oats
Peach seeds
Pear seeds
Plum seeds
Raspberries
Rye
Sesame seeds
Sprouts (all)
Strawberries
Whole wheat
Wheatgrass

Vitamin C (Ascorbic Acid)

Vitamin C is an antioxidant that helps repair tissue, gums, and adrenal glands. It aids in the production of interferon and antistress hormones, protects against the harmful effects of pollution, enhances immune system function, and improves the body's assimilation of iron.

Acerola cherries
Alfalfa sprouts
Asparagus
Avocados
Bananas
Blackberries
Black currants (fresh and dried)
Blueberries
Brazil nuts
Broccoli
Brussels sprouts
Cabbages
Cantaloupe
Cauliflower

Cherries
Green peppers
Guava
Hibiscus flowers
Honeydew melon
Kidney beans
Kiwi
Kumquats
Leafy green vegetables (especially
  collard greens, kale, kohlrabi,
  spinach, and watercress)
Lemons
Limes
Mangoes

Oranges
Papayas
Parsley
Pineapple
Radishes
Raspberries
Rose hips

Sauerkraut (unpasteurized)
Sorrel
Strawberries
Sweet potatoes
Tomatoes
Watermelon

Vitamin D

Vitamin D stimulates calcium absorption and supports blood clotting, nervous system function, and the growth of bones and teeth. For the most part, the body manufactures its own vitamin D through a process stimulated by exposure of the skin to ultraviolet rays (as from sunlight). Certain foods, however, provide small amounts of dietary vitamin D.

Alfalfa leaves
Basil
Chickweed
Bee pollen
Fenugreek seeds
Leafy green vegetables
  (especially watercress)
Horsetail

Mullein
Nettles
Papayas
Parsley
Shiitake mushrooms
Sunflower seeds and sunflower greens
Sweet potatoes
Wheatgrass

Vitamin E

Vitamin E is an antioxidant that improves circulation, aids tissue repair, promotes normal blood clotting, minimizes scarring, promotes fertility, and helps maintain healthy muscles, nerves, skin, and hair. Vitamin E also inhibits the oxidation of lipids, thus preventing the formation of destructive free radicals in the body.

Alfalfa sprouts and leaves
Apples
Asparagus
Beans (especially pea)
Blackberries
Broccoli
Cold-pressed oils (especially
  vegetable oils)
Cherries

Dandelion greens
Dulse
Flaxseeds
Leafy green vegetables (especially
  beet and turnip greens, lettuce,
  kale, spinach, and watercress)
Kelp
Leeks
Nettles

Nuts (especially almonds and
  hazelnuts/filberts)
Parsley
Parsnips
Peanuts
Purslane
Raspberry leaves

Rose hips
Strawberries
Sunflower seeds
Sweet potatoes
Tomatoes
Whole grains and their sprouts
  (especially oats and quinoa)

Essential Fatty Acids (EFAs)

All cells, including those involved in the production of hormones, need essential fatty acids (EFAs). These nutrients improve skin and hair, lower blood pressure and cholesterol levels, and reduce the risk of blood clots. EFAs are found in particularly high concentrations in the brain.

Gamma-Linolenic Acid (GLA)

Gamma-linolenic acid (GLA) helps lower cholesterol levels and blood pressure. GLA inhibits the formation of blood clots, improves mood, and can aid in weight loss.

Black currant seed oil
Borage seed oil

Evening primrose oil

Omega-3 Fatty Acids (Alpha-Linolenic Acids)

Omega-3 and omega-6 fatty acids are the only types of fatty acids that the body cannot synthesize itself. Omega-3 fatty acids are necessary for the production of anti-inflammatory prostaglandins and are found in cell membranes.

Beans (all)
Blue-green algae
Cabbages
Chia
Flaxseeds
Leafy green vegetables
  (especially spinach)
Hemp seeds
Pine nuts

Pumpkin seeds
Purslane
Sesame seeds
Soy
Sprouts (all)
Squash
Walnuts
Whole wheat

Omega-6 Fatty Acids (Linoleic Acids)

Like omega-3 fatty acids, omega-6 fatty acids cannot be synthesized in the body. A deficiency of omega-6 fatty acids can contribute to eczema, hair loss, liver degeneration, and susceptibility to infection, as well as infertility in men and miscarriage in women.

Beans (all)
Black currant seed oil
Borage seed oil
Corn
Evening primrose oil
Seeds (especially pumpkin and sesame)
Vegetable oils (all)
Whole grains (all)

Vitamin K

The "K" in this case comes from "the Koagulation vitamin" (there already was a vitamin C), in tribute to this vitamin's role in blood clotting. Vitamin K also aids in bone formation and in converting glucose into glycogen for storage in the liver. Intestinal bacteria normally synthesize half of the vitamin K that the body needs, and the rest must be ingested.

Alfalfa sprouts and leaves
Broccoli
Brussels sprouts
Cabbages
Cauliflower
Kelp
Leafy green vegetables
  (especially spinach, turnip
  greens, and watercress)
Nettles
Oats
Rye
Seaweeds
Shepherd's purse
Soy
Whole wheat

Vitamin U

Vitamin U is named after its ability to help heal ulcers.

Cabbages
Celery
Leafy green vegetables (all)

Boron

Boron helps the body metabolize calcium and magnesium and may promote bone integrity. It also enhances brain function and improves mental alertness.

Alfalfa leaves
Almonds
Apples
Beans (especially pea)
Cabbages
Carrots
Dates
Grapes and raisins
Hazelnuts/filberts
Kelp

Leafy green vegetables
(especially spinach)
Pears

Plums and prunes
Soy
Whole grains (all)

Calcium

Calcium helps the formation of bones, teeth, and muscles. It helps maintain a regular heartbeat, prevents muscle cramps, and enhances the transmission of nerve impulses.

Almonds
Beans (especially black, garbanzo, lentil, pinto, soy, and white)
Brazil nuts
Broccoli
Carob
Dandelion greens
Figs (fresh and dried)
Hazelnuts/filberts

Leafy green vegetables (especially beet, collard, mustard, and turnip greens, and kale)
Miso
Oats
Seaweeds (especially dulse, hiziki, kelp, kombu, and wakame)
Sesame seeds
Sunflower seeds
Yogurt

Cobalt

The mineral cobalt is a necessary component of a hemoglobin-type molecule that aids in the synthesis of vitamin B_{12}.

Alfalfa
Broccoli

Spinach

Chromium

Chromium aids in metabolism of glucose, fats, and proteins. By supporting the function of insulin, chromium helps stabilize blood sugar levels.

Apples
Bananas
Barley
Basil
Beans (all)
Beets
Black pepper
Broccoli
Carrots

Catnip
Cloves
Grapes and raisins
Horsetail
Licorice root
Mushrooms
Nettles
Nutritional Yeast
Nuts (especially walnuts)

Oatstraw

Oranges

Red clover flowers

Tomatoes

Whole grains (especially rye)

Yarrow

Chlorine

The digestive system uses chlorine in its secretions to cleanse, purify, and disinfect itself.

Beets

Blackberries

Cabbages

Carrots

Celery

Coconut

Cucumbers

Dandelion greens

Figs (fresh and dried)

Leafy green vegetables (especially spinach, Swiss chard, and watercress)

Mushrooms

Onions

Parsnips

Radishes

Sweet potatoes

Tomatoes

Copper

Copper helps in the formation of bones, collagen, elastin, and red blood cells.

Almonds

Apricots

Avocados

Beans (especially lentil)

Beets

Brazil nuts

Broccoli

Cauliflower

Garlic

Grapes and raisins

Leafy green vegetables (all)

Hazelnuts/filberts

Mushrooms

Pecans

Plums and prunes

Seaweeds

Soy

Sunflower seeds

Tomatoes

Walnuts

Whole grains and their sprouts (especially barley, buckwheat, millet, and oats)

Fluorine

Fluorine promotes hardness in the teeth and bones, and also helps the body resist infection.

Almonds

Avocados

Black-eyed peas

Brussels sprouts

Cabbages

Carrots

Cauliflower
Goat's milk (unpasteurized)
Green tea
Leafy green vegetables (especially
 beet greens and spinach)

Parsley
Rice
Rye
Seaweeds
Tomatoes

Germanium

Germanium improves immune system function and cellular oxygenation.

Aloe vera
Barley
Chlorella
Comfrey
Garlic

Ginseng (and eleuthero, formerly
 known as Siberian ginseng)
Oats
Shiitake mushrooms
Suma

Iodine

Iodine is a trace element necessary for thyroid health and the prevention of goiter. It helps curb weight gain.

Asparagus
Bee pollen
Beets
Cabbages
Carrots
Garlic
Leafy green vegetables (especially
 turnip greens and Swiss chard)

Onions
Pineapple
Sea salt
Seaweeds
Sesame seeds
Soy
Whole wheat

Iron

Iron is essential in the blood for oxygen transport and hemoglobin production. It also relieves fatigue.

Almonds
Apricots (fresh and dried)
Beans (especially black, garbanzo,
 lentil, lima, navy, pea, pinto, and soy)
Blackberries
Bran (especially wheat)
Burdock root
Carrots
Cherries

Dandelion greens
Deep-colored fruits
Dulse
Leafy green vegetables (especially
 beet and collard greens, kale,
 spinach, Swiss chard, and
 watercress)
Grapes and raisins
Green peppers

Jerusalem artichokes
Millet
Miso
Nettles
Oatmeal
Onions
Oysters
Parsley
Persimmons

Plums and prunes
Pumpkin seeds
Seaweeds (especially dulse, hiziki, kelp, kombu, and nori)
Sesame seeds
Shallots
Sprouted grass seeds
Squash (especially winter squash)
Sunflower seeds

Lithium

Lithium can help prevent depression (especially bipolar depression), violent behavior, violent impulses, and addiction, and it can improve fertility.

Dulse
Eggplant
Leafy green vegetables (all)

Kelp
Peppers
Tomatoes

Magnesium

Magnesium is necessary for bone structure and muscle and nerve function. It helps prevent and relax muscle spasms, and also prevents the bowel pockets that contribute to diverticulitis.

Alfalfa leaves
Apricots (fresh and dried)
Artichokes
Avocados
Bananas
Beans (especially black-eyed pea, kidney, lentil, lima, pea, and soy)
Broccoli
Cantaloupe
Carrots
Catnip
Cauliflower
Celery
Cloves
Corn
Dandelion greens
Dates

Fenugreek seeds
Figs (fresh and dried)
Leafy green vegetables (especially beet, collard, and mustard greens, spinach, Swiss chard, and watercress)
Mangoes
Mushrooms
Nettles
Nuts (especially almonds, Brazil nuts, cashews, pecans, pine nuts, and walnuts)
Oranges
Paprika
Parsley
Parsnips
Peaches
Peppermint

Peppers
Pineapple
Plums and prunes
Raspberry leaves
Red clover
Sage
Seaweeds (especially dulse, kelp, nori, and wakame)
Seeds (especially hemp, pumpkin, sesame, and sunflower)
Shepherd's purse
Squash
Strawberries
Sweet potatoes
Tomatoes
Triticale
Watermelon
Whole grains (especially barley, brown rice, buckwheat, millet, oats, quinoa, rye, and wild rice)
Yarrow
Yellow dock

Manganese

Manganese strengthens the tissues and linings of many structures in the body (including bones) and improves memory, brain, and nerve function. It is needed for blood sugar balance and immune system function.

Alfalfa leaves
Apples
Apricots (fresh and dried)
Avocados
Bananas
Beans (especially pea)
Bee pollen
Beets
Blueberries
Broccoli
Burdock root
Carrots
Catnip
Celery
Chamomile
Chickweed
Corn
Dandelion greens
Ginseng
Leafy green vegetables (all)
Hops
Lemongrass
Mullein
Nasturtium leaves
Nuts (especially almonds, pine nuts, and walnuts)
Parsley
Peppermint
Persimmons
Pineapple
Plums and prunes
Raspberry fruit and leaves
Red clover flower
Rose hips
Seaweeds
Seeds (especially fennel and fenugreek)
Soy
Sweet potatoes
Whole grains (especially oats and rye)
Yarrow
Yellow dock

Methyl-Sulfonyl-Methane (MSM)

Methyl-sulfonyl-methane (MSM) is an organic compound containing sulfur. MSM helps prevent skin eruptions, thickens and beautifies hair, improves athletic recovery time, supports tissue elasticity, and enhances brain function.

Aloe vera
Pine bark
Pine needles

Pine nuts
Rain-watered fruits and
  vegetables (unwashed)

Molybdenum

Molybdenum is needed in tiny amounts for the metabolism of nitrogen. It promotes normal cell function and a healthy libido.

Apricots (fresh and dried)
Beans (especially lentil, lima,
  pea, and soy)
Cantaloupe
Carrots
Garlic

Grapes and raisins
Leafy green vegetables (all)
Strawberries
Sunflower seeds
Whole grains (especially barley
  and buckwheat)

Phosphorus

Phosphorus is needed by all the organs of the body. It builds nerve strength, enhances mental capacity, and stimulates bone and hair growth. It helps generate cell energy and is a component of DNA. Phosphorus tends, however, to be overabundant in Western diets.

Asparagus
Beans (especially garbanzo, pea,
  and soy)
Broccoli
Corn
Garlic
Leafy green vegetables (especially
  collard greens and kale)

Nuts (especially almonds)
Parsnips
Pumpkin seeds
Sesame seeds
Seaweeds (especially dulse)
Whole grains (especially buckwheat,
  rye, and wheat)

Potassium

Potassium promotes tissue elasticity, supple muscles, regular heartbeat, and stable blood pressure. Cramps, muscle spasms, or a changeable personality can indicate a potassium deficiency.

Almonds
Apricots (fresh and dried)
Avocados
Bananas
Beans (especially lentils)
Beets
Black currants
Blueberries
Brown rice
Buckwheat
Cabbages
Cantaloupe
Carrots
Catnip
Dandelion greens
Dates
Dulse
Figs (fresh and dried)
Garlic
Grapes and raisins
Leafy green vegetables (especially
  beet greens, spinach, and
  Swiss chard)
Hops
Horsetail
Nettles
Onions
Oranges
Papayas
Peaches
Plantains
Pumpkin seeds
Red clover blossoms
Sage
Skullcap
Sunflower seeds
Tomatoes
Watermelon
Winter squash

Selenium

Selenium helps inhibit the oxidation of fats. It protects the immune system by preventing the formation of free radicals and aiding in the production of antibodies.

Alfalfa leaves
Asparagus
Beets
Black-eyed peas
Broccoli
Burdock root
Cabbages
Carrots
Catnip
Cayenne
Celery
Chamomile
Chickweed
Fennel seeds
Fenugreek seeds
Garlic
Ginseng
Hawthorn berries
Honey
Hops
Horsetail
Leafy green vegetables
  (especially spinach)
Nutritional yeast
Nuts (especially Brazil nuts and
  cashews)

Oatstraw
Onions
Parsley
Peppermint
Raspberry leaves
Rose hips
Seaweeds (especially kelp)
Soy

Sprouts
Squash
Sunflower seeds
Tomatoes
Whole grains (especially barley
  and brown rice)
Yarrow
Yellow dock

Silicon

Silicon is found in bodily structures such as nerve sheaths, blood vessels, cartilage, lungs, tendons, trachea, teeth, hair, nails, and ligaments. It is insulating, helps warm the body, and promotes the electrical flow of body energy by way of electrolytes. Silicon improves elasticity and agility. A silicon deficiency can cause uncoordination, wrinkles, susceptibility to fungal infections, and erectile dysfunction.

Almonds
Apples
Apricots (fresh and dried)
Asparagus
Barley
Beets
Burdock root
Carrots
Cauliflower
Celery
Cherries
Cucumbers
Dandelion greens
Figs (fresh and dried)
Grapes and raisins
Hemp seeds
Horseradish
Horsetail

Jerusalem artichokes
Kelp
Leafy green vegetables (especially
  lettuce, nettles, spinach, and
  Swiss chard)
Leeks
Oats
Parsnips
Peppers
Pumpkins
Radishes
Sprouts (especially alfalfa)
Strawberries
Sunflower seeds
Tomatoes
Watermelon
Wild rice

Sodium

Sodium purifies and cools the blood and helps in the formation of saliva, bile, and pancreatic fluids.

Apples
Apricots (fresh and dried)
Asparagus
Beets
Celery
Coconut
Dandelion greens
Garbanzo beans
Goat's milk (unpasteurized)
Grapes and raisins
  Leafy green vegetables (especially beet and mustard greens, spinach, romaine lettuce, Swiss chard, and watercress)

Millet
Okra
Olives
Plums and prunes
Seaweeds
Sesame seeds
Strawberries
Sweet potatoes
Tomatoes
Turnips

Sulfur

Sulfur aids in the digestion of fats and helps prevent blood platelet aggregation. It imparts a glow to the skin, improves skin elasticity and tissue repair, and prevents scarring. It also reduces lactic acid buildup and athletic recovery time. Sulfur competes for the same binding sites as parasites do, thus leaving parasites homeless. It promotes bodily warmth and is a disinfectant. Some sulfur-rich foods can be gas-forming, but eating them with sodium-rich foods can relieve this effect.

Apples
Apricots (fresh and dried)
Asparagus
Beans (all)
Blue-green algae
Broccoli
Brussels sprouts
Cabbages
Carrots
Cauliflower
Cayenne
Celery
Durians

Garlic
Leafy green vegetables (especially arugula, kale, mustard greens, nasturtium leaves, Swiss chard, and watercress)
Hemp seeds
Horseradish
Nuts (all)
Onions
Peaches
Plums and prunes
Spirulina
Turnips
Whole grains (all)

Vanadium

Vanadium is needed for the formation of teeth and bones. It aids growth, reproduction, and cellular metabolism.

Dill

Olives

Parsley

Radishes

Soy

String beans

Whole grains (especially buckwheat and oats)

Zinc

Zinc is needed for the production of sex hormones and fluids, fertility, and a strong immune system. It also improves one's sense of taste and smell. Adequate zinc is necessary to prevent or remedy acne, hair loss, skin disorders, low sperm count, poor wound healing, and poor eyesight.

Alfalfa sprouts and leaves

Almonds

Beans (especially adzuki and pea)

Bee pollen

Brazil nuts

Burdock root

Cashews

Cayenne

Chamomile

Chickweed

Coconut

Corn

Dandelion greens

Garlic

Fennel seeds

Hops

Kelp

Leafy green vegetables
  (especially spinach)

Macadamia nuts

Milk thistle seeds

Mushrooms

Nettles

Nutritional yeast

Onions

Parsley

Peanuts

Pecans

Pine nuts

Poppy seeds

Pumpkin seeds

Rose hips

Sage

Sarsaparilla

Sesame seeds

Soy

Sunflower seeds

Walnuts

Whole grains (especially buckwheat, brown rice, oats, and rye)

Chlorophyll

Chlorophyll is found in virtually every green, plant-source food, but the three superfoods listed below are exceptionally good sources of chlorophyll.

Blue-green algae   Spirulina   Wheatgrass

Coenzyme Q₁₀ (Ubiquinone)

Coenzyme Q_{10}, also known as Co-Q_{10} or ubiquinone, is an antioxidant that strengthens heart muscle, lowers blood pressure, reduces the effects of aging, and relaxes constricted blood vessels. It is synthesized in the cells of the body but can also be ingested.

Almonds   Spinach   Whole grains (all)

Super-Oxide Dismutase (SOD)

Super-oxide dismutase (SOD) is a scavenger enzyme (that is, it binds to free radicals). It reduces the rate of cell destruction and is considered to have anti-inflammatory, anti-aging, and antioxidant properties.

Barley grass   Leafy green vegetables (all)
Broccoli   Nutritional yeast
Cabbages   Wheatgrass

Amino Acids

Amino acids are the building blocks of protein. Eight of the amino acids are called "essential," meaning that they must be acquired through the diet because the body does not manufacture adequate amounts of them. The essential amino acids are:

Isoleucine   Phenylalanine
Leucine   Threonine
Lysine   Tryptophan
Methionine   Valine

▉*Arginine*

Arginine enhances immune function, improves liver function, is a component of seminal fluid, and accelerates the repair of tissue. It is also necessary for building muscle.

Apples   Pineapple
Apricots (fresh and dried)   Seeds (all)
Beans (all)   Strawberry
Berries (all)   Tomatoes
Coconut   Vegetables (all except celery and
Eggplant   turnips)
Nuts (all)   Whole grains (all)

▪Cysteine

Cysteine improves skin texture and is needed for B-vitamin utilization. It is considered an antioxidant, helping protect the body from the ravages of pollution.

Brazil nuts
Soy
Whole wheat

▪Glutamic Acid

Glutamic acid increases the firing of neurons. It also aids in the metabolism of fats and sugars, and helps potassium cross the blood-brain barrier.

Dates
Shiitake mushrooms

▪Glutamine

Glutamine elevates glutathione levels (see below) and is necessary for the production of RNA and DNA. It strengthens immune health, hastens recovery time, and rejuvenates muscles weakened by illness and stress. Glutamine also helps balance acid/alkaline levels and promotes mental alertness.

Oats
Parsley
Spinach

▪Glutathione

Glutathione is not a true amino acid but a tripeptide: a compound derived from three amino acids (in this case, cysteine, glutamic acid, and glycine). This antioxidant aids liver cleansing, helps prevent the formation of cataracts, supports carbohydrate metabolism, and is believed to have anti-aging properties.

Apples
Asparagus
Avocados
Broccoli
Cantaloupe
Carrots
Cauliflower
Garlic
Onions
Parsley
Peaches
Potatoes
Spinach
Sprouted seeds (all)
Strawberries
Tomatoes
Walnuts
Watermelon
Winter squash

Glycine

Glycine is needed for the synthesis of bile acids and is also used in the formation of RNA and DNA. High levels of glycine are found in the connective tissues and skin.

Avocados

Oats

Wheat germ

Whole wheat

Histidine

Histidine is a metal-chelating agent (combines with metals). It transports other nutrients and is needed to produce red and white blood cells.

Apples

Beans (all)

Nuts (all)

Papayas

Pineapple

Seeds (all)

Vegetables (all except celery, radishes, and turnips)

Isoleucine

Isoleucine helps make biochemical components that produce energy. Isoleucine is also needed for the production of hemoglobin and helps regulate blood sugar levels.

Apples

Apricots (fresh and dried)

Beans (especially lentil)

Dates

Figs (fresh and dried)

Nuts (especially almonds and cashews)

Peaches

Pears

Persimmons

Rye

Seeds (all)

Strawberries

Tomatoes

Vegetables (all except celery, lettuce, and radishes)

Leucine

Leucine is necessary for growth. It stimulates protein synthesis in muscles and also aids in healing wounds to the bones and skin.

Apples

Apricots (fresh and dried)

Dates

Figs (fresh and dried)

Nuts (all)

Peaches

Pears

Seeds (all)

Strawberries

Tomatoes

Vegetables (all except celery, lettuce, and radishes)

Whole grains (all)

■ Lysine

Lysine supports the absorption of calcium from the intestinal tract and helps in the production of antibodies, enzymes, hormones, collagen, and bones. It also inhibits the replication of sores caused by the herpes virus.

Aloe vera

Apples

Apricots (fresh and dried)

Avocados

Bananas

Beans (all)

Cantaloupe

Dates

Figs (fresh and dried)

Grapefruit

Nuts (all)

Oranges

Papayas

Peaches

Pears

Persimmons

Pineapple

Seeds (all)

Strawberries

Tomatoes

Vegetables (all)

Whole grains (especially quinoa)

Yogurt

■ Methionine

Methionine is an antioxidant that aids digestion, protects against radiation, minimizes fat buildup in the liver, and reduces histamine reaction.

Apples

Apricots (fresh and dried)

Avocados

Bananas

Brown rice

Cantaloupe

Chives

Dates

Figs (fresh and dried)

Garlic

Lentils

Nuts (especially Brazil nuts)

Oranges

Papayas

Peaches

Pears

Persimmons

Pineapple

Sesame seeds

Soy

Strawberries

Sunflower seeds

Tomatoes

Vegetables (especially Brussels sprouts, cabbages, cauliflower, onions, and watercress)

Whole grains (especially corn)

Yogurt

■ Phenylalanine

Phenylalanine helps in the formation of neurotransmitters, including norepinephrine. It can help relieve pain and depression.

Apples
Apricots (fresh and dried)
Avocados
Bananas
Beans (especially garbanzo,
  lentil, lima, and soy)
Figs (fresh and dried)
Nuts (especially almonds)
Parsley
Peaches

Pears
Persimmons
Pineapple
Seeds (all)
Strawberries
Tomatoes
Vegetables (all except lettuce and
  radishes; especially carrots and beets)
Whole grains (all)

▓Threonine

Threonine supports the health of tooth enamel, elastin, and collagen. It minimizes fat in liver and stimulates the immune system.

Apples
Apricots (fresh and dried)
Beans (all)
Dates
Figs (fresh and dried)
Nuts (all)
Peaches

Pears
Persimmons
Seeds (all)
Strawberries
Tomatoes
Vegetables (all except celery and lettuce
Whole grains (all)

▓Tryptophan

Tryptophan is needed for niacin (vitamin B_3) production. Because tryptophan works as a precursor for the neurotransmitter serotonin, it can encourage healthy sleep and elevate mood.

Alfalfa leaves
Avocados
Bananas
Beans (especially adzuki, mung,
  and soy)
Chives
Dates
Durians
Figs (fresh and dried)
Grapefruit
Nuts (especially cashews)
Oranges

Papayas
Peaches
Pears
Perisimmons
Pineapple
Seeds (especially pumpkin and
  sunflower)
Strawberries
Tomatoes
Vegetables (especially sweet potatoes)
Whole grains (all)

■ *Tyrosine*

Tyrosine is a precursor to the neurotransmitters norepinephrine and dopamine, which help mood regulation. It helps curb appetite, reduces body fat, and is needed for proper thyroid function.

Alfalfa leaves	Leeks
Almonds	Lettuce
Apples	Parsley
Apricots (fresh and dried)	Pumpkin seeds
Asparagus	Sesame seeds
Avocados	Sunflower seeds
Bananas	Spinach
Beans (all)	Spirulina
Beets	Strawberries
Bell peppers	Watercress
Carrots	Watermelon
Cherries	Wheat germ
Cucumbers	Whole wheat
Figs (fresh and dried)	Yogurt

■ *Valine*

Valine is stimulating and curbs addictions. It can help build muscles and aids in tissue repair.

Apples	Pears
Apricots (fresh and dried)	Persimmons
Beans	Seeds (all)
Dates	Strawberries
Figs (fresh and dried)	Tomatoes
Mushrooms	Vegetables (all except celery and lettuce)
Nuts (all)	
Peaches	Whole grains (all)

Alpha-Lipoic Acid

Alpha-lipoic acid is an antioxidant that improves the utilization of glucose, lowers cholesterol, and reduces oxidation of low-density lipoproteins (LDLs).

Broccoli	Spinach
Potatoes	

Allyl Sulfides

Allyl sulfides stimulate glutathione levels and help form S-transferase, a detoxifying enzyme.

Chives

Garlic

Leeks

Onions

Fructo-Oligosaccharides

Fructo-oligosaccharides are chains of sugar molecules that help support populations of beneficial bacteria in the intestines. Fructo-oligosaccharides also decrease putrefactive substances, promote bowel regularity, improve immune function, and support liver function.

Artichokes

Bananas

Barley

Burdock root

Chicory root

Dandelion root

Garlic

Jerusalem artichokes

Onions

Tomatoes

Indoles

Indoles are cancer-fighting compounds; they induce the formation of protective enzymes that deactivate estrogen.

Broccoli

Brussels sprouts

Cabbages

Cauliflower

Kale

Mustard greens

Radishes

Limonene

Limonene boosts the production of enzymes that help neutralize carcinogens and reduce tumors.

Caraway seed

Celery seed

Grapefruit

Lemons

Mint

Oranges

Tangerines

Lignins

Lignins are hormonelike substances that inhibit estrogen and block the formation of cancers and of unfriendly prostaglandins. Lignins also prevent damage by free radicals.

Flaxseeds

Pectin

Pectin is a type of soluble fiber that can help reduce cholesterol and inhibit diabetes by slowing the digestive and absorption of carbohydrates, thus preventing rapid blood sugar elevations. Pectin may also prevent malignant (cancerous) cells from clumping together.

Apples   Figs (fresh and dried)
Bananas   Grapefruit
Blueberries   Lima beans
Broccoli   Mustard greens
Brussels sprouts   Onions
Cabbages   Turnip greens
Carrots   Watercress
Cauliflower

Flavonoids

Flavonoids are sometimes referred to as vitamin P ("P" for "permeability") because they help increase capillary strength and absorption. This nutrient category contains over 5,000 powerful antioxidants. Flavonoids give many fruits, herbs, and berries their deep colors; fruits and vegetables contain more flavonoids than any other food group.

Anthocyanins

These antioxidant, polyphenol flavonoids give fruits a reddish pigment. They have anti-inflammatory properties and help protect small and large blood vessels from oxidation damage. Anthocyanins also inhibit cholesterol synthesis.

Black currants (fresh and dried)   Raspberries
Blueberries   Red cabbage
Cherries   Strawberries
Cranberries (fresh and dried)

Bioflavonoids

Bioflavonoids, another type of flavonoid, enhance the assimilation of vitamin C and thereby help protect the structure of cell membranes, capillaries, and other blood vessels. Bioflavonoids have an antibacterial effect, improve circulation, lower cholesterol, and stimulate bile production.

Apricots (fresh and dried)   Black currants (fresh and dried)
Blackberries   Blueberries

Buckwheat
Cantaloupe
Cherries
Citrus fruits and skins
  (the inner rinds)
Cranberries (fresh and dried)
Elderberries
Gooseberries
Grapefruit
Huckleberries
Lemon balm
Lemons
Onions (especially red)
Papayas

Parsley
Peppers (especially green and bell)
Persimmons
Pine bark and pine needles
Plums and prunes
Pomegranates
Raspberries
Red grapes (with seeds) and raisins
Rose hips
Salmonberries
Strawberries
Tomatoes
Walnuts

Catechin

Catechin has been found to inhibit viral infection. It also has antioxidant properties and helps protect against lipid peroxidation, thereby suppressing the growth of many types of cancer.

Berries (all)
Green and black tea

Rhubarb

Hesperidin

By lowering low-density lipoprotein (LDL) and elevating high-density lipoprotein (HDL) levels, hesperidin lowers cholesterol levels. This flavonoid also has an anti-inflammatory effect.

Berries (all)
Buckwheat
Grapefruits

Lemons
Oranges

Isoflavones

Isoflavones, a group of flavonoid compounds such as genistein, daidzein, and glycitein, block the absorption of estrogen by cells, thereby decreasing cancer risk.

Alfalfa sprouts
Berries (all)
Broccoli

Cabbages
Carrots
Soy

Kaempferol

The flavonoid kaempferol has anti-allergenic, anti-inflammatory, and anti-cancer properties.

Asparagus	Dill
Beets	Grapefruit
Cauliflower	Strawberries

Proanthocyanadins and Anthocyanosides

These flavonoids include cyanidin, delphinidin, malvidin, and petunidin. Proanthocyanadins and anthocyanosides strengthen capillaries and collagen, and prevent inflammation, allergic reactions, and varicosities.

Bilberries	Elderberries
Blackberries	Ginkgo
Blueberries	Grape seeds
Citrus fruit seeds	Pine bark
Cherries	Raspberries

Quercetin

Quercetin is an antioxidant with anti-inflammatory and antiviral properties. It is a component of the pigment in many plants.

Apples	Garlic
Blue-green algae	Green and black tea
Broccoli	Leafy green vegetables (all)
Buckwheat	Onions (yellow and purple)
Cherries	Pansy flowers
Citrus fruits	Ragweed pollen
Clover blossoms	Red grapes
Eucalyptus leaves	Rinds and barks from wild fruits

Rutin

Rutin is a flavonoid that enhances the elasticity of veins and the assimilation of vitamin C.

Apricots (fresh and dried)	Ginkgo
Blackberries	Hawthorn berries
Buckwheat	Rose hips
Cherries	Yarrow
Citrus fruit peels (the inner white portion)	

Curcumin

Curcumin is an anti-inflammatory antioxidant that helps protect against certain carcinogens.

Cumin seeds   Turmeric

Ellagic Acid

Ellagic acid is an antioxidant that competes with carcinogens for the same receptor sites and helps neutralize carcinogens before they can invade DNA. Ellagic acid also reduces DNA damage caused by molds and environmental pollutants.

Apples   Grapes and raisins
Black currants (fresh and dried) Pomegranates
Black walnuts   Raspberries
Cherries   Strawberries
Cranberries (fresh and dried)

Resveratrol

This compound has antioxidant and anticancer properties.

Grape skins   Grape leaves

Sulforaphane

Sulforaphane stimulates cancer-fighting enzymes and blocks carcinogens from damaging healthy cells.

Broccoli   Cauliflower
Brussels sprouts   Kale
Cabbage   Turnips

Lecithin

Lecithin is a phospholipid that prevents the buildup of arterial plaque by metabolizing fat molecules so they are small enough to be carried in the blood to the cells.

Beans (all)   Whole grains (all)
Nutritional yeast

Ribonucleic Acid (RNA)

Ribonucleic acid (RNA) is involved in the control of cellular chemical activities. In layman's terms, RNA carries genetic information, signals, and messages from DNA out into cells and throughout the body.

Asparagus

Beets

Leafy green vegetables (all)

Lentils

Mushrooms

Nuts (all)

Radishes

Glossary

Achene: A small, dry, one-seeded fruit that remains closed at maturity (e.g., a sunflower seed).

Allergenic: Likely to cause an allergic reaction.

Alterative: Alters one's condition; restores bodily functions. Increases blood flow to tissues, detoxifies, aids assimilation of nutrients, stimulates metabolism, and promotes excretion and elimination of waste.

Amino acid: An organic compound that is a component of protein.

Analgesic: Relieves pain.

Anaphrodisiac: Curbs sex drive.

Anesthetic: Deadens sensation.

Anodyne: Lessens pain by diminishing nerve excitability.

Antibiotic: Inhibits or destroys disease-causing microorganisms.

Anticoagulant: Prevents clotting of blood.

Antidepressant: Elevates mood and counteracts depression.

Anti-emetic: Reduces or relieves nausea and vomiting.

Antifungal: Inhibits growth of fungal organisms.

Antigalactagogue: Suppresses lactation (milk production).

Anti-inflammatory: Reduces inflammation.

Antimutagenic: Prevents cellular mutations.

Antinutrient: Inhibits proper absorption or production of nutrients.

Antioxidant: Prevents free-radical damage that is believed to contribute to cancerous growths.

Antiparasitic: Inhibits parasites.

Antipyretic: Lowers fever. Also known as *febrifuge*.

Antirheumatic: Eases pain, swelling, and stiffness in joints and muscles.

Antiscorbutic: Prevents scurvy.

Antiseptic: Prevents bacterial growth, inhibits pathogens, and counters sepsis.

Antispasmodic: Prevents or eases cramps or spasms.

Antitumorigenic: Suppresses the growth of tumors.

Antitussive: Relieves coughing.

Antiviral: Inhibits viral replication.

Aphrodisiac: Increases sexual desire and potency.

Aromatic: Is fragrant or pungent; improves flavor of bitter herbs; often stimulates digestive tract.

Assimilable: Enhances the use of nutrients.

Astringent: Tightens, tones, and dries. (See also "The Five Flavors," beginning on page 271.)

Bitter: Stimulates flow of digestive secretions, as well as those of pituitary gland, liver, and duodenum (first section of small intestine). (See also "The Five Flavors," beginning on page 271.)

Bronchodilator: Relaxes bronchial muscles, thus allowing easier breathing.

Calyx: The cuplike green petals (sepals) found at the base of a flower.

Carbohydrate: A group of carbon compounds including sugars, starches, and cellulose.

Carcinogen: Can contribute to the formation of cancer.

Carminative: Decreases or prevents gas.

Cholagogue: Promotes bile flow from gallbladder.

Cholesterol: A fatty substance produced by the liver and needed to build cellular membranes, insulate the nervous system, form bile acids, lubricate the skin, and aid hormonal production; may cause arteriosclerosis.

Deaminated: Having its amino group removed; lacking life force.

Demulcent: Soothes irritated tissues, especially of mucous membranes.

Denatured: Having a molecular structure that has been modified (e.g., by heat) so that original properties (i.e., biological activity, vital nutrients) are destroyed or diminished.

Deobstruent: Removes obstructions.

Dextrinized: Having starches "stuck together" as a thickening agent.

Diaphoretic: Promotes perspiration.

Diuretic: Increases secretion and expulsion of urine by promoting activity of kidneys and bladder.

Emmenagogue: Stimulates uterus; normalizes female reproductive system.

Emollient: Soothes or softens.

Endogenous: Originating inside the body.

Enzyme: A complex protein created by living cells that activates chemical changes within the body.

Estrogenic: Has estrogenlike effects or helps the body produce estrogen.

Exogenous: Originating from outside the body.

Expectorant: Aids in the expulsion of mucus from the lungs.

Fatty acid: The basic component of fats.

Flavonoid: A compound that is brightly colored, contributing to the colors found in fruits; also has a capillary-strengthening effect.

Galactagogue: Increases production of mother's milk.

Hemostatic: Arrests or slows bleeding.

High-density lipoprotein (HDL): The type of cholesterol that is considered beneficial.

Hypertensive: Increases blood pressure.

Hypoglycemic: Helps lower blood sugar levels.

Hypotensive: Reduces blood pressure.

Laxative: Stimulates bowel movements.

Low-density lipoprotein: The type of cholesterol that is considered harmful to the body.

Mineral: An inorganic element that is essential to human nutrition and helps regulate body fluids, build structures such as bones and teeth, and make up enzymes.

Mucilaginous: Produces a smooth coating that lubricates, soothes, and heals.

Mucolytic: Reduces viscosity of mucus.

Mucopolysaccharide: A chain of sugar molecules that produces a mucilaginous (lubricating) effect.

Mutagenic: Causes cellular mutations.

Nervine: Calms and nourishes nerves.

Nutritive: Supplies nutrients to build and tone the body.

Peristalsis: Wavelike contractions that propel matter along the alimentary canal; associated with the urge to move the bowels.

Photosensitive: Sensitive to light.

Phytoestrogenic: Provides raw (plant-source) materials that help the body make its own estrogen or promote an estrogenlike effect.

Polysaccharide: A chain of sugar molecules.

Purgative: Strongly laxative.

Refrigerant: Cools body temperature.

Regeneration: Repair of bones, flesh, cartilage, and other tissues.

Rejuvenative: Renews body, mind, and spirit; can counteract stress and increase endurance.

Restorative: Helps rebuild a depleted condition and restores normal bodily functions.

Rubefacient: Increases blood flow to surface of skin; draws out deep impurities.

Saturated fat: Fats that are solid at room temperature, such as those found in dairy products, lard, and coconut oil; they provide warmth and energy for the body.

Sedative: Slows bodily functions; quiets nerves.

Starch: A type of carbohydrate.

Stigma: The part of the flower pistil on which pollen grains are both received and germinated.

Stimulant: Quickens various bodily functions and improves circulation.

Stomachic: Encourages healthy stomach activity.

Sudorific: Induces perspiration.

Tonic: Promotes general health and well-being; builds energy, blood, and *chi*.

Trans fat: Manufactured fats, including hydrogenated and partially hydrogenated oils, that are considered harmful to the body. They are not easily broken down and have a chemical structure similar to that of plastic.

Unsaturated fat: A type of fat used by the body for energy that are solid at cold temperatures. Monounsaturated fats, such as olive oil, do not go rancid quickly. Polyunsaturated fats, such as sunflower and sesame oils, go rancid quickly, especially upon exposure to light and heat.

Vasodilator: Expands blood vessels, thereby reducing blood pressure.

Vermifuge: Causes worms to be expelled.

Vitamin: An organic substance which in minute amounts is essential to the growth, metabolism, and health of the body.

Volatile oil: A component of plants, also known as essential oil, that evaporates quickly and with aromatic and various other properties, depending upon the type. Many volatile oils have antiseptic, antifungal, and circulatory-stimulating properties.

Bibliography

Alexander, Joe. *Blatant Raw Foodist Propaganda*. Nevada City, CA: Blue Dolphin Publishing, 1990.

Anderson, Rich. *Cleanse and Purify Thyself: The Clean-Me-Out Program*. Tucson, AZ: Arise and Shine, 1988.

Arlin, Stephen. *Raw Power*. San Diego, CA: Maul Brothers Publishing, 2000.

Arlin, Stephen, Dini Fouad, and David Wolfe. *Nature's First Law: The Raw Food Diet*. San Diego, CA: Maul Brothers Publishing, 1996.

Avery, Phyllis. *The Garden of Eden Raw Fruit and Vegetable Recipes*. Vista, CA: Hygeia Publishing, 2000.

Baker, Arthur. *Awakening Our Self-Healing Body: A Solution to the Health Care Crisis*. Los Angeles, CA: Self Health Care Systems, 1994.

Baker, Elton, and Elizabeth Baker. *The Uncook Book: Raw Food Adventures to a New Health High*. Indianola, WA: Drelwood Publications, 1992.

Boutenko, Victoria. *Twelve Steps to Raw Foods: How to End Your Addiction to Cooked Food*. Ashland, OR: Raw Family Publishing, 2001.

Bragg, Paul C. *Build Powerful Nerve Force*. Santa Barbara, CA: Health Science, 1992.

Bragg, Paul C. *The Miracle of Fasting*. Santa Barbara, CA: Health Science, 1979.

Bragg, Paul, and Patricia Bragg. *Toxicless Diet*. Santa Barbara: CA: Health Science, 1994.

Bragg, Paul C., and Patricia Bragg. *Healthful Eating without Confusion*. Santa Barbara, CA: Health Science, 1992.

Bushkin, Estitta, and Gary Bushkin. *All about Green Food Supplements*. Garden City Park, NY: Avery Publishing Group, 1999.

Calabro, Rose Lee. *Living in the Raw: Recipes for a Healthy Lifestyle.* Santa Cruz, CA: Rose Publishing, 1998.

Carper, Jean. *Food—Your Miracle Medicine.* New York, NY: Harper Collins, 1993.

Carper, Jean. *The Food Pharmacy.* New York, NY: Bantam Books, 1988.

Christopher, John R. *Dr. Christopher Talks on Rejuvenation through Elimination.* Provo, UT: self-published, 1976.

Cichoke, Anthony J. *Enzymes and Enzyme Therapy: How to Jumpstart Your Way to Lifelong Good Health.* New Canaan, CT: Keats Publishing, Inc., 1994.

Clement, Anna Maria, and Brian Clement. *Children: The Ultimate Creation.* West Palm Beach, FL: A. M. Press, 1994.

Clement, Brian R. *Hippocrates Health Program: A Proven Guide to Healthful Living.* West Palm Beach, FL: Hippocrates Books, 1989.

Cousens, Gabriel. *Conscious Eating.* Patagonia, AZ: Essene Vision Books, 1997.

Cousens, Gabriel. *Spiritual Nutrition and the Rainbow Diet.* San Rafael, CA: Cassandra Press, 1986.

Diamond, Harvey, and Marilyn Diamond. *Fit for Life.* New York, NY: Warner Books, 1987.

Diamond, Harvey, and Marilyn Diamond. *Fit for Life II: Living Health, The Complete Health Program.* New York, NY: Warner Books, 1987.

Dina, Jamey, and Kim Sproul. *Uncooking with Jamey and Kim.* Encinitas, CA: Healthforce Publishing, 2000.

DuBelle, Lee. *Proper Food Combining Works: Living Testimony.* Phoenix, AZ: self-published, 1994.

Ehret, Arnold. *Physical Fitness through a Superior Diet, Fasting, and Dietetics.* Beaumont, CA: Ehret Literature Publishing Company, 1975.

Elliot, Rose, and Carlo de Paoli. *Kitchen Pharmacy.* New York, NY: William Morrow, 1991.

Fathman, George, and Doris Fathman. *Live Foods: Nature's Perfect System of Human Nutrition.* Beaumont, CA: Ehret Literature Publishing Company, 1973.

Fife, Bruce. *The Healing Miracle of Coconut Oil.* Colorado Springs, CO: Healthwise, 2001.

Flowerdew, Bob. *The Complete Book of Fruit.* New York, NY: Penguin USA, 1996.

Freedom, David, and Tierra True. *Nature's Path to Supreme Health: A Story of Living Nutrition.* Kearney, NE: True Freedom Press, 1998.

Fry, T. C., and David Klein. *Your Natural Diet: Alive Raw Foods.* Sebastopol, CA: Living Nutrition Publications, 2001.

Gallo, Roe. Perfect Body: *Beyond the Illusion.* San Mateo, CA: Roe Gallo Publishing, 1997.

Goldbeck, Nikki, and David Goldbeck. *The Goldbecks' Guide to Good Food.* New York, NY: New American Library, 1987.

Graham, Douglas N. *The High Energy Diet Recipe Guide.* Key Largo, FL: self-published, 2001.

Graham, Douglas N. *Grain Damage.* Marathon, FL: self-published, 1998.

Griggs, Barbara. *The Food Factor: An Account of the Nutrition Revolution.* New York, NY: Penguin Group, 1988.

Hagiwara, Yoshihide. *Green Barley Essence: Health Benefits of Nature's Ideal Fast Food.* New Canaan, CT: Keats Publishing, 1986.

Heinerman, John. *Heinerman's Encyclopedia of Fruits, Vegetables and Herbs.* West Nyack, NY: Parker Publishing Company, 1988.

Holdstock, Sharon. *Shazzie's Detox Delights.* London, England: Raw Creation, 2001.

Hotema, Hilton. *Man's Higher Consciousness.* Pomeroy, WA: Health Research, 1962.

Howell, Edward. *Enzyme Nutrition: The Food Enzyme Concept.* Wayne, NJ: Avery Publishing Group, 1985.

Jensen, Bernard. *Foods that Heal.* Garden City Park, NY: Avery Publishing Group, 1988.

Jensen, Bernard. *Food Healing for Man.* Escondido, CA: Bernard Jensen Enterprises, 1983.

Jensen, Bernard. *Nature Has a Remedy: It Can Be Physical, Mental or Spiritual.* Escondido, CA: Bernard Jensen Enterprises, 1978.

Jubb, Annie, and David Jubb. *The LifeFood Recipe Book.* New York, NY: Excellence Incorporated, 2000.

Juliano. Raw: *The Uncook Book.* New York, NY: Harper Collins, 1999.

Kadans, Joseph. *Encyclopedia of Fruits, Vegetables, Nuts and Seeds for Healthy Living.* West Nyack, NY: Parker Publishing Company, Inc., 1973.

Kalson, Stanley Steven. *Holistic H.E.L.P. Handbook: Guide to Healthy Living.* Prescott, AZ: International Holistic Center, Inc., 1997.

Kirschner, H. E. *Nature's Healing Grasses.* Riverside, CA: H. C. White Publications, 1975.

Krok, Morris. *Golden Path to Rejuvenation.* Freemont, CA: Custodian Publishing Company, 1986.

Kulvinskas, Viktoras. *Survival into the Twenty-first Century.* Wethersfield, CT: Omangod Press, 1975.

Levin, James, and Natalie Cederquist. *Vibrant Living: Over 250 Heart Healthy Live Food Recipes.* La Jolla, CA: GLO, Inc., 2001.

Lopez, D. A., R. M. Williams, and K. Miehlke. *Enzymes: The Fountain of Life.* Charleston, SC: Neville Press, 1994.

Lu, Henry C. *Chinese Foods for Longevity.* New York, NY: Sterling Publishing, 1990.

Lu, Henry C. *Chinese System of Food Cures: Prevention and Remedies.* New York, NY: Sterling Publishing Company, 1986.

Lust, John B. *About Raw Juices.* Sussex, England: Lewes Press Wightman and Company, 1968.

MacManiman, Geb. *Dry It—You'll Like It!* Seattle, WA: Evergreen, 1980.

Markowitz, Elysa. *Warming up to Living Foods.* Summertown, TN: Book Publishing Company, 1998.

Markowitz, Elysa. *Living with Green Power. A Gourmet Collection of Living Food Recipes.* Burnaby, British Columbia, Canada: Alive Books, 1997.

Meyer, Clarence. *Vegetarian Medicines.* Glenwood, IL: Meyerbooks, 1981.

Meyerowitz, Steve. *Water: The Ultimate Cure.* Summertown, TN: Book Publishing Company, 2000.

Meyerowitz, Steve. *Wheat Grass: Nature's Finest Medicine.* Great Barrington, MA: Sproutman Publications, 1999.

Mindell, Earl R. *Earl Mindell's Food as Medicine.* New York, NY: Simon and Schuster, 1994.

Montgomery, Beth. *Transitioning to Health: A Step by Step Guide for You and Your Child.* San Diego, CA: Montgomery, 2001.

Montgomery, Beth. *Introducing Living Foods to Your Child: Guidebook for Babies through Two Years.* San Diego, CA: Nature's First Law, 2000.

Murray, Frank. *Yoshihide Hagiwara: Pioneer of Better Living.* New Canaan, CT: Keats Publishing, 1990.

Murray, Michael T. *The Healing Power of Foods.* Rocklin, CA: Prima Publishing, 1993.

Nees, Mary Helen, Nedra Carroll, and Diane Louise Gallina. *Optimum Health Institute of San Diego: Optimal Living Recipes.* Lemon Grove, CA: Optimum Health Institute of San Diego, 2000.

Nison, Paul. *The Raw Life.* New York, NY: 343 Publishing Company, 2000.

Olive, Diane. *Think Before You Eat.* Glendale, CA: Griffin Publishing, 1994.

Onstad, Dianne. *Whole Foods Companion.* White River Junction, VT: Chelsea Green Publishing, 1996.

Parham, Barbara. *What's Wrong with Eating Meat?* Denver, CO: Ananda Marga Publications, 1979.

Patenaude, Frederic. *The Sunfood Cuisine: A Practical Guide to Raw Vegetarian Cuisine.* San Diego, CA: Genesis 1:29 Publishing, 2002.

Pitchford, Paul. *Healing with Whole Foods.* Berkeley, CA: North Atlantic Books, 1993.

Polunin, Miriam. *Healing Foods: A Practical Guide to Key Food for Good Health.* New York, NY: Dorling Kindersley Publishing, Inc., 1997.

Raso, Jack. *Mystical Diets: Paranormal, Spiritual and Occult Nutrition Practices.* Buffalo, NY: Prometheus Books, 1993.

Reader's Digest Association. *Foods that Harm, Foods that Heal.* Pleasantville, NY: Reader's Digest Association, Inc., 1997.

Rhio. *Hooked on Raw.* New York, NY: Beso Entertainment, 2000.

Robbins, John. *Diet for a New America: How Your Food Choices Affect Your Health, Happiness and the Future of Life on Earth.* Walpole, NH: Stillpoint Publishing, 1987.

Romano, Rita. *Dining in the Raw: Groundbreaking Natural Cuisine that Combines the Techniques of Macrobiotic, Vega, Allergy-Free, and Raw Food Disciplines.* New York, NY: Kensington Publishing Corporation, 1992.

Safron, Jeremy. *Dining from an Empty Bowl: A Fasting Handbook.* Paia, HI: Raw Truth Press, 1999.

Salaman, Maureen. *Foods that Heal.* Menlo Park, CA: Statford Publishing, 1989.

Sarno, Chad. *Vital Creations: An Organic Life Experience.* Patagonia, AZ: Vital Creations, 2002.

Schmid, Ronald F. *Traditional Foods Are Your Best Medicine: Health and Longevity with the Animal and Sea Vegetable Foods of Our Ancestors.* Stratford, CT: Ocean View Publications, 1987.

Scott, William D. *In the Beginning God Said, Eat Raw Food.* Coeur d'Alene, ID: North Idaho Publishing, 1999.

Seibold, Ronald. *Cereal Grass: What's in It for You!* Lawrence, KS: Wilderness Community Education Foundation, 1990.

Shannon, Nomi. *The Raw Gourmet.* Vancouver, Canada: Alive Books, 1999.

Shelton, Herbert M. *Health for the Millions*. Tampa, FL: American Natural Hygiene Society, 1996.

Shelton, Herbert M. *Superior Nutrition: Eat Better, Live Longer!* San Antonio, TX: Willow Publishing, Inc., 1994.

Soria, Cheria. *Angel Foods: Healthy Recipes for Heavenly Bodies*. Santa Barbara, CA: Heartstar Productions, 1996.

Tobe, John H. *Eat Right and Be Healthy*. St. Catherine's, Ontario, Canada: Modern Publication, 1965.

Vetrano, Vivian Virginia. *Errors on Hygiene: T. C. Fry's Devolution, Demise and Why*. Barksdale, TX: GLH Publishing, 1999.

Walker, Norman.W. *Raw Vegetable Juices: What's Missing in Your Body*. Phoenix, AZ: Norwalk Press, 1970.

Walker, Norman W. *Become Younger*. Phoenix, AZ: Norwalk Press, 1995.

Wigmore, Ann. *Recipes for Total Health and Youth*. San Fidel, NM: self-published, 1999.

Wigmore, Ann. *You Are the Light of the World*. Boston, MA: self-published, 1989.

Wigmore, Ann. *Why You Do Not Need to Grow Old*. Boston, MA: self-published, 1985.

Wigmore, Ann. *The Hippocrates Diet and Health Handbook*. Wayne, NJ: Avery Publishing Group, Inc., 1984.

Wigmore, Ann. *Be Your Own Doctor: Nature's Way Is the Organic Way*. St. Paul, MN: Dan Pilla Printing and Engraving, 1975.

Wolfe, David. *Eating for Beauty*. San Diego, CA: Maul Brothers Publishing, 2002.

Wolfe, David. *The Sunfood Diet Success System*. San Diego, CA: Maul Brothers Publishing, 2001.

Wood, Rebecca. *The Whole Foods Encyclopedia*. New York, NY: Prentice Hall Press, 1988.

Resources

Educational and Retreat Centers

All Life Sanctuary
P.O. Box 2853
Hot Springs, Arkansas 71914
800-927-2527
www.naturalUSA.com/retreat/
Raw lifestyle, live-foods preparation, and indoor gardening.

Angel's Nest Retreat
P.O. Box 2009
El Prado, New Mexico 87529
310-488-1847
www.angelsnestretreats.com
Offers lodging, workshops, healing therapies, and a raw and organic foods menu.

The Ann Wigmore Foundation
P.O. Box 399
San Fidel, New Mexico 87049
505-552-0595
www.wigmore.org
Educational live-food retreats.

Ann Wigmore Institute
Ruta 115, Km 20
Barrio Guayabo
Aguado, Puerto Rico 00743
787-868-6307
Mailing address:
P.O. Box 429
Rincon, Puerto Rico 00677
www.annwigmore.org
Classes on living foods, and a retreat center.

Assembly of Yahweh Wellness Center
7881 Columbia Highway
Eaton Rapids, Michigan 48827
517-633-1637
www.assemblyofyahweh.com
A live-foods, residential healing program.

British Natural Hygiene Society
3 Harold Grove
Frinton-on-the-Sea, Essex
England
Sells health-related books and videos, holds conferences.

Canadian Natural Hygiene Society
P.O. Box 235, Station T
Toronto, Ontario M6B 4A1
Canada
*Sells health-related books and
videos, holds conferences.*

Creative Health Institute
918 Union City Road
Union City, Michigan 49094
517-278-6260
*Health educators, classes based on
Ann Wigmore program. Offers one-
to three-week detoxification programs
based on wheatgrass and live foods.*

Hippocrates Health Institute
1443 Palmdale Court
West Palm Beach, Florida 33411
561-471-8876
www.hippocratesinst.com
Spas and alternative education center.

**Hippocrates Health Centre
of Australia**
Elaine Avenue
Mudgeeraba 4213
Gold Coast, Queensland
Australia
01-075-530-2860
*One- to six-week Wigmore educa-
tion programs and retreats.*

Hippocrates Health Resort of Asia
"The Farm" at San Benito
Isle of Luzon
Philippines
800-827-2527, ext. 202
www.thefarm.com.ph
A raw foods resort facility.

Kwatamani Holistic Institute
P.O. Box 2514
Arcadia, Florida 34265
850-258-9684
www.livefoodsunchild.com
*Organic gardens, spiritual retreat,
raw foods.*

**Naples Institute for Optimum
Health and Healing**
2329 Ninth Street North
Naples, Florida 34103
800-243-1148, 941-649-7551
www.naplesinstitute.com
*Wheatgrass, living foods, cleansing,
education, and healing retreat center.*

National Health Association
P.O. Box 30630
Tampa, Florida 33630
813-855-6607
*Publishes Health Science magazine,
sells health-related books and
videos, and holds conferences.*

New Life Retreat
R.R. #4, 453 Dobbie Road
Lanark, Ontario K0G 1K0
Canada
613-259-3337
www.newliferetreat.com
*Offers programs on juicing, fasting,
live foods, and spiritual support.*

Nonpareil Natural Health Retreat
R.R. #3
Stirling, Ontario K0K 3E0
Canada
613-395-6332
www.3sympatico.ca/nonpareil
*Detoxification programs, fasting,
yoga, and healing therapies.*

Optimum Health Institute
6970 Central Avenue
Lemon Grove, California
　91945-2198
800-993-4325

R.R. #1, Box 339-J
Cedar Creek, Texas 98612
512-303-1239
www.optimumhealth.org
Retreat center and one- to three-week educational programs on wellness through living foods.

Rest of Your Life Health Retreat
P.O. Box 102
Barksdale, Texas 78828
830-234-3488
Provides restful, raw, healing retreats.

Shinui Living Foods Retreat
　and Learning Center
1085 Lake Charles Drive
Roswell, Georgia 30075
770-992-9218
www.shinuiretreat.com
Raw foods retreats, training, demonstrations, and books.

Tree of Life Rejuvenation Center
P.O. Box 1080
Patagonia, Arizona 85624
520-394-2520, 800-720-2520
www.treeoflife.nu
Live-foods, spiritual retreat center.

Educators

Victoria and Igor Boutenko
P.O. 172
Ashland, Oregon 97529
www.rawfamily.com
541-488-8865
Workshops, books, and raw supplies.

Suzanne Alex Ferrara
www.chefsuzannealexferrara.com
Raw workshops and lectures.

Doug Graham, D.C.
www.doctorgraham.cc/
Invite Dr. Graham to speak at your convention, school, professional or business meeting, health conference, athletic organization, or private seminar.

Professor Rozalind Gruben
1 Cassidy Place
New Town Road
Storrington, West Sussex RH20 4EY
UK
01-903-746572
healthyunlimited@aol.com
Fitness, health, and nutrition consultant; one of England's premier natural-health lecturers and fitness trainers.

Healthful Living International
P.O. Box 7383
San José, California 95150
866-HLI-3HLI
www.healthfullivingintl.org
A collective of top natural-hygiene speakers.

Juliano
609 Broadway
Santa Monica, California 90403
310-587-1552
www.rawjuliano.com
Exquisite living-food workshops.

Living Light House
1457 12th Street
Santa Monica, California 90401
310-395-6337
Raw periodicals, education.

Living Light Culinary Arts Institute
704 North Harrison
Fort Bragg, California 95437
800-484-6933, ext. 6256
www.rawfoodchef.com
Cherie Soria, author of Angel Foods, teaches workshops and certificate programs for raw foods chefs.

Elaina Love
51 Ord Street
San Francisco, California 94114
415-558-1624
elaine@purejoylivingfoods.com
Classes, workshops, videos, and recipe book, Elaina's Pure Joy Kitchen.

Viktaras Kulvinskas
L.O.V.E.-I.N.G.
P.O. Box 1556
Mount Ida, Arkansas 71957
870-867-4521
www.naturalusa.com/viktor/
   sanctuary.html
Raw foods classes and books.

Brigitte Mars
1919 D 19th Street
Boulder, Colorado 80302
303-442-4967
www.brigittemars.com
Raw foods workshops, herb walks, and private consultations.

Raw Foods Festival
503-293-3039
www.rawfoods.com/festival
This ultimate raw foods festival in Portland, Oregon brings together many raw teachers, workshops, great food, and beautiful people.

Rhio's Raw Energy Hotline
P.O. Box 2040
Canal Street Station
New York, New York 10013
212-343-1152
www.rawfoodinfo.com
Raw food support, classes, and workshops.

Jeremy Safron
P.O. Box 790358
Paia, Hawaii 96779
808-878-8091
www.lovingfoods.com
Raw workshops, yoga, and classes on diagnostic techniques.

Chad Sarno
Vital Creations
P.O. Box 1153
Patagonia, Arizona 85624
888-276-7170
www.rawchef.org
Raw classes, books, and chef training.

Transformation Institute
214-796-6930
www.transformationist.org
Home-study courses in natural hygiene.

David Wolfe
888-RAW-FOOD
www.davidwolfe.com
Lectures, workshops, books, and raw foods excursions. The phone number is for Nature's First Law, which handles bookings.

Periodicals

Boletin Crudivegano
Lista de Correos
18960 Almunecar (Granada)
Spain
01-619-78-85-70
A Spanish raw foods magazine.

Die Wurzel (The Roots)
    Magazine
Torwartstrasse 22
90480 Nurnberg
Germany
01-0049-911-4089116
A German raw foods magazine.

Fresh Network News
c/o Nature's First Law
P.O. Box 900202
San Diego, California 92190
A United Kingdom raw foods magazine.

Fruitarian Network News
P.O. Box 293
Trinity Beach, Queensland 4879
Australia
An Australian raw foods magazine.

Living Nutrition Magazine
P.O. Box 256
Sebastopol, California 95473
707-829-0362
www.livingnutrition.com
A natural-hygiene magazine.

Just Eat an Apple
P.O. Box 900202
San Diego, California 92190
888-RAWFOOD (888-729-3663)
www.sunfood.net/jeaa
A great raw foods magazine.

Internet Resources

www.colitis-crohns.com
Colitis and Crohn's Health Recovery Services; features raw author David Klein.

www.e3live.com
Offers super green food.

www.fruitariannetwork.com
Source webpage for fruitarian raw foods interests.

www.fresh-network.com
Lists raw products and events.

www.gardenofhealth.com
Books, products, events, and recipes.

www.highvibe.com
Super foods, raw food appliances, green foods, books, and natural cosmetics.

www.living-foods.com
Networking, community, articles, and recipes.

www.lovewisdom.org
Website about Johnny Lovewisdom, pioneer fruitarian.

www.matthewgrace.com
Website for Matthew Grace, author of A Way Out.

www.organicbox.com
Ships organic produce.

www.radicalhealth.com
Raw stories, articles, research.

www.rawfoods.com
An educational website devoted to raw foods.

www.rawfoodnews.com
Information and articles.

www.raw-passion.com
Raw Passion events, with speakers on raw foods and natural hygiene.

www.rawganique.com
Organic, hemp clothes and food.

www.rawtimes.com
Chat group, books, recipes, and resources.

www.rawvegan.com
Latest research, connections to other raw foodists.

www.sunfood.net
Recipes and articles.

www.thegardendiet.com
Raw vegan news articles, links.

Product Suppliers

Acme Equipment
1024 Concert Avenue
Spring Hill, Florida 34609
800-882-0157
Sells dehydrators, wheatgrass juicers, Greenlife Champion juicers, and much more.

The Date People
P.O. Box 808
Niland, California 92257
760-359-3211
Sells high-quality, low-temperature-dried dates.

Diamond Organics
P.O. Box 2159
Freedom, California 95019
888-ORGANIC (888-674-2642)
www.diamondorganics.com
Organic produce and dehydrated foods. Ships overnight.

Excalibur Dehydrator
6083 Power Inn Road
Sacramento, California 95824
800-875-4254, 916-381-4254
The very best in food dehydrators.
Also carries Teflex sheets.

Glaser Organic Farms
19100 SW 137th Avenue
Miami, Florida 33012
305-238-7747
www.glaserorganicfarms.com
Raw food products, as well as
on-site classes and an organic
farmer's market.

Gold Mine Natural Food
   Company
7805 Arjons Drive
San Diego, California 92126
800-475-FOOD, 858-537-9830
Sells pickle presses and fine, organic
foods.

Grain and Salt Society
273 Fairway Drive
Ashville, North Carolina 28805
800-867-7258
Sells Celtic salt.

Hallelujah Acres
P.O. Box 2388
Shelby, North Carolina 28151
800-915-9355
Christian, raw foods organization
offering newsletter, products, home-
study course, books, and videos.

Island Herb
P.O. Box 25
Waldron Island, Washington
   98297
360-739-4035
www.partnereartheducationcenter.
   com
Seaweeds and excellent, wildcrafted,
organic herbs. Send a self-addressed,
stamped envelope for a catalog.

Jaffee Brothers Natural Foods
P.O. Box 636
Valley Center, California 92082
619-749-1133
Organically grown fruits, nuts, and
nut butters. No minimum order.

Living Tree Community
P.O. Box 10082
Berkeley, California 94709-5082
800-260-5534, 510-526-7106
www.livingtreecommunity.com
Mail-order foods, specializing in
organic nuts and low-temperature-
dried fruit.

Miracle Exclusives, Inc.
64 Seaview Boulevard
Port Washington, New York 11050
800-645-6360
Sells juicers, wheatgrass juicers,
dehydrators, sprouters, and pickle
presses.

Nature's First Law
P.O. Box 900202
San Diego, California 92190
619-645-7282, orders:
     619-596-7979, 888-RAWFOOD
     (888-729-3663)
www.rawfood.com
*Excellent source for books and
raw-food supplies.*

Norwalk Juicers
808 South Bloomington
Lowell, Arkansas 72745
800-643-8645
www.norwalkjuicers.com
Sells the ultimate hydraulic-press juicer.

Omega Juicers
800-633-3401
P.O. Box 4523
Harrisburg, Pennsylvania 17111
Sells powerful juicers.

Organic by Nature
1542 Seabright Avenue
Long Beach, California 90813
800-452-6884
www.organicbynaturetrading.com
Whole-foods nutritional products.

Pines Wheatgrass
P.O. Box 1107
Lawrence, Kansas 66044
800-MY-PINES (800-697-4637)
www.wheatgrass.com
*Sells wheatgrass in tablet and
powdered form.*

The Raw World
c/o Paul Nison
405 Montgomery
Ojai, California 93023
866-RAW-DIET (866-729-3438)
www.therawworld.com
*A source for raw books, videos,
foods, and appliances.*

Rejuvenative Foods
Box 8464
Santa Cruz, California 95061
831-462-6715
www.rejuvenative.com
Really raw nut butters, sauerkraut.

**Sundance Wheateena Wheatgrass
     Juicer**
P.O. Box 1446
Newburgh, New York 12551
914 565-6065
Great wheatgrass juicers.

Sweet Wheat, Inc.
639 Cleveland Street, Suite 210
Clearwater, Florida 33755
888-22-SWEET (888-227-9338)
www.sweetwheat.com
Freeze-dried wheatgrass juice.

Tribest Corporation
P.O. Box 4089
Cerritos, California 90703
888-618-2078
www.tribest.com
*Books and equipment for a raw
lifestyle, including Green Power
juicers and Freshlife sprouters.*

Tropical Traditions
PMB #219
823 S. Main Street
West Bend, Wisconsin 53095
1-866-311-2626
Really raw coconut oil.

Vitalities Incorporated
P.O. Box 652
Kilauea, Kauai, Hawaii 96754
808-828-0600
www.vitalities.org
Sells excellent selection of raw foods videos.

Vita Mix Household Division
8615 Usher Road
Cleveland, Ohio 44138
800-848-2649
www.vitamix.com
Sells a highly durable and versatile blender.

Welles Enterprises
6565 Balboa Avenue, Suite A
San Diego, California 92111
619-473-8011
Sells juice presses and slantboards.

RAW RESTAURANTS & JUICE BARS

The rawvolution is happening! Raw restaurants are springing up throughout planet. Support these places. We all know restaurants come and go, so be sure to call first and let us know about new restaurants. Some of these listings simply offer some raw fare and on certain days. Also be sure to check out organic and vegetarian restaurants, which often offer some live fare.

UNITED STATES

Alabama

TBO Deli
5510 Highway 280
Birmingham, AL
205-995-8888

Alaska

Organic Oasis Restaurant
& Juice Bar
2610 Spenard Road
Anchorage, AK
907-277-7882

Arizona

Botanica Restaurant
(Opening Soon)
330 East Seventh Street
Tucson, AZ
520-623-0913
www.anjali.com

Sedona Raw Café
1595 West Highway 89A
Sedona, AZ
928-282-2997

Tree of Life Café
771 Harshaw Road
Patagonia, AZ
520-394-2589, 520-394-2520

California

Alive! Café
1972 Lombard Street
San Francisco, CA
415-923-1052
www.AliveVeggie.com

Au Lac Vegetarian Restaurant
Mile Square Plaza, 16563
   Brookhurst
Fountain Valley, CA
714-418-0658
www.aulac.com

Beverly Hills Juice Club
8382 Beverly Boulevard
Los Angeles, CA
323-655-8300

Cafe Gratitude (#1)
2400 Harrison Street
San Francisco, CA
415-824-4652 x1
www.withthecurrent.com

Cafe Gratitude (#2)
1336 9th Avenue
San Francisco, CA
415-824-4652 x2
www.withthecurrent.com

Cafe Gratitude (#3)
1730 Shattuck
Berkeley, CA
415-824-4652 x3
www.withthecurrent.com

Cafe Gratitude (#4)
2200 4th Street
San Rafael, CA
415-824-4652 x4
www.withthecurrent.com

Café La Vie
429 Front Street
Santa Cruz, CA
831-429-ORGN
www.lavie.us

Cafe Muse (at UC Berkeley Art
   Museum)
2625 Durant Avenue
Berkeley, CA
510-548-4366

Castle Rock Inn
5827 Sacramento Avenue
Dunsmuir, CA
530-235-0782

Champions
7523 Fay Avenue
La Jolla, CA
858-456-0536

Cilantro Live (#1)
315 3rd Avenue
Chula Vista, CA
619-827-7401
www.cilantrolive.com

Cilantro Live (#2)
300 Carlsbad Village Drive
Carlsbad, CA
760-585-0136

Cilantro Live (#3)
7820 Broadway
Lemon Grove, CA
619-433-0680
www.cilantrolive.com

Cru
1521 Griffith Park Boulevard
Los Angeles, CA
323-667-1551

Elixir Teas and Tonics
8612 Melrose Avenue
West Hollywood, CA
310-657-9310

Erehwon Natural Foods Market
7660 Beverly Boulevard
West Hollywood, CA
323-937-0777
www.Erewhonmarket.com

Euphoria Loves Rawvolution
2301 Main Street
Santa Monica, CA
310-392-9501
www.rawvolution.com/?q=raw
    volution_store

Good Mood Food Café
5930 Warner Avenue
Huntington Beach, CA
714-377-2028
www.goodmoodfood.com/Cafe.htm

Good Mood Food Café
  (at "Apple a Day" Vitamin Shop)
Heritage Plaza
14310 Culver Drive, Suite E
Irvine, CA
949-552-1444
www.goodmoodfood.com/Cafe.htm

Green Life Evolution Center
410 Railroad Avenue
Blue Lake, CA
707-668-1781

The Inn of the Seventh Ray
128 Old Topanga Canyon Road
Topanga, CA
310-455-1311

Juicy Lucy's
703 Columbus Avenue
San Francisco, CA
415-786-1285

Juliano's Raw
609 Broadway
Santa Monica, CA
310-587-1552
www.rawplanet.com

Kung Food
2949 5th Avenue
San Diego, CA
619-298-7302
www.kung-food.com

Leaf Cuisine #1
11938 West Washington
    Boulevard
Culver City, CA
310-390-6005
www.leafcuisine.com

Leaf Cuisine #2
14318 Ventura Boulevard
Sherman Oaks, CA
818-907-8779
www.leafcuisine.com

Leaf Cuisine #3
8365 Santa Monica
    Boulevard
West Hollywood, CA
323-301-4982
www.leafcuisine.com

Madeleine Bistro
18621 Ventura Boulevard
Tarzana, CA
818-758-6971
www.madeleinebistro.com

Millenium Restaurant
  (at the Savoy Hotel)
580 Geary Street
San Francisco, CA
415-345-3900

Mother's Market & Kitchen
19770 Beach Boulevard
Huntington Beach, CA
714-963-6667

Mother's Market & Kitchen
225 East 17th Street
Costa Mesa, CA
949-631-4741

Mother's Market & Kitchen
2963 Michelson Drive
Irvine, CA
949-752-6667

Mother's Market & Kitchen
24165 Paseo De Valencia
Laguna Woods, CA
949-768-6667

Naked Apples
784 Coast Highway
Laguna Beach, CA
949-715-5410

**Parawdise Raw Organic Cuisine
  Restaurant**
587 Post Street, Union Square
San Francisco, CA
415-346-8935
www.RawInTen.com

People's Food Co-op
4765 Voltaire Street
San Diego, CA
619-224-1387

Rancho's Natural Foods Market
3918 30th Street
San Diego, CA
619-298-3339

**Raw Energy Organic Juice
  & Café**
2050 Addison
Berkeley, CA
510-665-9464
www.rawenergy.net

Sunfood Nutrition
11653 North Riverside Drive
Lakeside, CA
619-596-7979, 1-888-RAWFOOD
www.rawfood.com

The Taste of the Goddess Café
  (at Prive Hair Salon & Spa)
7373 Beverly Boulevard
Los Angeles, CA
323-933-1400, 323-874-7700
www.TasteOfTheGoddess.com

Terra Bella Living Cuisine Café
1408 South Pacific Coast
  Highway
Redondo Beach, CA
310-316-8708
www.TerraBellaCafe.com

Voila! Juice Bar and Café
510 Derby Avenue
Oakland, CA
510-261-1138
www.voilajuice.com

Zephyr Vegetarian Café
340 East 4th Street
Long Beach, CA
562-435-7113

Colorado

Cafe Prasad (at the Boulder Coop)
1904 Pearl Street
Boulder, CO
303-447-COOP
www.bouldercoop.com

Turtle Lake Refuge (at the Rocky
  Mountain Retreat)
848 East 3rd Avenue
Durango, CO
970-247-8395
www.turtlelakerefuge.org

Connecticut

The Alchemy Juice Bar Café
203 New Britain Avenue
Hartford, CT
860-246-5700
www.alchemyjuicebar.com

Blue Green Organic Juice Café
  (at the Equinox Gym)
72 Heights Road
Darien, CT
203-662-9390
www.bluegreenjuice.com

The Stand
31 Wall Street
Norwalk, CT
203-956-5670

Delaware

Main Squeeze Juice Bar
280 East Maine Street

Newark, DE
302-455-1022

District of Columbia

Source of Life Juice Bar (at the
  Everlasting Life Health Food
  Supermarket)
2928 Georgia Avenue NW
Washington D.C.
202-232-1700
www.everlastinglife.net

Florida

Glaser Farms Organic Market
  (open on Saturdays)
SW corner of Grand & Margaret
  in Coconut Grove
Miami, FL
305-238-7747
www.glaserorganicfarms.com

Grassroots Organic Restaurant
2702 North Florida Avenue
Tampa, FL
813-221-ROOT

Health Station
2500 North Highway A1A
Indialiantic, FL
321-773-5678

The Present Moment Café
224 West King Street
St. Augustine, FL
904-827-4499
www.thepresentmomentcafe.com

S & L Fruit Stand
7805 West Irlo Bronson Memorial
  Highway
Kissimmee, FL
407-396-1026

Vee Raw Food Underground (at the Silver Tray Café)
601 West Indiantown Road
Jupiter, FL
561-745-5433 or 561-901-8097
www.rawfoodunderground.com

Georgia

Cafe Life (at the Life Grocery)
1453 Roswell Road
Marietta, GA
770-977-9583

Lov'n It Live
2796 East Point Street
East Point, GA
404-765-9220
www.lovingitlive.com

Lush Life Café
1405 Ralph D. Abernathy
    Boulevard
Atlanta, GA
404-758-8737

**Mutana Health Cafe and
    Marketplace**
1392 Ralph D. Abernathy
    Boulevard SW
Atlanta, GA
404-753-5252

R Thomas Deluxe Grill
1812 Peachtree Street NW
Atlanta, GA
404-872-2942
www.rthomasdeluxegrill.com

RAW
878 Ralph D. Abernathy Boulevard
Atlanta, GA
404-758-1110

Hawaii

Blossoming Lotus
4504 Kukui Street
Kapaa, Kauai, HI
808-822-7678
www.blossominglotus.com

Joy's Place
1993 South Kihei Road
Kihei, Maui, HI
808-879-9258

Mandala Garden Juice Bar and Deli
Baldwin Avenue
Paia, Maui, HI
808-579-9500

Westside Natural Foods
193 Lahainaluna
Lahaina, Maui, HI
808-667-2855

Idaho

Akasha Organics
    (at the Chapter One Bookstore)
160 North Main Street
Ketchum, ID
208-726-4777

Illinois

Charlie Trotters
816 West Armitage
Chicago, IL
773-248-6228
www.charlietrotters.com

Chicago Diner
3411 North Halsted
Chicago, IL
773-935-6696
www.vegiediner.com

Cousins Incredible Vitality
3038 West Irving Park Road
Chicago, IL
773-478-6868
www.cousinsiv.com

Karyn's Fresh Corner
1901 North Halsted
Chicago, IL
312-255-1590
www.karynraw.com

Maryland

The Yabba Pot
2433 St. Paul Street
Baltimore, MD
410-662-8638

Zia's Café
13 Allegheny Avenue
Towson, MD
410-296-0799
www.ziascafe.com

Massachusetts

Basil Chef Cuisine
   (at Body and Soul Center)
13 R Bessom Street, Village Plaza
   Shopping Center
Marblehead, MA
781-631-7286

Organic Garden Restaurant
   & Juice Bar
294 Cabot Street
Beverly, MA
978-922-0004
www.organicgardencafe.com

Minnesota

Ecopolitan
2409 Lyndale Avenue
South Minneapolis, MN
612-874-7336
www.ecopolitan.net

Nevada

Go Raw Café West
2910 Lake East Drive
Las Vegas, NV
702-254-5382
www.gorawcafe.com

Go Raw Café East
2381 East Windmill Lane
Las Vegas, NV
702-450-9007
www.gorawcafe.com

New Jersey

Down to Earth
7 Broad Street
Red Bank, NJ
732-747-4542

East Coast Vegan
313-A West Water Street
Toms River, NJ
732-473-9555
www.eastcoastvegan.com

The Energy Bar Vegetarian Café
307C Orange Road
Montclair, NJ
973-746-7003
www.kheperfoods.com/energybar.
   html

New Mexico

Whole Body Cafe
(at the Body Center)
333 Cordova Road
Santa Fe, NM
505-986-0362
www.bodyofsantafe.com/body_
cafe.html

New York

Blue Green Organic Juice Café
248 Mott Street
New York, NY
212-334-0805
www.bluegreenjuice.com

Blue Green Organic Juice Café
203 East 74th Street
New York, NY
212-744-1460
www.bluegreenjuice.com

Blue Green Organic Juice Café
(at The Plant in Dumbo)
25 Jay Street
Brooklyn, NY
718-722-7541
www.bluegreenjuice.com

Bob's Natural Foods
(and Juice Bar)
104 West Park Avenue
Long Beach, NY
516-899-8955
www.bobsnaturalfoods.com

Bonobo's Vegetarian Restaurant
and Store
18 East 23rd Street
New York, NY

Candle 79
154 East 79th Street
New York, NY
212-537-7179

Caravan of Dreams
405 East 6th Street
New York, NY
212-254-1613
www.caravanofdreams.net

Counter Vegetarian Restaurant
105 First Avenue
New York, NY
212-982-5870

Exotic Superfoods
185-02 Horace Harding
Expressway
Fresh Meadows, NY
718-353-4807
www.exoticsuperfoods.com

Jandi's Natural Market & Organic
Cafe & Deli
3000 Long Beach Road
Oceanside, NY
516-536-5535
www.jandis.com

Jubb's Longevity LifeFood Store,
Organic Juice Bar & Patisserie
508 East 12th Street
New York, NY
212-353-5000
www.lifefood.com

Juice and Roots Bar
(at the Safmink Holistic Center)
446B Dean Street
Brooklyn, NY
718-638-8250

Kate's Joint
58 Avenue B
New York, NY
212-777-7059

Lifethyme Natural Market
410 Sixth Avenue
New York, NY
212-420-9099

Liquiteria
170 Second Avenue
New York
212-358-0300

Organic Soul Café
  (at the Sixth Street Center)
638 East 6th Street
New York, NY
212-677-1863
www.sixthstreetcenter.org/cafe

Pure Food and Wine
54 Irving Place
New York, NY
212-477-1010
www.purefoodandwine.com

Pure Juice and Takeaway
1251/2 East 17th Street
New York, NY
212-477-7151

Quintessence
263 East 10th Street
New York, NY
646-654-1823

Raw Foods Eatery and Everything
  Wellness Bookstore
118 South Cayuga Street
Ithaca, NY
607-254-6074

Raw Soul Catering & Restaurant
348 West 145th Street
New York, NY
212-491-5859
www.rawsoul.com

Sacred Chow
227 Sullivan Street
New York, NY
212-337-0863

24 Carrots Organic Juice Bar
244 West 72nd Street
New York, NY
212-595-2550

North Carolina

Good OM Kitchen
  (at the Namaste Yoga
  & Healing Center)
Broadway
Asheville, NC
828-253-6985

Ohio

Healthy Harvest
8785 Mentor Avenue
Mentor, OH
440-255-3468

Oregon

The Blossoming Lotus
  (at the Yoga in the Pearl)
925 NW Davis
Portland, OR
503-525-YOGA
www.blossominglotus.com

Pennsylvania

Arnold's Way Vegetarian Raw Café
319 West Main Street, Store #4 Rear
Lansdale, PA
215-361-0116
www.arnoldsway.com

Kind Café
724 North 3rd Street
Philadelphia, PA
215-922-KIND
www.kindcafe.com

Loving Life Café
109 Carlisle Street
New Oxford, PA
717-476-LOVE
www.lovinglifecafe.com

Maggie's Mercantile
320 Atwood Street
Pittsburgh, PA
724-593-5056

Maggie's Mercantile #2
1262 Route 711
Stahlstown, PA
724-593-5056

Oasis Living Cuisine
134 Lancaster Avenue
Frazer, PA
610-647-9797
www.oasis-pa.com

Texas

Blueberry Market
2819 Sandage Avenue
Fort Worth, TX
817-703-3438
www.blueberrymarket.com

Pure Café
2720 Greenville Avenue
Dallas, TX
214-824-7776

Sunfired Foods
4915 MLK Boulevard
Houston, TX
713-643-2884
www.sunfirehealthfoods.com

Utah

Living Cuisine Raw Food Bar
  (at Herbs for Health)
1100 East Highland Drive
Sugarhouse, UT
801-467-4082

Sage's Café
473 East 300 Street
South Salt Lake City, UT
801-322-3790
http://sagescafe.com

Washington

The Chaco Canyon Café
4759 Brooklyn Avenue NE
Seattle, WA
206-522-6966
www.chacocanyoncafe.com

Wyoming

Harvest Natural Foods Bakery
  & Cafe
130 West Broadway
Jackson, WY
307-733-5418

CANADA

Live Health Café
258 Dupont Street
Toronto, ON
416-515-2002

The Living Source Café (in the
  Melting Pot Gallery)
1111 Commercial Drive
Vancouver, BC
604-254-3335
www.livingsourcecafe.ca

Papaya Island
513 Yonge Street
Toronto, ON
416-960-0821

Raw Health Café
1849 West 1st Avenue
Vancouver, BC
604-737-0420

**Super Sprouts (Wheatgrass Juice
  Bar, Sprouts, and Bookstore)**
720 Bathurst Street
Toronto, ON
416-977-7796
www.supersprouts.com

Tout Cru dans l'Bec
129 7e rue Rouyn-Noranda, QC
819-764-9843

**W.O.W. Wild Organic Way Café
  & Juice Bar**
22 Carden Street
Guelph, ON
519-766-1707

ENGLAND

VitaOrganic Wholistic Restaurant
279c Finchley Road
London
020-7435-2188

JAMAICA

Ashanti Foods Monthly Brunch
C/O Yvonne Hope
876-944-3316

Earl's Juice Garden
16 Derrymore Road
Kingston
876-906-4287, 876-920-7009

Earl's Juice Garden (2nd location)
Shop #6, 6 Red Hills Road
Kingston 10
876-754-2425

SPAIN

Organic Café
de la Junta de Comera 11
Barcelona
(011) (34) 93-301-0902
www.organic.es

THAILAND

Rasayana Raw Food Café
57 Soi Sukhumvit39 (Prom-mitr)
  Sukhumvit Road
Klongton-Nua Wattana 10110
Bangkok
66-2662-4803-5

Index

Acacia, 98
Achene, 315
Acidity, 261–264
Acidosis, 262
Acid-producing foods,
    263–264
Acrylamide, 6–7
Aflatoxin, 83
Agar, 92–93, 235
Air drying foods, 130
Alfalfa leaf, 19
    juice, 127
Alfrawdo Sauce, 205
Alkalinity, 261–265
Alkali-producing foods,
    264–265
Alkalosis, 262
All-American theme
    dinner, 258
Allergenic, 315
All-Raw Apple Pie, 237
Allspice, 105–106
Allyl sulfides, 309
Almond Cheese, 143
Almond Crackers, 226
Almond Mayonnaise,
    180
Almond Milk, 144
Almond Ricotta Cheese,
    142
Almond Shortbread, 226
Almond Yogurt, 145
Almonds, 21, 78–79
Alpha-carotene, 281

Alpha-linolenic acids. *See*
    Omega-3 fatty acids.
Alpha-lipoic acid, 308
Alterative, 315
Amaranth, 72, 87–88
Amazing Cake, 244
American Cancer Society,
    1, 28
American Heart Institute, 1
*American Journal of
    Surgery,* 95
Amino acids, 6, 9, 18,
    303–308, 315
Analgesic, 315
Anaphrodisiac, 315
Anchusa, 98
Anesthetic, 315
Anise, 21, 106
Anise hyssop, 98
Anodyne, 315
Anthocyanins, 310
Anthocyanosides, 312
Antibiotic, 315
Anticoagulant, 315
Antidepressant, 315
Anti-emetic, 315
Antifungal, 315
Antigalactagogue, 315
Anti-inflammatory, 315
Antimutagenic, 315
Antinutrient, 316
Antioxidant, 316
Antiparasitic, 316
Antipyretic, 316

Antirheumatic, 316
Antiscorbutic, 316
Antiseptic, 316
Antispasmodic, 316
Antitumorigenic, 316
Antitussive, 316
Antiviral, 316
Aphrodisiac, 316
Apple-Ginger Juice, 151
Apple-Raisin Scones, 223
Apples, 25–27, 98,
    255–256
    juice, 127
Applesauce, 180
Apricot Ice Cream, 249
Apricot Pudding, 246
Apricots, 19, 28, 255
    juicing supplements,
    128
April produce, 137
Arame, 93
Arginine, 303
Aromatic, 316
Arugula, 28, 98
Ascorbic acid. *See*
    Vitamin C.
Asian Cucumber Salad,
    153
Asian Dressing, 164
Asian Noodle Bowl, 215
Asian Salad, 154
Asparagus, 28–29
    juice, 127
Assimilable, 316

Astringent, 316
August produce, 137
Avocados, 19, 26, 29, 162, 219, 253, 255
  juicing supplements, 128
Ayurvedic medicine, 271

Babies, 255–256
Bachelor's buttons, 98
Banana Shake, 150
Banana Split, 250
Bananas, 19, 29–30, 98, 256
  juicing supplements, 128
Banana-Sesame Smoothie, 150
Banana-Strawberry Rush, 150
Barbecue Sauce, 181
Barley, 72
Basil, 21, 98, 106, 219
Beans, 19
Bee products, 110
Beebalm, 98
Beets, 30–31, 219
  juice, 127–128
Begonia, 98
Berries, 19, 253, 255–256
Berries and Nut Cream, 230
Berry Good Scones, 223
Beta-carotene, 282
Better-than-bread unbakery, 220–228
Better-Than-Crab Cakes, 216
Beverages, 147–152
  cleansing, 277–278
Bibliography, 321–327
Bioflavonoids, 310–311
Biotin, 286
Bitter flavor, 272, 316

Black foods, 270
Black sesame seeds, 22
Blackberries, 32
Blender, 117
Blood-building tonic, 129
Blue foods, 268–269
Blueberry, 32–33
Blueberry Pie, 238
Blue-green algae, 19, 94
Borage, 98
Boron, 292–293
Borscht (Beet Soup), 167
Brazil Nut-Banana Pancakes, 139
Brazil nuts, 79
Breakfast, 138–141
Breakfast for Champions, 138
Breakfast Patties, 139
Breakfast Pudding, 141
British Royal Navy, 49
Broccoli, 19, 21, 33, 98
Bronchodilator, 316
Brussels sprouts, 19, 33–34
Buckwheat, 19, 21, 73
  lettuce, 253
  sprouts, 120
Burdock, 88
Busk, Leif, 7
Buttered Noodles, 204
Butterscotch Puddings, 247
Butterscotch Sauce, 188

Cabbages, 19, 21, 26, 34
  juice, 127
Cacti juicing supplements, 128
Caesar Salad, 156
Calcium, 293
Calendula, 99
Calyx, 316
Canapes, 252

Canary creeper, 99
Cancer, 9
Cantaloupe, 26, 35–36
Caraway, 106
Carbohydrates, 6, 316
Carcinogen, 316
Cardamom, 21, 22, 106
Caribbean theme dinner, 258
Carminative, 316
Carnation, 99
Carob, 36
Carob Brownies, 230
Carob Crunch Balls, 231
Carob Frosting, 245
Carob Layer Cake, 242
Carob Pudding, 248
Carob Sauce, 186
Carotenoids, 281–283
Carrot Salad, 154
Carrot-Ginger Soup, 168
Carrots, 19, 26, 36, 219, 253
  juice, 127–128
Cashews, 79
Catalyst, 9
Catechin, 311
Catnip, 99
Cattail, 99
Cauliflower, 19, 37, 253
Cayenne and jalapeño pepper, 22, 23, 106–107
Celery, 26, 37–38, 107
Celery Soup, 169
Chamomile, 99
Chapatis, 222
Charlemagne, 82
Chayote, 38
Cherimoya, 38–39, 255
Cherries, 19, 39, 255
  juicing supplements, 128
Cherry Soup, 168

Chervil, 99
Chewing food, 271
Chi, 27, 46, 48, 69
Chia seed, 79–80
Chickweed, 88, 99
   juice, 127
Chicory, 99
Children and raw diet,
   255–258
Chile Rellenos, 211
Chili powder, 115
Chive, 39–40, 99
Chlorine, 294
Chlorophyll, 94–98, 302
   benefits of, 95
Cholagogue, 317
Cholesterol, 317
Choline, 287
Chromium, 293
Chrysanthemum, 99
Cichoke, Anthony J., 16
Cilantro. *See* Coriander/
   cilantro.
Cinnamon, 21, 22, 107
Cinnamon Buns, 141
Citrus fruit, 253
   juice, 127
Citrus Juice Cleanser, 278
Citrus juicer, 117
Citrus vs scurvy, 49
Classic herb mix, 115
Cleansing beverages,
   277–278
Clove, 107–108
Clove dianthus, 99
Clover
   blossoms, 19
   sprouts, 120
Cobalt, 293
Coconut, 19, 80–81, 255
Coconut Bacon, 201
Coconut Crisps, 215
Coconut Milk, 149
Coconut oil, 104

Coconut Pudding, 248
Coconut Soup, 166
Coconut Yogurt, 146
Coenzyme Q_{10}, 303
Colanders, 117
Coldness in winter,
   21–23
Cole Slaw, 155
Collard. *See* Kale and
   collard.
Color therapy, 265–270
Cooking, detriments of,
   4–7
Cool Cucumber-Mint
   Salad, 155
Copper, 294
Coriander/cilantro, 99,
   108, 219
Corn, 19, 26, 73
Corn Bread, 224
Corn Chips, 222
Corn on the Cob, 179
Corn Salad, 157
Corn Soup, 169
Cosmic Carob Fudge,
   231
Cowslip, 99
Cranberry, 40
Cranberry Sauce, 182
Creamed Asparagus
   Soup, 167
Creamy Carob-Coffee
   Pie, 242
Cryptoxanthin, 282
Cucumber Soup, 168
Cucumbers, 19, 26,
   40–41, 162, 252, 253
   juice, 127
Cumin, 21, 108
Curcumin, 313
Curried Cauliflower
   Soup, 170
Curry, 22
   powder, 116

Curry Sauce, 182
Cyanocobalamin. *See*
   Vitamin B_{12}.
Cysteine, 304

Dairy products, 142–146
Dandelion, 88–89, 99
   juice, 127
Date Chutney, 182
Date Sauce, 185
Dates, 19, 26, 41–42, 253
Day lily, 99
Deaminated, 317
December produce, 137
Dehydrating, 129–132
   times for fruits and
   vegetables, 132
Deluxe Frosting, 245
Demulcent, 317
Denatured, 317
Deobstruent, 317
Desserts, 229–250
Detox reaction, 14–15, 24
Dextrinized, 317
Diaphoretic, 317
Diet, 14
Digestion, 20–21
Dill, 99, 108
Dinner parties, 252–254,
   258–260
Dips and pâtés, 190–194,
   252
Disease, 14
Diuretic, 317
Doctrine of Signatures,
   274
Donaldson and
   colleagues, 17
Dressing for a Large
   Group, 165
Dried-Fruit Jam, 189
Drying food, 130–132
Dulse, 93
Durians, 19, 42

Easy Cheese Spread, 144
EFAs. *See* Essential fatty
   acids, 291
Eggplant, 19, 42–43
Elder, 99
Electrolyte beverage, 129
Elimination, 6, 15
Ellagic acid, 313
Emmenagogue, 317
Emollient, 317
Emotions, 15
Enchiladas, 208
Endive and escarole,
   43–44
   juice, 127
Endogenous, 317
Endorphins, 12
Energy Soup, 172
English daisy, 99
Entrées, 195–219
Enzyme, 317
Enzymes, 5, 9–11
   digestive, 10–11, 20–21
   endogenous, 10–11
   exogenous, 10–11
   metabolic, 11
   therapy, 9
Essene Bread, 227
Essential fatty acids,
   291–292
Estrogenic, 317
Exercise, 12, 15
Exogenous, 317
Expectorant, 317

Falafel Balls, 210
Family and raw diet,
   254–258
Fasting, 275–278
   breaking, 278
   when not to, 276
Fats, 4, 6
Fats and oils, 103–105
Fatty acid, 317

February produce, 137
Feces, 15
Fennel, 21, 99, 108
   juice, 127
Fenugreek sprouts, 120
Fermenting, 131–132
Fiber, 6
Figs, 26, 44
Five flavors, 271–273
Flavonoids, 310–312, 317
Flax Crackers, 221, 252
   variations, 221
Flaxseed, 81–82
Flaxseed Burrito, 209
Flower Sun Teas, 102
Flowers, edible, 98–102,
   253
Fluorine, 294
Folic acid, 286
Food colorings, natural,
   246
Food combining,
   278–279
Food dehydrator,
   117–118, 130–132
Food processor, 118
Foods, 19–23, 25–70
   acid-producing,
      263–264
   alkali-producing,
      264–265
   preparation, 117–133
   warming, 22
Free radicals, 5, 7, 104
Freezing foods, 133
French Dressing, 163
French theme dinner, 258
Fructo-oligosaccharides,
   309
Fruit Aspic, 234
Fruits, 19, 25–71
   dehydrating times, 132
   fondue, 253
   slices, 253

Fuchsia, 99

Galactagogue, 317
Gamma-carotene, 282
Gamma-linolenic acid,
   291
Gandhi, Mahatma, 82,
   275
Garam masala, 116
Garbanzo beans, 19
Garlic, 23, 26, 99, 109
   juice, 127
Garlic Butter, 184
Garlic chive, 99
Garlic Toast, 225
Garnishes, 253
Gazpacho, 171
Geranium, 99
German theme dinner,
   258
Germanium, 295
Ginger, 21, 23, 109
Gingerroot, 219
GLA. *See* Gamma-
   linolenic acid.
Gladiolus, 99
Glass jars, 118
Glore, Mrs., 86
Glutamic acid, 304
Glutamine, 6, 304
Glutathione, 304
Glycine, 305
Goji berry. *See* Lycium
   berry.
Grains, 71–76
   sprouting, 124–126
Grapefruit, 44–45
Grapes, 20, 26, 45–46
Green Bean Scene, 174
Green foods, 268
Green Goddess Dressing,
   163
Green superfoods, 94–98
Groovin' Granola, 140

Guacamole, 192, 252, 253

Hawthorn, 99
Hazelnut/filbert, 82
Healing foods, 261–279
Hemmings, W. A., 10
Hemoglobin, 6
Hemostatic, 317
Hemp seeds, 20, 82
Herb Pesto, 206
Herbal Butter, 184
Herbed Turnips, 178
Herbs, 105–116, 253
   fresh vs dried, 105
Hesperidin, 311
Hey Beetnik!, 154
Hibiscus, 99
High-density lipoprotein (HDL), 317
Histidine, 305
Hiziki, 93
Holiday Frosting, 245
Holiday Mushroom Loaf, 202
Holiday theme dinner, 259
Hollyhock, 99
Holy Molé, 186
Honey, 109–110, 256
Honeydew melon, 21
Honey-Lemon Dressing, 163
Honeysuckle, 99
Hop, 99
Horseradish, 23, 109
   juice, 127
Howell, Edward, 10, 16
Hummus, 193
Hunger, 21
Hydrochloric acid, 3
Hypertensive, 318
Hypoglycemic, 318
Hypotensive, 318

Hyssop, 100

I Can't Believe It's Not Feta, 143
Ice cream maker, 118
If You Like Piña Colada, 149
Illness, 14
Immune system, 2, 9, 95
Indian theme dinner, 259
Indigo foods, 269
Indoles, 309
Inositol, 287
Intestinal motility, 6
Iodine, 295
Iron, 285–296
Isoflavones, 311
Isoleucine, 305
Italian Dressing, 164
Italian Salad, 157
Italian theme dinner, 259

Jalapeño. *See* Cayenne and jalapeño pepper.
January produce, 137
Jasmine, 100
Jicama, 46–47, 178
Jicama Crunch Sticks, 177
Johnny-jump-up, 100
Journal of Nutrition, 17
Juicer, 118
Juices, 277
Juicing, 126–129
   combinations, 128–129
   pulp disposal, 129
Juicing supplements, 128
July produce, 137
June produce, 137

Kaartinen and colleagues, 17
Kaempferol, 312

Kale (or Collard Green) Salad, 161
Kale and collard, 21, 47, 100
Kamut, 73–74
Kelp, 93
Key Lime Pie, 239
Kitchen aids, 117–133
Kitcheree, 212
Kiwi, 47–48
   juicing supplements, 128
Knives, 118
Knotweed, 89
Kombu, 93–94
Kuhne, Willy, 9
Kumquat, 48

Laetrile. *See* Vitamin B_{17}.
Lamb's-quarter, 89
   juice, 127
Lasagna, 196
Lavender, 100
Laxative, 318
Leafy green vegetables, 19
Lecithin, 313
Leeks, juice, 127
Lemon balm, 100, 110
Lemon Delight, 234
Lemon geranium, 100
Lemon Pudding, 247
Lemon verbena, 100
Lemons, 26, 48–49, 100, 253
Lentils, 19
Lettuce, 49–50
Leucine, 305
Leukocytosis, 18
Lignins, 309
Lilac, 100
Lime Pudding, 247
Limeade, 147
Lime-Avocado Ice Cream, 249

Limes, 50
Limonene, 309
Lind, James, 49
Linden, 100
Ling and colleagues, 17
Linoleic acids. *See*
   Omega-6 fatty acids.
Lipase, 12
Litchee, 50–51
Lithium, 296
Live Holiday Nuts, 236
Livestock, 4
Lopez, D.A., 16
Lovage, 100
Low-density lipoprotein,
   318
Lungs, 15
Lutein, 282
Lycium berry, 51
Lycopene, 283
Lysine, 6, 306

Macadamia nut, 83
Macadamia-Apricot
   Cookies, 233
Magnesium, 296
Magnolia, 100
Mallow, 100
Malva, 89–90
Manganese, 297
Mango, 51–52, 255–256
   juicing supplements, 128
Mango Chutney, 183
Mango Lassi, 148
Mango-Papaya Ice
   Cream, 250
March produce, 137
Marigold, 100
Marjoram, 100
Mashed Parsnips, 179
Master Cleanser, 277
Max Planck Institute for
   Nutritional Research,
   5, 18

May produce, 137
McCarrison, Robert, 16
Meadowsweet, 100
Meat, detriments of, 3–4
Mediterranean Salad, 160
Melons, 20, 255–256
Mermaid Salad, 156
Methionine, 6, 306
Methyl-sulfonyl-methane,
   298
Mexican Pâté, 191
Mexican Salad, 157
Mexican theme dinner,
   259
Middle Eastern theme
   dinner, 260
Miehlke, K., 16
Millet, 19, 74
Mineral, 318
Mint, 100
Mint Chutney, 183
Miso, 110
Miso Soup, 171
Miso-Tahini Sauce, 185
Molybdenum, 298
Monoterpenes, 283
Mucilaginous, 318
Mucolytic, 318
Mucopolysaccharide, 318
Mullein, 100
Mung beans, 19
Mushrooms, white, 63
Mustard, 90, 100, 110
   greens juice, 127
   sprouts, 120
Mustard Sauce, 188
Mutagenic, 318
Mutation Research, 95

Nama Shoyu Gravy, 184
Nasturtium, 100
Nectarines, 26
   juicing supplements,
   128

Nervine, 318
Nettle, 90–91
   juice, 127
Niacin. *See* Vitamin B$_3$.
Nobel Prize, 10
NoodleRoni and Cheese,
   204
Nori, 93–94
Nori Rolls, 218, 253
   fillings, 219
Not Fried Rice, 214
November produce, 137
Nut "Meat" Balls, 195
Nut Burgers, 199
Nut Nog, 150
Nut Pyramids, 220
Nut Stuffing, 198
Nutcracker, 118
Nutmeg, 110–111
Nutrient loss, 7, 12
Nutrients, 281–313
Nutrition and Food
   Science, 17
Nutritional yeast, 111
Nutritive, 318
Nuts, 19, 26, 76–86, 253
   oils, 77
   sprouting, 124–126
Nutty Fruitcake, 229

Oat, 74
October produce, 137
Oils, 103–104
   concerns about, 104
Okra, 20, 52, 100
   juicing supplements,
   128
Olive oil, 103
Olive Pesto, 207
Olive Spread, 192
Olives, 52–53, 219, 253
Omega-3 fatty acids, 291
Omega-6 fatty acids,
   291–292

Onions, 53, 100, 219
  juice, 127
On-the-Road-Again Bars, 228
Orange blossom, 100
Orange foods, 266–267
Orange Frosting, 246
Orange Sunshine, 148
Orange-Berry
  Un-Gelatin, 232
Oranges, 20, 53–54, 162
Oregano, 100, 111
Oriental Broccoli, 176
Oriental medicine, 271
Oriental Noodles, 214
Oriental theme dinner, 260
Oxalic acid, 6
Oxeye daisy, 100

PABA. *See* Para-aminobenzoic acid.
Pad Thai, 218
Palak (Creamed Spinach Curry), 212
Pangamic acid. *See* Vitamin B_{15}.
Pansy, 100
Pantothenic acid. *See* Vitamin B_5.
Papaya Soup, 172
Papayas, 20, 26, 54–55, 255
  juicing supplements, 128
Paprika, 111
Para-aminobenzoic acid, 286–287
Parsley, 20, 111
  juice, 127
Parsnip, 55–56
  juice, 127
Party-on Onion Dip, 194
Passionflower, 100

Pasta Primarawva, 203
Pâtés, 190–194, 252
Peaches, 20, 26, 56–57, 255–256
  juicing supplements, 128
Peanuts, 26, 83
Pears, 20, 26, 57, 255–256
Peas, 20, 56, 100, 255
Pecan Cauliflower Pâté, 192
Pecan Parsnips, 175
Pecan Pie, 240
Pecans, 83
Pecan-Spinach Quiche, 202
Pectin, 310
Peony, 100
Pepper, 23, 112
Peppermint, 100, 112
Peppermint geranium, 101
Peppers (bell peppers and others), 20, 26, 31–32
Peristalsis, 318
Persimmon, 57–58
Pesticides, 26
Pets and raw diet, 257
Petunia, 101
pH, 261
Phenylalanine, 306–307
Phosphorus, 298
Photosensitive, 318
Phytoene, 283
Phytoestrogenic, 318
Phytofluene, 283
Pine nuts, 83
Pineapple, 58
Pineapple guava, 101
Pineapple sage, 101
Pink Lemonade, 147
Pinks, 101

Pistachio, 83–84
Pizza, 206, 253
Plantains juicing supplements, 128
Plums, 59, 101, 255–256
Polysaccharide, 318
Pomegranates, 59
  seeds, 253
Poppy, 101
  seeds, 84
Poppyseed Pastry, 232
Potassium, 298–299
Pottenger, Francis M., 16
Poultry seasoning, 115
Preserving food, 129
Primrose, 101
Proanthocyanadins, 312
Produce, seasonal, 136–137
Proteins, 5, 9, 18–20
  caloric contents, 21
  sources of, 19–21
Pumpkin, 21, 59–60
  seeds, 19, 84
Pumpkin Pie, 241
Pungent (Spicy) flavor, 273
Purgative, 318
Purple Haze, 148
Purslane, 91, 101
Pyridoxine. *See* Vitamin B_6.

Quercetin, 312
Quinoa, 19, 74

Radish, 60–61, 101, 253
  juice, 127
  sprouts, 120
Rainbow Salad, 158
Raisins, 46
Ranch Dressing, 165
Raspberry, 61
Raw Carob Milk, 145

Raw foods diet, 1–2, 3–7, 9–24, 25–116, 117–133, 135–250, 251–260, 261–279, 281–314
  children and, 255–258
  digestibility, 20–21
  family and, 254–258
  frequently asked questions, 18–24
  how to start, 23–24
  pets and, 257
  preparation, 135–136
  recipes, 135–250
  research studies, 15–17
  transition eating, 23–24
Raw Ketchup, 181
Raw-Style Ribs, 219
Rawvioli, 197
Recipes, 135–250
Red, White, and Blue Fruit Salad, 241
Red blood cells, 6, 95
Red clover, 91, 101
Red foods, 265–266
Red pepper, 162, 219, 253
  juice, 127
Red Pepper Sauce, 186
Redbud, 101
Refrigerant, 318
Regeneration, 318
Rejuvelac, 138, 147, 151–152
Rejuvelac Recharger, 152
Rejuvenative, 318
Resources, 329–341
Restaurants, 251–252, 337–341
Restorative, 319
Resveratrol, 313
Rhubarb, 61–62
Riboflavin. *See* Vitamin B$_2$.

Ribonucleic acid, 314
Rice, 75
Rice replacements, 178
RNA. *See* Ribonucleic acid.
Rocket, 101
Romaine lettuce juice, 127
Roots Rock Reggae, 201
Rose geranium, 101
Rose of Sharon, 101
Rose, 101
Roselle, 101
Rosemary, 21, 101, 112
Rosewater, 112
Rubefacient, 319
Runner bean, 101
Russian Dressing, 162
Rutabaga, 62, 178
Rutin, 312
Rye, 75

Safflower, 101
Saffron, 112
Saffron crocus, 101
Sage, 101, 112
Salad burnet, 101
Salad dressings, 162–165
  commercial, 162
Salads, 153–165
Salsa, 193
Salt, 113
Salty flavor, 273
Samosas, 216
Sandwich ideas, 227
Saturated fat, 319
Sauces and condiments, 180–189
Sauerkraut, 159
  additions to, 159
Savory, 101
Savory Veggie Burgers, 200
Scallion, 113

Scandinavian Journal of Rheumatology, 17
Scurvy, 49
Sea palm, 94
Seasonal eating, 136
Seasonings, 105–116
Seaweeds, 92–94
  juicing supplements, 128
Secretions, 15
Sedative, 319
Seeds, 76–86, 253
  oils, 77
  sprouting, 124–126
Selenium, 299
September produce, 137
Sesame seeds, 19, 84–85
Sesame-Spirulina Bars, 236
Shiitake mushroom, 62–63
Shish kabobs, 252
Shungiku, 101
Signatures, Doctrine of, 274
Silicon, 300
Simple Fruit Leather, 235
  variations, 235
Sleep, 14–15
Snapdragon, 101
SOD. *See* Superoxide dismutase.
Sodium, 300
Sorrel, 101
Soups, 166–173
Source foods, 281–314
Sour Dream Cream, 146
Sour flavor, 272
Soursop, 63
Southern theme dinner, 260
Southwestern Pâté, 190
Soy foods, 19
Spanish Rice, 209

Spearmint, 21, 101, 113
Spelt, 75
Spice blends, 115–116
Spicy flavor. *See* Pungent flavor.
Spinach, 21, 26, 63–64, 255
  juice, 127
Spinach Dip, 194
Spinach Soup, 173
Spiral slicer, 118
Spiralizer, 203
Spirulina, 20, 94
Spleen, cold and damp, 21–22
Spring Green Rolls, 213
Sprouting, 119–126
  bags, 118
  guide, 124–126
  jars, 118–118, 120
  paper towel, 121
  problems, 122
  trays, 122–123
Sprouts, 20, 118–126, 219, 253
Squash, 101
Star fruit, 64, 253
Starch, 319
Stigma, 319
Stimulant, 319
Stomachic, 319
Strainers, 119
Strawberries, 26, 64–65, 162
Strawberry Shake, 149
String beans, 20, 26, 65, 255
  juice, 127
Stuffed Mushrooms, 176
Sudorific, 319
Sulforaphane, 313
Sulfur, 301
Summer squash, 20, 65–66, 256

Summer Squash Supreme, 177
Summer, James, 10
Sunburgers, 200
Sun-cured olives, 20
Sunflower Pâté, 191
Sunflower Power Balls, 233
Sunflower, 101
  greens, 19, 253
  seeds, 85, 162
  sprouts, 120
Superoxide dismutase, 303
Super Sesame Bars, 237
Sweat, 15
Swedish National Food Administration Research and Development Department, 7
Sweet and Sour Sauce, 187
Sweet cicely, 102
Sweet flavor, 272–273
Sweet Mint Sauce, 185
Sweet Potato Casserole, 175
Sweet Potato Pie, 238
Sweet Potato Soup, 172
Sweet potatoes, 20, 26, 66–67, 178, 255
  juice, 127
Sweet woodruff, 102
Swiss chard, 67

Tabouli, 160
Tahini Dressing, 164
Tahini Sauce, 187
Take-It-with-You Bar, 228
Tamari, 113
Tamarind, 113
Tandoori Nut Balls, 213

Tarragon, 114
Teff, 75
Thai Vegetables, 217
Theme dinners, 258
Thiamine. *See* Vitamin B_1.
Thistle, 102
Threonine, 307
Thyme, 21, 102, 114
Tiger lily, 102
Tomato Cream Soup, 170
Tomato Sauce, 205
Tomatoes, 20, 26, 67–68, 162
  cherry, 253
Tonic, 319
Tonic gomashio, 116
Tostadas, 224
Toxins, 7, 14–15
Trans fat, 319
Trans-fatty acids, 6
Traveling, 254
Trays, 119
Tryptophan, 307
Tufts Medical School, 12
Tulip, 102
Turmeric, 21, 114
Turnip, 68–69, 178
  greens, 20
  juice, 127
Turnip Greens, 178
Tyrosine, 308

Ubiquinone. *See* Coenzyme Q_{10}.
University College of North Wales, 10
University of Kuopio, Finland, 17
University of Texas, 43
Unsaturated fat, 319
Uric acid, 4
Urine, 15

Valine, 308
Vanadium, 302
Vanilla, 114
Vanilla Pudding, 248
Vasodilator, 319
Vegetable chips, 252
Vegetable dishes, 174–179
Vegetable Kabobs, 210
Vegetable pasta, 203
Vegetable Pot Pie, 198
Vegetables, 5–6, 25–71
  brush, 119
  dehydrating times, 132
  fondue, 253
  marinated, 253
  steamed, 5–6
Vermifuge, 319
Very Vanilla Cake, 243
Vinegar, 115
Violet, 91, 102
  juice, 127
Violet foods, 269–270
Violet Honey, 188
Vitamin A, 5
Vitamin B-complex, 283–289
Vitamin B_1, 5, 284
Vitamin B_2, 5, 284
Vitamin B_3, 284–285
Vitamin B_5, 287
Vitamin B_6, 285
Vitamin B_{12}, 288
Vitamin B_{15}, 288
Vitamin B_{17}, 289

Vitamin C, 5, 289–290
Vitamin D, 5, 290
Vitamin E, 5, 290–291
Vitamin K, 5, 292
Vitamin U, 292
Vitamins, 319
  loss of, 5
Volatile oil, 319

Wakame, 94
Walnuts, 21, 85–86, 162
Washington Post, 6
Water, 276–277
Water filter, 119
Water lily, 102
Watercress, 20, 21, 69–70, 102, 253
  juice, 127
Watermelon, 26, 70
  boat, 252
Weight gain, 13
Weight loss, 12–13
Weight management, 11–12
Western lifestyle, 11, 14
Wheat, 75
Wheatgrass, 96–98, 123
  benefits, 96–97
  juicer, 119
White blood cells, 6, 18
White foods, 270
Wild edibles, 86–91
  gathering guidelines, 86–87
  juice, 127

Wild greens, 219
Wild oregano, 102
Wild rice, 76
Wild Thing Pesto, 207
Williams, R.M., 16
Winter Cereal, 140
Winter Solstice Salad, 158
Winter squash, 26, 70–71, 255
Winter Squash Soup, 173
Winter Waldorf Salad, 158
World Health Organization, 7, 255
Wound healing, 96

Yams, 67
Yang, 27, 53, 261, 266–267, 271
Yarrow, 102
Yellow foods, 267
Yellow squash, 255
Yin, 26–27, 30, 50–51, 57, 59, 65–66, 261, 268–269, 271–272
Yogananda, 79
Yucca, 102

Zeaxanthin, 283
Zeta-carotene, 283
Zinc, 302
Zucchini, 20, 21, 178, 252, 255

About the Author

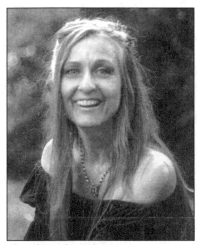

Photo by Andee Smits

Brigitte Mars is an herbalist and nutritional consultant from Boulder, Colorado. She has been working with natural medicine for more than thirty years and teaches herbal medicine through Esalen, Boulder College of Massage Therapy, and Naropa University. She is a professional member of the American Herbalist Guild. Visit her website, www.brigittemars.com, for information about private consultations and herb classes.

Other Publications by Brigitte Mars

▇Books

Addiction Free Naturally: Liberating Yourself from Sugar, Caffeine, Food Addiction, Tobacco, Alcohol and Prescription Drugs (Healing Arts Press, 2001)

Dandelion Medicine: Remedies and Recipes to Detoxify, Nourish and Stimulate (Storey Books 1999)

The Desktop Guide to Herbal Medicine (Basic Health Publications, Inc., 2007)

Herbs for Healthy Skin, Hair and Nails: Banish Eczema, Acne and Psoriasis with Healing Herbs that Cleanse the Body Inside and Out. (Keats Publishing, 1998)

Natural First Aid: Herbal Treatments for Ailments and Injuries, Emergency Preparedness and Wilderness Safety (Storey Books, 1999)

The HempNut™ Health and Cookbook: Ancient Food for a New Millennium (HempNut, 2000) (Richard Rose, coauthor)

▇Audiotapes

The Herbal Renaissance: How to Heal with Common Plants and Herbs. Louisville, CO: Sounds True, 1990.

Natural Remedies for a Healthy Immune System. Louisville, CO: Sounds True, 1990.

You can order these tapes directly from Sounds True by calling their mail-order number: 1-800-333-9185.

▇Computer Software Program

The Herbal Pharmacy: The Interactive CD-Rom Guide to Medicinal Plants. Boulder, CO: Hale Software, 1998.